THE COMPETITIVE EDGE
Advanced Marketing for Dietetics Professionals
Third Edition

■ KATHY KING

CEO, Publisher

Helm Publishing

Lake Dallas, Texas

 Wolters Kluwer | Lippincott Williams & Wilkins

Health

Philadelphia · Baltimore · New York · London
Buenos Aires · Hong Kong · Sydney · Tokyo

Acquisitions Editor: David Troy
Managing Editor: Linda G. Francis
Project Manager: Cindy Oberle
Manufacturing Manager: Margie Orzech
Marketing Manager: Zhan Caplan
Design Coordinator: Teresa Mallon
Production Service: Maryland Composition/ASI

© **2010 by LIPPINCOTT WILLIAMS & WILKINS, a WOLTERS KLUWER business**

530 Walnut Street
Philadelphia, PA 19106 USA
LWW.com

Printed in the USA

Library of Congress Cataloging-in-Publication Data

The competitive edge : advanced marketing for dietetics professionals /
[edited by] Kathy King. —3rd ed.
    p. ; cm.
  Includes bibliographical references.
  ISBN 978-0-7817-9896-9 (alk. paper)
  1. Dietetics—Marketing. 2. Dietetics—Practice. I. Helm, Kathy King.
  [DNLM: 1. Dietetics—organization & administration. 2. Marketing of Health Services—methods. 3. Office Management. WB 400 C737 2010]
  RM218.5.C66 2010
  613.2068′8—dc22

                                                                        2008033860

To purchase additional copies of this book, call our customer service department at **(800) 638-3030** or fax orders to (301) 223-2320. International customers should call **(301) 223-2300.**

Visit Lippincott Williams & Wilkins on the Internet: at **LWW.com.** Lippincott Williams & Wilkins customer service representatives are available from 8:30 am to 6 pm, EST.

10 9 8 7 6 5 4 3 2 1

DEDICATION

I dedicate this new edition to God's flowers in my garden, my husband, Dr. Larry Gilbert; my precious daughters, Savannah and Cherokee; and my godson, Mophat Chongo. I also want to dedicate it to all the wonderful dietitians who have taught me so much along the way as we prodded and stretched our profession into new frontiers.

CONTRIBUTORS

CHAPTER AUTHORS

Chris Biesemeier, MS, RD, LDN, FADA
Manager, Clinical Services and Nutrition Outcomes Research
Vanderbilt University Medical Center
Nashville, Tennessee

Mona Boyd Brown, MS, RD
Owner
Nutrition Communication Services
New York, New York

Felicia Busch, MPH, RD
President
Felicia Busch and Associates
St. Paul, Minnesota

Amelia Catakis, MBA, RD
Retired
Marriott Corporation
Chevy Chase, Maryland

Mary Lee Chin, MS, RD
President
Nutrition Edge Communications
Denver, Colorado

Nancy Clark, MS, RD, CSSD
Private Practitioner, Sports Dietitian
Healthworks
Chestnut Hill, Massachusetts

Neva Hudiburgh Cochran, MS, RD, LD
Nutrition Consultant
Writer and Researcher, *Woman's World*
Advisory Board Member and Contributor, *Maximum Fitness*
Dallas, Texas

Nancy DiMarco, PhD, RD, CSSD, LD
Director
Institute for Women's Health
Texas Women's University
Denton, Texas

Becky Dorner, RD, LD
President
Becky Dorner and Associates, Inc.
Akron, Ohio

Michele M. Fairchild, MA, RD, LDN, FADA
Regional Vice President
Morrison Management Specialists
Naperville, Illinois

Denice Ferko-Adams, RD
President
Denice Ferko-Adams and Associates
Coopersburg, Pennsylvania

Ruth B. Fischer, MS
Former President
NutriSmart, Inc.
Rochester, New York

Linda Gay, MS, RD
Lifestyle Counselor
Weight Control and Diabetes Research Center
Providence, Rhode Island

Betty Goldblatt, MPH, RD
Former Executive Editor
Environmental Nutrition Newsletter
New York, New York

Sue Goodin, MS
CEO
Progressive Health Center
Denver, Colorado

Linda Hachfeld, MPH, RD
CEO
Appletree Press, Inc.
Mankato, Minnesota

Elizabeth Hamilton, RD
President
Elizabeth Hamilton & Associates Inc.
Winnipeg, MB, Canada

Savannah Helm, BBA
Vice President of Marketing
Helm Publishing
Golden, Colorado

Mindy G. Hermann, MBA, RD
President
The Hermann Group, Inc.
Mount Kisco, New York

Mary Abbott Hess, LHD, MS, RD, LD, FADA
Partner, Culinary Nutrition Associates, LLC
Past President, The American Dietetic Association
Chicago, Illinois

Mary Ann Hodorowicz, RD, LDN, MBA, CDE
Owner
Mary Ann Hodorowicz Consulting, LLC
Palos Heights, Illinois

Joan Horbiak, MS, RD
Alexandria, Virginia

Sharon O'Melia Howard, MS, RD, CDE, FADA, LDN
Private Practitioner
Kennett Square, Pennsylvania

Kaye Jessup, MS, RD
Dallas, Texas

Mary Kimbrough, RD, LD
Dallas, Texas

Kathy King, RD, LD
Publisher
Helm Publishing
Lake Dallas, Texas

Tara Liskov, MS, RD
Private Practitioner
Trumbull, Connecticut

Linda McDonald, MS, RD, LD
Editor, *Supermarket Savvy*
Houston, Texas

Diana Noland, MPH, RD, CCN
Burbank, California

Julie Mattson Ostrow, MS, RD
Felicia Busch and Associates
St. Paul, Minnesota

Teresa Pangan, PhD, RD, LD
Founder and President
Web Noxious
Flower Mound, Texas

Kathy Peterson, DTR, MD
Anderson Cancer Center
Houston, Texas

Catharine Powers, MS, RD, LD
Medina, Ohio

Patti Steinmuller, MS, RD, CSSD, LN
Sports Dietitian and Nutrition Educator
Gallatin Gateway, Montana

Jean Storlie, MS, RD
Marketing Manager for Health
Big G Cereral Division, General Mills
Mabel, Minnesota

Celia Topping, MNS, RD, CDE
Nutrition Consultant
Rochester, New York

Evelyn Tribole, MS, RD
Nutrition Therapist and Author
Beverly Hills, California

CASE STUDY AUTHORS

Rebecca Bitzer, MS, RD
Greenbelt, Maryland

Carolyn Brown, RD
The Colony, Texas

Mona Boyd Brown, MS, RD
New York, New York

Jean R. Caton, MS, MBA, RD
St. Louis, Missouri

Holly Deitrick
Lake Dallas, Texas

Becky Dorner, RD, LD
Akron, Ohio

Mark Haley
Dallas, Texas

Melissa Hooper, MS, RD, LD
Newport Beach, California

Barbara Ann Hughes, PhD, MPH, RD, LDN
Raleigh, North Carolina

Tendai Kaisa, MS, RD, LDN
Jenkintown, Pennsylvania

Mary Kimbrough, RD, LD
Dallas, Texas

Joan Lichten, PhD, RD
Marietta, Georgia

Maye Musk, RD
New York, New York

Jan Patenaude, RD
Carbondale, Colorado

Robin Plotkin, RD, LD
Dallas, Texas

Manette Richardson, RD
Jeffersonville, Pennsylvania

Jessica Setnick, MS, RD, LD
Dallas, Texas

Katherine Tallmadge, MS, RD
Washington, DC

Liz Weiss, MS, RD
Lexington, Massachusetts

Barbara Williams, MS, RD
Philadelphia, Pennsylvania

Theresa Wright, MS, RD, LDN
East Norriton, Pennsylvania

Global Perspective Authors

Jane Badham, RD (SA)
Johannesburg, South Africa

Susan Chung, MS, RD
Hong Kong, China

Reiko Hashimoto, RD
Tokyo, Japan

Paula Hunt, Bsc, RD
London, England

Yaakov Levinson, MS, Nutritionist
Jerusalem, Israel

Sanirose Orbeta, MS, RD, FADA
Manila, Philippines

Najat Yahia, PhD, RD
Mt. Pleasant, Michigan

FOREWORD

What do authors Isaac Bashevis Singer and Raymond Chandler, inventor Thomas Edison, artist Pablo Picasso, and entertainer Cher have in common? All of them offer advice on how to achieve competitive advantage. The common denominator of this advice—that success takes knowledge, motivation, and action—is what *The Competitive Edge* is all about.

> *"For those who are willing to make an effort, great miracles and wonderful treasures are in store."*
> **—Isaac Bashevis Singer**

The third edition of *The Competitive Edge*, edited and co-written by noted marketer Kathy King, provides essential information to help you prepare for the future. More than 60 noted practitioners have contributed their expertise, giving dietetics professionals information, strategies, and tools to achieve professional success.

> *"Ability is what you're capable of doing. Motivation determines what you do. Attitude determines how well you do it."*
> **—Raymond Chandler**

In today's world, knowledge alone is not enough. Dietitians must seize every opportunity to market themselves, their products, and their services. Dietetics professionals work in diverse settings within and beyond traditional health care. Many areas of practice—such as sports nutrition, food and culinary nutrition, wellness and community dietetics, and school foodservice—require specialized knowledge. Contributing authors from these and other areas of practice share strategies that have made them successful.

For too long, too many dietitians have done excellent work quietly, with neither recognition nor appropriate financial reward. This state of affairs has created opportunities for others to provide services that belong within our scope of practice. As a profession, we believe that dietitians are the food and nutrition experts; marketing ourselves based on this belief is the key to our success.

> *"A genius is a talented person who has done his homework."*
> **—Thomas Edison**

To excel in such a competitive marketplace, dietitians must understand marketing trends and master techniques to promote our products and services. We work hard; there is no doubt about that. But we need to focus on working smarter. Each of us must become what Thomas Edison called a "genius." The first two sections of *The Competitive Edge* provide essential marketing information, tools, and strategies to turn our talents into genius, increasing not only our value in the marketplace but also our incomes.

> *"Action is the foundational key to all success."*
> **—Pablo Picasso**

Learning about marketing is just the first step. Building on that foundation, dietitians must develop business skills in networking, negotiation, fee setting, promotion, media relations, and other essential business skills. A successful marketing plan sets a goal and identifies a sequence of steps to get there. Clearly establishing a goal is essential to the process, and only you can determine your goal. Reaching it will require time, effort, and resources. *The Competitive Edge* is a key resource.

> *"If you really want something, you can figure out how to make it happen."*
> **—Cher**

Effective communication is also essential to achieving competitive advantage. Chapters 20 to 40 describe how to write, publish, publicize, approach varied audiences, and create the buzz to effectively market yourself, your services, or your product. These chapters provide case studies, tools, and examples of best practices to maximize time, energy, and resources. Use these tools to bring your marketing plan to life.

Now it is time to read and reflect on valuable information collected in this book. Take action and become the success you deserve to be.

Mary Abbott Hess, LHD, MS, RD, LD, FADA
Partner, Culinary Nutrition Associates, LLC
Past President, The American Dietetic Association,
1990 to 1991

ABOUT THE EDITOR

Kathy King, RD, LD, has been an entrepreneurial nutritionist since 1972, when she quit her traditional hospital job to start a private practice in Denver, Colorado. She specialized in weight loss, sports nutrition, and prevention. She has been a counselor to over 6,000 patients, as well as to the Greenhouse Spa and the Denver Broncos Football team. As a speaker, she has given over 800 presentations on such topics as marketing, counseling, entrepreneurship, and to the lay public on nutrition. Kathy has given over 600 media interviews as the Denver NBC-TV "NoonDay Nutritionist," in Dallas as host of her own nationally syndicated nutrition radio talk show, for food companies as a media spokesperson, and as a guest on "Nightline" and "Connie Chung's 1986" show. She has been an international speaker in Israel, Germany, South Africa, Australia, and Asia.

Kathy began Helm Publishing in 1991 in Lake Dallas, Texas, to fill a niche in outpatient and complementary nutrition continuing education courses and books. She has been the author, co-author, or publisher of over 50 self-study tests and 21 books.

Kathy is past President of the Colorado Dietetic Association, former ADA Chair of the Council on Practice, and past member of the Board of Directors and House of Delegates for the American Dietetic Association.

PREFACE

The concept of a marketing book for the dietetics profession was first proposed by James Rose, MS, RD, and I to the Publications Committee of The American Dietetic Association in 1984, and it was approved. Shortly thereafter, ADA made teaching its members about marketing a high priority and sponsored national seminars and gave each member a free copy of that first edition. I was the editor and one of 65 contributing authors of the popular second edition in 1995, published by ADA. Many dietetic instructors are still using portions of that book even though it went out of print in 2001. Today, Lippincott Williams & Wilkins is the publisher and I am again the editor and contributing author along with over 60 creative, innovative practitioners from around the world.

This book fills a niche by teaching students and practitioners how to attract and "sell" nutrition knowledge and food products to their "buying" target markets—whether in a clinic, school cafeteria, or locker room. It teaches dietetics professionals how to be more successful.

The information in this book is basic, especially now, over 25 years later—with the universal acceptance of marketing's role in business and the recognition that even in health care we are in business. But, it is also new and advanced because many marketing skills and techniques are difficult, challenging, or expensive—not for the novice. Marketing is not an exact science; it is often a process of trial and error to see what works. It is fluid because what worked one time may not work the same way if the market changes or a new competitor arrives. There are times when we do everything we know to do and it just doesn't work. There are other times when we simplify our message, use testimonials from satisfied customers, and our phone doesn't stop ringing. This book covers it all through its chapters and case studies.

This third edition begins by covering the most current trends and market conditions that are shaping and impacting our profession. The authors cover the most necessary marketing skills and knowledge that a practitioner needs to know, like how to market yourself and network,

how to create great customer service, how to set fees and negotiate contracts, how to get on the media, or how to write a marketing plan. This is followed by discussion and case studies on the ways marketing is used in different practice areas: culinary and food, acute care and outpatient settings, wellness and health promotion, and as dietetic technicians. I wanted this edition again to have practical, hands-on samples and how-to information, so we have 21 short chapters in our How-to section on such things as how to sell; how to self-publish; how to write a proposal, pitch letter, or press release; and how to market yourself in supermarkets, sports dietetics, or in complementary medicine markets.

This new edition is totally updated with new trends chapters, plus new chapters on customer service, marketing food and food services, selling, marketing sports dietetics and entering the complementary nutrition market, marketing a website, selling a newspaper column, and becoming a consultant. There is supplemental information online with more extensive marketing plan financial forms and all the URLs mentioned in the book. In addition, purchasers of the text can access the searchable Full Text online by going to the *The Competitive Edge* website at http://thePoint.lww.com/King-Comp3e. See the inside front cover of this text for more details, including the passcode you will need to gain access to the website.

I would like to acknowledge my friend, Jim Rose, whom I dearly miss. Also, my appreciation goes to my copy editors, Dollie Parsons and Savannah Helm, who read my revisions with their critical eyes wide open. My thanks go to Steven Brunson, who runs my business so that I can spend my time in solitary confinement writing for long spans of time. I want to thank David Troy at Lippincott for his consistent interest and support for my books. And, a special appreciation to my editor at Lippincott, Linda Francis.

Kathy King, RD, LD

TABLE OF CONTENTS

Contributors   v
Foreword   ix
   Mary Abbott Hess, LHD, MS, RD, LD, FADA
About the Editor   xi
Preface   xiii

PART I   Introduction to Marketing   **1**
      1   Marketing in the New Millennium *Kathy King, RD, LD*   3
      2   Trends: You, Food, and Health Care *Kathy King, RD, LD*   9

PART II   Marketing   **15**
      3   Marketing 101 *Kathy King, RD, LD*   17
      4   Marketing You *Evelyn Tribole, MS, RD, and Kathy King, RD, LD*   27
      5   Marketing a Service *Kathy King, RD, LD, and Denice Ferko-Adams, RD*   35
      6   Marketing a Product *Kathy King, RD, LD*   43
      7   Customer Service *Kathy King, RD, LD*   49
      8   Evaluating Your Competition *Mindy G. Hermann, MBA, RD*   55

PART III Business Skills and Marketing Plan   **61**
      9   Marketing through Networking *Sharon O'Melia Howard, MS, RD, CDE, FADA, LDN* 63
     10   Negotiating Agreements *Felicia Busch, MPH, RD, and Julie Mattson Ostrow, MS, RD* 69
     11   Setting Prices and Fees *Elizabeth Hamilton, RD, and Kathy King, RD, LD*   75
     12   Marketing and Business Ethics *Mindy G. Hermann, MBA, RD, and Kathy King, RD, LD* 83
     13   Promotion: PR, Advertising, Websites, and Other Strategies *Kathy King, RD, LD* 89
     14   Pursuing the Potential of the Media *Mary Lee Chin, MS, RD, and Joan Horbiak, MS, RD* 103
     15   Writing a Marketing Plan *Kaye Jessup, MS, RD, and Kathy King, RD, LD*   113

PART IV   Application to Practice   **121**
     16   Marketing Healthy Food and the Food Industry *Catharine Powers, MS, RD, LD,* 123
           Mary Abbott Hess, LHD, MS, RD, LD, FADA, and Mary Kimbrough, RD, LD
     17   Marketing Health Care: Acute and Outpatient Settings *Chris Biesemeier, MS, RD, LDN, FADA* 135
     18   Marketing Wellness and Health Promotion *Kathy King, RD, LD, and*   143
           Jean Storlie, MS, RD
     19   Marketing Dietetic Technicians *Kathy Petersen, DTR, MD*   157

PART V   Quick "How to" Reference   **161**
     20   How to Sell *Kathy King, RD, LD*   163
     21   How to Market Nutrition in the Supermarket *Linda McDonald, MS, RD, LD*   169
     22   How to Enter the Functional Medicine Nutrition Market *Diana Noland, MPH, RD, CCN* 179
     23   How to Market Sports Dietetics *Nancy DiMarco, PhD, RD, CSSD, LD, and*   183
           Patti Steinmuller, MS, RD, CSSD, LN
     24   How to Market a Website *Teresa Pangan, PhD, RD, LD*   189

25   How to Market Yourself as a Speaker *Becky Dorner, RD, LD*   195

26   How to Use a Book to Grow Your Career *Nancy Clark, MS, RD, CSSD*   201

27   How to Self-Publish and Market Your Book *Linda Hachfeld, MPH, RD*   205

28   How to Write a Marketing Brochure *Tara Liskov, MS, RD*   213

29   How to Write a Resume, CV, and Bio *Michele M. Fairchild, MA, RD, LDN, FADA*   217

30   How to Write a Proposal *Linda McDonald, MS, RD, LD*   225

31   How to Obtain Publicity for Your Special Event *Sue Goodin, MS*   229

32   How to Write a Press Release *Mona Boyd Browne, MS, RD*   233

33   How to Write a Query or Pitch Letter *Neva Hudiburgh Cochran, MS, RD, LD*   237

34   How to Develop a Press Kit *Amelia Catakis, MBA, RD*   241

35   How to Market at Conventions and Trade Shows *Ruth B. Fischer, MS*   243

36   How to Write Effectively to Physicians *Linda Gay, MS, RD*   247

37   How to Market a Newsletter *Betty Goldblatt, MPH, RD*   251

38   How to Create and Use Focus Groups *Ruth B. Fischer, MS, and Savannah Helm, BBA*   255

39   How to Write a Nutrition Newspaper Column *Celia Topping, MNS, RD, CDE*   259

40   How to Become a Consultant *Mary Ann Hodorowicz, RD, LDN, MBA, CDE*   261

Index   267

INTRODUCTION TO MARKETING

MARKETING IN THE NEW MILLENNIUM

Kathy King, RD, LD

MARKETING: THE BOTTOM LINE IN BUSINESS

Twenty-five years ago, marketing was seen as the functions businesspeople performed to promote and sell their products and services. We discussed logos, color palettes, brochures, ad layouts, dressing for success, the features of the service or product, and how to give a sales pitch.

Today, we see marketing as an integral part of the entire business process. Marketing involves everything it takes to make the customer want our product or service more than any other, and with today's cluttered media and fast-paced living that is really a challenge. In other words, when we instruct the secretary how to answer the phone better, serve fresh fruit in a colorful new bowl to the kids at the daycare, change the weight-loss group to a room on the first floor because it's easier to find, or arrive on clinical service an hour earlier to attend patient rounds with the physicians and interns, we are paying attention to details that make our products or services more responsive, attractive, and needed by our target markets.

We are trying to please our customers. Why? Because it makes good sense. It increases demand, which usually increases our income and power, and it improves our image. These usually heighten the value that customers place on our products and services. It also makes good sense because satisfied customers will return to buy again, and they will send their friends.

THE CHALLENGES

It is well known that people buy services and products from people, companies, and brands they trust or have a relationship with in some way (1). Individual dietitians, dietetic technicians, and small businesses do not have unlimited marketing money or other resources, which means they must work smart—starting with relationship-building. Loyal customers return to buy again—and we are all selling something—whether it is food, nutrition therapy, nutrition advice in a book or on the media, management expertise, or a nutrition course at a college.

Until recently, most small businesses and local hospitals only had to worry about local competitors within 10 to 20 miles and the majority of their customers came from that same geographic area. Products like a self-published book on weight loss often were sold to a regional or national market, but services like nutrition counseling sold locally. Speaking, media work, and consulting to businesses were three exceptions. In the last 10 years or so with the use of the Internet, email, low cost telephone calling, cell phones, and overnight delivery, technology is setting up communication channels that make a home-based business run by a dietitian in Omaha as accessible to world markets as a multinational company.

Marketing is changing for large businesses as well. They can afford mass advertising, but it doesn't work as well as it used to. There are too many products, too much clutter and overkill in advertising, too many telemarketers, too many discount stores (which promote low prices and less brand loyalty), and TV networks have lots of competition. Other reasons mass advertising doesn't work as well as it used to are the changing demographics and lifestyles of consumers, which affect us all.

Demographics show that more women, the primary food buyers around the world, are working away from home or in home-based businesses and have little free time. In 2005, the most common household arrangement in the United States was not the traditional family with both parents and two kids, but instead it was married childless couples at 28% of all households (2). There is a dramatic increase in homes run by single parents and people living alone. This creates the next great problem: lack of personal time, which has contributed to the interest in buying through catalogs, direct mail, home shopping networks, and one-stop-shopping stores. As Rapp and Collins state, "Advertisers must almost literally run down the street to catch up with and button-hole the hurrying customers" (1). On top of this, the marketplace now includes more minorities, teenagers, and golden-agers that do not want or need the same things as the former "average" consumer. So now, the "one size fits all" mass message and many utilitarian products are not as attractive to customers as they used to be. That means that nutrition messages can't be geared for the masses; they must be individualized as much as possible.

Since lifestyle influences what people eat, these changes as well as economic considerations greatly affect the dietetic profession. Instead of wives and mothers buying the groceries and making family nutrition decisions, it may be the children or husbands or a widower who has never cooked. More meals are eaten away from home, plus we are eating already-prepared food at home. Fewer meals are made from scratch, and, therefore, fewer people know how to cook. Consumers want fast, healthy food that tastes good. However, most Americans' food choices are more influenced by taste and abundant availability than by wise words of advice, as seen in the obesity epidemic. Also, a too-high percentage of the population is going hungry every day or they live in urban areas where convenience stores are the only grocery stores, and making adequate healthy food available to them is also our concern.

CREATING OPPORTUNITIES

As dietetic professionals, we are answering these changes with changes of our own. A growing number of dietitians and dietetic technicians work with the manufacturers and producers of food. We own, consult for and work as chefs at restaurants, spas, and corporate food services. We bring nutrition education to students in school systems and to consumers in grocery stores and on the media. We created "social marketing" campaigns like "Fruits & Veggies—More Matters" (formerly 5-A-Day) and "Project LEAN" to educate consumers. We invent or help market new, healthier foods. We conduct weight-loss classes, and manage food pantries and hunger programs. This book will present you with role models who display the skills needed to successfully pursue these markets.

THE LARGER ECONOMIC PICTURE

This new millennium has not disappointed those looking for change, and it has made others long for "the good ole days" of even 10 to 15 years ago when life was more innocent and predictable. If there was any doubt that globalization would export jobs, cost for traditional health care could bankrupt families, or our American food supply could become contaminated and injure thousands, that doubt is gone.

In fact, we do not have to wait for historians to tell us this is a memorable time that will change our lives forever. Worldwide, population migration is at an all-time high and people are concerned about terrorism, the environment, global warming, high energy costs, and the spread of poverty and diseases like AIDS and tuberculosis. The fast food industry is having monumental influence on American agriculture, and restaurants of all types are affecting family eating habits and the nutritional intake of those who eat there regularly.

On the positive side, productivity is at an all-time high and new drugs and health awareness are extending life expectancy. Up to the past couple years, middle-income Americans have had more disposable income and higher educations. As pointed out by financial columnist Scott Burns, the past 35 years have been good economically (for most Americans) (see Table 1.1) (3–5). Burns goes on to describe our

TABLE 1.1. CHANGES IN AMERICA		
	1970 (3,5)	**Updates**
Median household income	$9,870	$43,318 (2006) (15)
Median household net worth (real $)	$24,217	$48,201 (2006) (16)
Annual paid vacation and holidays	15.5 days	22.5 days (1990) (5)
Women in the work force	31.5%	56.6% (2006) (17)
Adult softball teams	29,000	>240,000 (2007) (17)
Recreational golfers	11.2 million	37.9 million (2004) (19)
Attendance at symphonies and orchestras	12.7 million	43.6 million (1990) (5)
Americans finishing 4 years of college	13.5%	31% (2006) (6)
Life expectancy at birth	70.8 years	77.9 years (2006) (20)

problem, first described by author Barry Schwartz as the "Cadillac problem—we forget, while fretting about the worn windshield wiper on the Cadillac, that we've got a Cadillac to fret about" (4).

Between 1967 and 2005, median household income rose 30.6% in constant dollars up to $43,318, mainly because of dual wage earners (6). However, although the U.S. has one of the highest median incomes in the world, it is not at the top of all the best lists. There are approximately 37 million Americans below the poverty line today, which is 4 million more than in 2001 (6). A 2007 UNICEF study of children's well-being in 21 industrialized nations, ranked the U.S. next to last (7). The infant mortality rate ranks the U.S. at 42nd out of 221 countries (8) and our life expectancy rank has dropped from 11th to 42nd in the world over the past 20 years (9). Our obesity rate is the highest in the industrialized world with 33% of adult Americans overweight and another 33% obese—doubling in just in the past 25 years (10). Diabetes is at epidemic levels.

Average Americans watch almost 5 hours of television (11) and listen to two-and-a-half hours of radio per day—more than anyone else in the world—and that doesn't count computer time (12). Twelve million Americans keep a blog (13). The most popular websites are eBay, MySpace, Amazon.com, The New York Times, and Apple (14).

And if these changes are not enough, the total American health care industry—our profession's largest employer—is in a state of flux unparalleled in history. Changes in the delivery and payment of health care are being debated in Congress and at every hospital and medical office in the United States. Hospital visits are getting shorter; locations for care are changing to outpatient services; primary care for the uninsured is taking place in the most expensive place possible—hospital emergency rooms. Prevention and wellness may finally start to take their rightful place in health care. The food industry, our other big employer, is exploding with interest in culinary skills, nutrition, organic foods, food safety, and how to meet the needs of its changing health-conscious customer base—while pleasing the other end of the spectrum that wants tasty, quick meals in abundance.

CREATING OPPORTUNITIES

What does this mean for the average dietetic professional? Look at the numbers and see what you can find. More people have disposable income for enjoyment and material possessions; what can you sell them that would improve their nutrition or lower their weight? Personal coaching on nutrition and fitness, culinary classes, private shopper grocery tours, home-cooked healthy cuisine, and sports nutrition consultation come to mind. People are living longer; others are becoming obese and thus there are more chronic diseases. Everyone should be trying to address the growing obesity problem along with its collateral diseases: diabetes, heart disease, and certain cancers.

Could you specialize in wellness, nutrition genomic counseling, geriatric nutrition, weight loss, diabetes, heart disease, or pediatric weight control? These job ideas fit the larger picture, but where you live there may be better niches to pursue. For example, the local schools may need someone to work with adolescents with eating disorders, a local physician may need a nutrition therapist to work with patients needing gluten-free diets, or the local television station may want a hospital nutritionist to offer a weekly "Food Fax" spot. They may call you, or you may see the need, bring it to their attention, and help them create the job for you.

INFORMATION AGE

As Tom Peters, author and business analyst, stated 15 years ago, "We are coping with the biggest economic change in 2 centuries (the Information Age). Amazingly, the chum caused by the Industrial Revolution just ended. We needed 150 years to work through the last big upheaval—even though most of the core technologies were put in place during the first 25 years or so. It may only take 25 years to get the new Information Age technological advancements in place, but it may take society 100 more years to adapt to the shakeout" (21).

See Table 1.2 on the recent worldwide explosion of technology and knowledge. "Each year, the world adds mountains of new information in computer files and on paper, film, and compact disc—enough to fill 37,000 Libraries of Congress with its 17 million volumes" (22). That's each year! Technology is facilitating the spread, collection, and management of information among people around the world.

The technological revolution that is presently taking place is eliminating jobs and job security (software has been and will continue to replace workers). New technologies and research make keeping up with the current body of nutrition knowledge a full-time challenge.

CREATING OPPORTUNITIES

What does this mean for dietetic professionals? First, these numbers show how important staying open-minded, flexible, intellectually curious, and well read is to remaining professionally viable. Nutrition information that set us apart as highly recognized

TABLE 1.2.   WORLD KNOWLEDGE INDICATORS

	Now	Then
College degree holders, world total	212 million	82 million (1980)
Bachelor's degree graduates	9.1 million	4.3 million (1980)
Doctoral degree graduates	293,085	114,808 (1981)
College professors worldwide	8.5 million	3.8 million (1980)
Human genome base pairs decoded	all 3.1 billion	0 (1990)
Wikipedia articles	5.3 million	0 (2001)
Personal computers	898 million	131 million (1990)
Landline phones	1.2 billion	333 million (1980)
Cell phones	2.7 billion	11.2 million (1990)
Countries connected to the Internet	209	20 (1990)
Secure Internet servers	401,050	0 (1990)
Internet websites	110 million	9,300 (1990)
Digital video recorders	17.4 million	0 (1990)
Portable memory storage (megabytes)	16,384	1.44 (1990)
Processor speeds (millions of operations per second)	21,600	16 (1990)
International telephone traffic (minutes)	145 billion	8.7 billion (1980)
Internet users	1.02 billion	2.6 million (1990)
E-mail accounts	1.4 billion	0 (1985)

(From http://dallasfed.org/fed/annual/2006/ar06c.cfm. Accessed July 15, 2007.)

experts even 10 years ago is common knowledge today—or is easily accessible on the Internet. However, our practical application and clinical experience with patients and clients set us apart from those who only know the information.

So what are dietitians and dietetic technicians doing with this knowledge? They are web designers, content experts, and online nutrition consultants. They use the technology to stream video education programs, teleconference, teach online, market their businesses, sell products, and more easily follow patients' progress.

GLOBALIZATION

The improved ability to communicate and transmit information instantaneously along with lower transportation costs has created the globalization of services and products. Globalization gives entrepreneurs around the world history's largest customer base (22). It has lead to agreements, collaborations, and productivity that were unknown and unimaginable just a decade ago (23). For example, in 2001 a surgeon in New York removed the gallbladder of a patient 3,870 miles away in Strasbourg, France, which was made possible by robotic surgical tools and high-speed communications. Now, doctors perform thousands of remote surgeries a year, including heart bypasses, kidney transplants, and hysterectomies (23).

According to the 2006 Annual Report of the Federal Reserve Bank of Dallas, "The Industrial Age limited companies' efficiency. As long as raw materials had to be trucked in and workers had to be on site, production functions rarely extended beyond a region or crossed national borders" (22). This meant employees had leverage to negotiate better salaries and benefits, consumers had to settle for what was available in local markets, monopolies could more easily exist, and prices could be raised without much competition. With globalization of goods, U.S. manufacturers have been forced to get lean—close plants, trim payrolls, and become more productive. Annual productivity per worker has risen from $52,000 in 1990 to $108,000 in 2006 (23). We had to learn how to make goods more cheaply and deliver them for less to remain competitive. (For many companies that also meant cutting retirement and health care insurance of their workers, which has created another set of problems.)

"In the past decade, U.S. prices fell for TV sets, toys, dishes, computers, clothing and many other products facing significant import competition. Prices rose for many products untouched by globalization—cable TV service, hospital services, sports tickets, rent, car repair and others," says the Federal Reserve Bank (23).

Service providers were largely insulated in their local markets because of the nature of services; they are consumed as they are delivered like nutrition counseling or teaching a culinary class. Services can't be stored in inventory, and, until recently, they couldn't be sold around the world because of the cost of communication. However, the Internet, email, and lower phone costs have changed all that. Language isn't even the barrier it once was. As we think of new ways we can use our nutrition expertise to reach world markets, be assured that people in other parts of the world are thinking of the same thing about the potential American markets. For example, U.S. professors can teach online to students in Europe, Asia, and the Americas—anywhere there is computer access (22).

Some globalization benefits include (22–24):

- Stronger competition improves productivity (for those who remain in business). Production becomes more efficient.
- Globalization stimulates creativity and innovation.
- Globalization lowers prices on goods by eroding market power and dissolving monopolies.
- More people around the world have improved standards of living and become consumers of more goods and services.
- Consumption of TV and Internet is less rivalrous than for material goods; use by new consumers does not mean former ones cannot use it. Thus, profits increase because more consumers have access. Increases in demand do not drive up prices.
- There is greater specialization: "We do what we do and trade for the rest."
- Greater knowledge spillover—as information is shared, it sparks ideas and opens doors to innovation.

CREATING OPPORTUNITIES

What can dietetic practitioners do with this information? Dietitians are working for companies that are expanding into overseas markets. Ellyn Luros-Elson, RD, has taken her Computrition software products into food service operations worldwide. This author was contacted by Reiko Hashimoto, a successful private practice dietitian in Japan, and for the past 10 years there has been a Japanese translation of her book, *The Entrepreneurial Nutritionist*. Dietitians of various ethnic backgrounds are finding ready markets in the U.S. working with nutrition needs of people in their ethnic groups, thus using familiarity with language and customs to create products and services. As we get to know each other better, there will be more global collaborations and sharing of ideas. Enjoy the "Global Perspective" insights from various countries at the ends of Chapters 2 to 8.

ADAPTING TO CHANGE

So what do the experts suggest we do to survive while all of this is going on? The consensus is that we should remain flexible, develop a tolerance for ambiguity, and become more independent and entrepreneurial. "Business schools are finally discovering entrepreneurship . . . how to create a new product, start a business, nurture it, and see it grow. Students are demanding it. Applications for MBA programs are down because fewer good jobs exist in large industries. Many MBA programs are adapting to this change in the marketplace by making their programs teach practical business skills and instinctive approaches, like when to take risks, listening to customers, and making business deals. The result will be graduates with broader skills, more real know-how" (25). This change in business started in the last decade and continues today.

People who anticipate trends, react quickly to changes in the marketplace, offer excellence in their products and services, and expect to remain responsible for their own careers will still prosper in today's markets. As you will read throughout this book, the dietetic profession has a wealth of dynamic, creative individuals who fit that description. Their interest and proficiency in marketing helped them reach their customers better, which in turn opened new doors and generated more revenue and self-satisfaction.

SUMMARY

Change is happening at an alarming rate, but core values and ethics need not change. In fact, they become even more important, often serving as the stable foundation while chaos reigns all around.

Throughout this book, we will discuss trends that particularly affect a topic. Three trends bear further investigation: you (self-marketing), our food (the growing interest in all facets of our food), and health care in the United States. These trends and others will be discussed in detail in the next chapter.

REFERENCES

1. Rapp S, Collins T. *The Great Marketing Turnaround.* Englewood Cliffs, NJ: Prentice Hall; 1990.
2. Williams B, Sawyer S, Wahlstrom C. *Marriages, Families and Intimate Relationships.* Boston, MA: Pearson; 2005.
3. Burns S. Steve reaches for the sky. *Denton Record-Chronicle* (Denton, TX). October 2, 2005.
4. Schwartz B. *The Paradox of Choice: Why More Is Less.* New York: HarperCollins; 2004.

5. These Are the Good Old Days: A Report on U.S. Living Standards. *1993 Annual Report—Federal Reserve Bank of Dallas*. Available at: http://www.dallasfed.org/fed/annual/1999p/ar93.html. Accessed July 15, 2007.

6. *Poverty Remains Higher, and Median Income for Non-Elderly is Lower Than When Recession Hit Bottom: Poor Performance Unprecedented for Four-Year Recovery Period.* Washington DC: Center for Budget and Policy Priorities (Sept. 1, 2006). Wikipedia retrieved on June 24, 2007.

7. *Child Poverty in Perspective: An Overview of Child Well-Being in Rich Countries.* Florence, Italy: UNICEF; 2007. Available at: http://www.unicef-irc.org/cgi-bin/unicef/title_down.sql?Title=Child+Well-being+in+Rich+Countries&submit=Search. Accessed January 16, 2008.

8. Rank Order—Infant Mortality Rate. *The World Factbook.* CIA. June 14, 2007. Available at: http://www.umsl.edu/services/govdocs/wofact2007/rankorder/2091rank.html Accessed January 16, 2008.

9. MacAskill E. US Tumbles Down the World Ratings List for Life Expectancy. *Guardian.* August 13, 2007. Available at: http://www.guardian.co.uk/world/2007/aug/13/usa.ewenmacaskill. Accessed January 16, 2008.

10. *Prevalence of Overweight and Obesity Among Adults: United States, NHANES 2003–2004.* Centers for Disease Control and Prevention, National Center for Health Statistics. Available at: http://cdc.gov/nccdphp/dnpa/obesity/. Accessed January 16, 2008.

11. Broadband and Media Consumption. *eMarketer.* June 7, 2007. Available at: http://www.emarketer.com/SiteSearch.aspx?arg=Broadband+and+Media+Consumption&src=search_go_welcome. Accessed January 16, 2008.

12. TV Fans Spill into Web Sites. *eMarketer.* June 7, 2007. Available at: http://www.emarketer.com/SiteSearch.aspx?arg=Broadband+and+Media+Consumption&src=search_go_welcome. Accessed January 16, 2008.

13. Digital Fact Pack 2007. *Advertising Age.* April 23, 2007: 21. Available at: http://adage.com/digital/article.php?article_id=116136. Accessed January 16, 2008.

14. Digital Fact Pack 2007. *Advertising Age.* April 23, 2007: 18–20. Available at: http://adage.com/digital/article.php?article_id=116136. Accessed January 16, 2008.

15. *Median Household Income in U.S. 2006.* Available at: http://en.wikipedia.org/wiki/Median_household_income. Accessed October 27, 2007.

16. *Median Household Net Worth in U.S. 2006.* Available at: http://en.wikipedia.org/wiki/Median_household_income. Accessed October 27, 2007.

17. *Women in the Labor Force: A Databook (2007 Edition)* U.S. Department of Labor. U.S. Bureau of Labor Statistics; September 2007; Report 1002. Available at: http://www.bls.gov/cps/wlf-table2-2007.pdf. Accessed January 16, 2008.

18. Amateur Softball Association. Available at: http://www.asasoftball.com/. Accessed January 16, 2008.

19. Number of Golfers is Growing. *Grounds Maintenance.* Penton Media. 2007. Available at: http://www.grounds-mag.com/news/number-golfers-growing/. Accessed January 16, 2008.

20. *CDC Life expectancy at birth in 2005 for the total U.S. population.* Center for Disease Control and Prevention. Available at: http://www.cdc.gov/nchs/deaths.htm. Accessed January 16, 2008.

21. Peters T. In search of excellence. *Dallas Business Journal.* September 17, 1993.

22. The Best of All Worlds: Globalizing the Knowledge Economy. *2006 Annual Report—Federal Reserve Bank of Dallas.* Available at: http://dallasfed.org/fed/annual/2006/ar06c.cfm. Accessed July 15, 2007.

23. Tallying the Benefits of Global Markets. *2006 Annual Report—Federal Reserve Bank of Dallas.* Available at: http://dallasfed.org/fed/annual/2006/ar06c.cfm. Accessed July 15, 2007.

24. Living Standards on the Rise. *2006 Annual Report—Federal Reserve Bank of Dallas.* Available at: http://dallasfed.org/ fed/annual/2006/ar06c.cfm. Accessed July 15, 2007.

25. *The Kiplinger Washington Letter.* December 29, 1993:1.

TRENDS: YOU, FOOD, AND HEALTH CARE

2

Kathy King, RD, LD

WHAT ARE TRENDS AND WHY DO WE CARE?

Trends are ideas that are shared by a large portion of society. They may be positive or negative, depending on your opinion. They may change the way people think forever or for a year or two. If they are very short-term, we usually call them fads. Some trends are so big that any products or services that do not follow the trend cannot thrive. For example, because of consumer interest and outside pressure, there are trends toward schools addressing the child obesity problem and hospital kitchens providing room service.

Although it may seem that the best health-related ideas stay popular forever, that is not entirely true. Consumers like to choose between the options, and sometimes it does not matter how well you do your job; other options just strike the fancy of consumers more. You might think that if you have a highly promoted, world-renowned health clinic with a popular weight loss program, you would be insulated from fads or trends. But listen to this. Years ago, I asked Georgia Kostas, former Director of Nutrition at Cooper's Aerobic Center in Dallas, Texas, how its traditional weight loss programs were doing since Oprah announced she had lost so much weight on the liquid protein-sparing fast diet. Georgia replied they had really been affected initially, and that was at a highly promoted, very visible program.

You can imagine how the trend toward liquid diets for weight loss affected other dietetic professionals. Some dietitians working in hospitals that embraced the diet found themselves in popular, revenue-generating centers while the trend thrived. Other dietitians who did not agree with the concept found themselves either highly respected by the institution (that may or may not have adopted the program) or marginalized—some even quit or were fired—because they were seen as rigid and not sympathetic to the bottom line of the employer. Do you know what stopped the trend almost overnight? A few women in Florida on one of the liquid diets started having gall bladder problems and their plight hit the media. Overnight, the programs started to disappear.

As you can tell by the above example, you have several options when faced with an overwhelming trend: you can lead the trend, embrace it and ride the wave to its natural conclusion, influence it, refute it, deny it, fight it, or of course, wait until it goes away, if it ever does. Shelley Case, a Canadian dietitian known as a gluten-free expert, became interested in celiac disease and gluten-free foods when helping first her patients and then herself cope. In 2001, she wrote and self-published a book, *Gluten-Free Diet*. Between promoting herself for speeches to colleagues and the public, selling her books, and being an expert at conferences, Shelley is not only riding the wave, but she is also increasing the size of the trend toward greater awareness of celiac disease. Her name and reputation will be forever linked in people's minds with "gluten-free." She is branded as the "gluten-free expert," and when someone wants a speaker, book, pamphlet, or expert witness on the topic, she will be one of the first people who come to mind. That is how to use a trend in a positive manner!

HOW TRENDS GET STARTED

Most individuals and businesses will never experience what it feels like to start a trend—at least they probably will never get credit for it. Trends can start in several ways:

- *People start talking about an idea because it sounds logical and the right thing to do, like saving the planet or the preventing chronic disease through better lifestyle choices.* Groups of individuals and businesses embraced wellness in the 1970s; others wanted more research; still others said, "I do not see any profit in it." When the economy got bad in the mid-1980s, wellness was the first to go in corporate settings because many businesses only offered it as a perk to the executives. Today, it is back in a big way because with rising health care costs, all employees, not just executives, need better health habits to lower health insurance premiums. The timing is right. The critical mass of people who believe in wellness has grown and everyone wonders why it took so long to catch on. Finally, the "hundredth monkey" believed wellness was important and it became an important ideological breakthrough trend.

■ *A huge event happens that coalesces people into agreement on an issue and a trend is created.* As an example, new high-quality research comes out that shows omega-3s are good for the heart and the trend to incorporate more omega-3s into American diets is born. Fishermen switch their catch; fish farms add more salmon to their ponds; dietitians answer questions in the media about omega-3s; food companies assess product levels of omega-3s or add them to food products; and marketers look for ways to add omega-3s to labels and advertising. Consumers read articles and labels to find out more about omega-3s and they buy more foods rich in omega-3s.

■ *Marketing can play a very big role in enticing people into wanting a "hot" new concept or a "breakthrough" product and thus create a trend.* Consider this example: a new book comes out with the hottest new weight loss diet. A movie star endorses it and shows how much thinner she is than the last time she appeared in public. The dietitian author and movie star hit all the talk shows. An infomercial shows

| BOX 2.1 | *The Hundredth Monkey Phenomenon* |

The Hundredth Monkey Phenomenon means that when only a limited number of monkeys (or people) know or believe something, it remains the conscious property of only those people. But there is a point at which if only one more person tunes in to this new awareness, the field is strengthened so much that this awareness is picked up by almost everyone. The added energy of this hundredth person somehow creates an ideological breakthrough! (Go to the original source to read the full monkey story in the book *The Hundredth Monkey* by Ken Keyes, Jr. Available at: http://www.worldtrans.org/pos/monkey.html. Accessed November 14, 2007.)

| BOX 2.2 | *Breakthrough* |

A breakthrough is often thought of as a one-time event, a new product, or technological invention; it is a quantum leap that moves us "outside the box."

the star exercising and eating a healthy diet heavy in fruits and vegetables, whole grains, and small portions of protein foods. The infomercial total package includes the "hot" book, a cookbook written by the star's personal chef, an exercise DVD, a small dinner plate with lines drawn to divide it into the correct food portions, a motivational CD to watch on the computer that also explains the supporting research and shows even more movie stars who have lost weight using the program, and finally, email support by a staff of dietitians 24 hours a day to help customers through the rough times. The public is gushing with excitement for the new concept. The infomercial phones can barely keep up with sales (three monthly payments of $39.95). Grocery stores are selling out of their healthiest foods and obesity drops 10% nationwide the first year. Why hasn't someone done this? We know the formula and it works for all the fad diets. Marketing can create trends.

PRODUCT LIFE CYCLE

Trends go through the various stages of the Product Life Cycle, just like products, services, businesses, careers, and people. They progress through birth and growth, usually stay a while at maturity, and then decline. With the speed of communication today and development of new technology, that progression can be greatly accelerated. This concept is so integral to business that it will be mentioned several times in the book in different context.

For the purposes of this discussion, the Product Life Cycle will illustrate a trend in business. There are four stages or phases to the Life Cycle as seen in Figure 2.1.

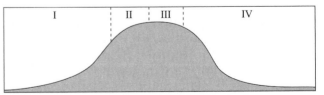

FIGURE 2.1. ■ The four stages of the Life Cycle.

In the first stage, introduction or infancy, the idea is new and the competition is light and not well established. Not many people are working in the trend area and the idea does not have mass appeal yet. The hundredth monkey has come on board, but the trend is just beginning. Little money is required to become established at this point. Lots of time may be invested in speaking to groups and networking with like-minded people who open doors for you and you do likewise. True entrepreneurs love this stage. They thrive on the untapped potential of the emerging trend.

In the second stage, growth begins when the trend becomes more popular and customers demand the best ideas, services, products, and people from stage one. Profits rise and the trend starts to attract the attention of other possible providers. Excitement builds and competitors improve on the best ideas and add marketing dollars to the mix. A good, analytical manager is needed at this stage to make the hard decisions because it is time to get rid of the dead weight and ineffective or marginal services, products, staff, and marketing strategies. The venture needs to be honed to a lean, well-functioning, revenue-generating business. As profits rise and leaders in this trend start to emerge, it becomes more expensive for newcomers to enter the field.

In the third stage, maturity, the trend is still strong but profits begin to top out and saturation becomes a problem. There are lots of customers who want the trend but there are also lots of competitors vying for a piece of the market. Sales are at the highest level since the trend began, but growth begins to decline. As Jim Rose stated in his Cooper Lecture, "During stage three the business becomes fairly routine, so many entrepreneurs lose interest. A person with good management skills is needed at this stage to keep the product or service consistent in quality and efficiently produced." Marketing is especially crucial with each competitor trying to attract the same shrinking target markets. The trend is no longer cutting edge. Businesses look for niches and untapped target markets that have not reached the full potential of the trend yet.

Finally, in the fourth stage, decline arrives. There are fewer new customers who want the trend. It can happen slowly over years, or, as in the earlier example of the liquid diet, the growth surge can happen almost overnight and so can the decline stage. In the decline stage, sales drop but competitors also leave, which can be a good thing. There are at least three viable options at this stage. First is to continue selling services and products for as long as they are profitable. The second is to reformulate and introduce a "new and improved" service or product, or to pursue and develop another niche market that was formerly untapped.

For example, if you have a successful healthy foods grocery tour that private clients love, why not approach the grocery chain about hiring you to represent their stores on the media and conduct tours for their customers? The third option is to invest a percentage of the business resources in a new, upcoming trend that is still in stage one or early stage two. Additional options that could work for some services or products is finding new outside grant or capital funding to reposition and advertise more, or selling out to another business or competitor before sales drop too much.

THE NEXT BIG TRENDS

In the last edition of this book, the growth in globalism and entrepreneurship were highlighted; both proved to be world-changing trends. The three trends that will be explored in more detail in this edition are self-marketing, food, and health care.

MARKETING YOURSELF

When discussing how to achieve success in your life and chosen career, all the best advice on education and credentials will not help if you do not first learn how to market yourself. With employers pulling out of the employee caretaking business, and with downsizing, mergers, and relocations, your jobs will change. You also may quit your job to go after another that is more challenging or fun.

Education and credentials will get your foot in the door for a job interview or proposal presentation, but what you are really "selling" is yourself. Meryl Streep once lamented, "I thought life would be like college, but it is not, life is like high school" (1). As we go through school, we are told that mastering our academics is the most important contributor to success, when in fact it is your attitude and popularity (1). People are attracted to others who have a passion, who are optimistic, and who give first without expecting something in return. But the most important reason people value someone is because he or she makes them feel good—your interpersonal skills. In the service professions, first place does not go to superior competence nor more years of experience (although these are near the top as well), but it is the feeling you give to people that makes you win in business and personal life (1). You show respect, interest, positive regard, humor, and honesty to other people to engender that feeling.

When marketing yourself, remember that people seek out specialists, masters of their trade, not jacks of all trade, so learn how to describe who you are and what you do in a single, memorable sentence.

Have a firm handshake, try to remember names, write thank you notes, and be known for the quality of your output—go that extra mile. See Chapter 4 on marketing yourself and your career.

MARKETING FOOD

It took a long time, but finally, food is becoming recognized for the wondrous carrier of nutrients, health, pleasure, and socialization that dietetic professionals know it to be. The public has always embraced good-tasting food. Chefs on the Food Network are celebrities and the channel is one of the fastest growing. Cookbooks are selling at record rates, culinary classes are filling up, and Americans are eating out more meals per day than ever before. Along with this interest in food comes the problem of over-consumption and its requisite solutions: diets, medications, and surgeries.

Organic food is coming into mainstream groceries and farmers markets in a big way. Genetically altered plants and hormone-altered milk and meats are in the grocery stores and have been for years—albeit not without controversy. The recent Congressional effort to significantly reform the U.S. Farm Bill away from the most subsidized farm commodities like beef, poultry, cotton, and some grains to more fruits and vegetables is not expected to pass, but the discussion was hotly debated. Considering the impact that large farming operations and the fast food industry have on the U.S. farming environment and the quality of our food supply, we as nutrition professionals need to know more about these issues in order to form opinions and advocate for the public good. See Chapter 16 on food and culinary.

MARKETING HEALTH CARE AND WELLNESS

Changes will be coming to health care in the United States because of the growing cost of insurance coverage, the cost of medical care, the ever-expanding number of uninsured Americans, and the Baby Boomers soon hitting the Medicare system. As mentioned earlier, U.S. health care is the most expensive in the world. Prevention and wellness will be used to help delay, control, or avoid chronic illness. Beauty and anti-aging through nutrition should become big businesses.

Complementary, alternative, or integrative health care—whatever you want to call it—will become even more popular in the future. Each year, more Americans visit an alternative practitioner than see a traditional medical practitioner (2). In years to come, there will be a blurring of lines or an integration of therapies, so that descriptions like "alternative" will not be needed.

Money is being allocated for nutrition research at levels never seen before. Many members of the medical profession are finally acknowledging the results of nutrition research and embracing the significant health contributions that good food, nutrient balance, gut and organ function, and nutrition-related genetic expression play. Functional medicine with its major emphasis on nutrition is expected to be a wave of the future (see Chapter 22).

🌐 GLOBAL PERSPECTIVE: SOUTH AFRICA

Jane Badham

The Association for Dietetics in South Africa (ADSA) turns 21 in 2008. There are just over 1,400 dietitians registered with the Health Professional Council of South Africa with the majority also members of the Association. There is no doubt that the profession is now entering its maturity because it is well established within the health professions and is gaining increased visibility amongst the media and general population. The Association's vision is to represent and develop the dietetics profession to contribute toward achieving optimal nutrition for all South Africans.

Diversity and Poverty

Optimum nutrition is a challenge in a country of great diversity, and a population of around 48 million with a high unemployment rate with an estimated 40 million living in poverty. Forty-six percent of the population has an estimated monthly household income of less than US $200.00. Although there has been an increase in the number of people receiving basic services, one third still live in informal and traditional dwellings, only a third have piped water, and only half have access to a flush or chemical toilet.

South Africa has the unfortunate reality of a quadruple burden of disease—infectious disease/diarrhea and micronutrient malnutrition; chronic disease; trauma and injury; and HIV/AIDS. The Medical Research Council recently completed the first South African Comparative Risk Factor Assessment, which estimates the contributions made by the 17 leading risk factors for disease and injury in South Africa. This further highlights the challenges faced by the public health services in delivering

continued

continued

treatment and simultaneously the need to improve risk management in primary care and to deliver much needed health promotion activities.

Seventeen Leading Risk Factors for Deaths in South Africa:

- Unsafe sex
- High blood pressure
- Tobacco smoking
- Alcohol harm
- High BMI
- Interpersonal violence
- High cholesterol
- Diabetes
- Physical inactivity
- Low fruit and vegetable intake
- Unsafe water, sanitation, and hygiene
- Childhood and maternal underweight
- Urban air pollution
- Vitamin A deficiency
- Indoor air pollution
- Iron deficiency anemia
- Lead exposure

Opportunities

All of these challenges also offer unique opportunities for dietitians and our specialized nutrition expertise—from policy making and public health nutrition to clinical and private practice and research that can match standards found anywhere in the world. There are also dietitians that work for or consult to the food industry as the focus of products, in line with global trends, shifts towards offering real nutrition solutions to match our diverse public health needs.

Nutrition, from under-nutrition to over-nutrition and from food security to food labeling, is undoubtedly one of the spotlight topics and it is therefore increasingly critical for dietitians to remain firmly grounded in evidence-based practice. Earning annual points to remain registered is now mandatory and there is on-going work to also have nutritionists registered. The main competitor to the dietitian is the self-styled and usually unqualified (or dubiously qualified) nutritionist who is usually highly skilled at marketing and so often becomes a media darling and is trusted by the consumer.

Marketing

Dietitians need to continue to market themselves in innovative ways in order to emphasize the vital roles we play and to ensure that our multiple roles and unique training are recognized. The challenge for dietitians, in a world where nutritional fiction abounds and

quackery makes plenty of money, is to reach out to the consumer with information and advice that understands the trends, recognizes what consumers want, and is relevant and enticing—without ever losing our grounding in evidence-based practice. To this end, the Association for Dietetics has begun a campaign, "If it's about nutrition ask a dietitian," through which it hopes to further highlight the role of the dietitian. The essence of the message is that nutrition is a science, and dietitians are the recognized experts in the field of evidence-based nutrition.

I firmly believe that South African dietitians—despite our unique working environment—like our colleagues around the world, must now more than ever before remain strong in our values and core competencies. We need to take ownership of our brand of evidence-based nutrition, and nurture and promote it.

It is exciting to be a dietitian in a country of such extremes and to see the professional Association and the profession itself come of age—I look forward to the next 21 years as we continue to grow and adapt to the needs and challenges of the community.

ABOUT THE AUTHOR

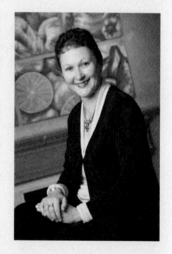

Jane Badham is a registered dietitian with a Masters Degree in Nutrition (cum laude) and a Post-Graduate Diploma in Marketing Management (cum laude). She first worked for a private hospital group and was then Public Relations Officer for the Association for Dietetics in South Africa before starting her own health communication and strategy business, JB Consultancy, in 1992. JB Consultancy focuses on advising the media, food manufacturers, and pharmaceutical industry on nutrition issues and trends, food labeling, and fortified and functional foods. Jane is well-known in the media and regularly comments on nutrition matters.

Jane is a member of FLAG (the Food Legislation Advisory Group to the Minister of Health), is the CEO of the 5-A-Day for Better Health Trust that encourages the increased consumption of vegetables and fruit, and is also in demand as a motivational speaker and strategy facilitator. Jane has contributed to a number of books and recently co-edited the guidelines for the eradication of nutritional anemia for the organization Sight and Life. Jane is involved in an exciting project, the African Nutrition Leaders Programme that aims to develop and network young leaders in the field of nutrition in Africa.

SUMMARY

The next chapters and case studies will discuss or illustrate many of the trends and principles discussed in this chapter, as well as other trends specific to areas of practice.

Once you learn how to recognize and assess a trend, it will become easier to create services and products that capitalize on that trend or even influence the direction and size of the trend. Trends create opportunities and threats that must be figured in to business planning.

REFERENCES

1. Beckwith H, Clifford Beckwith C. *You, Inc.: The Art of Selling Yourself.* New York: Warner Business Books; 2007.
2. Higher percentages of Americans use alternative medicine. *Managed Health care Executive.* February 1, 2005. Available at: http://www.managedhealthcareexecutive.com/mhe/article/articleDetail.jsp?id=146114&sk=&date=&%0A%09%09%09&pageID=2. Accessed January 15, 2008.

MARKETING

MARKETING 101

Kathy King, RD, LD

WHAT DOES MARKETING DO?

Marketing is defined as the aggregate of functions used to move goods or services from the producer to the consumer (1). A common adage is that marketing ascertains consumers' needs and wants, and then fills them. In reality, it is also the reverse: businesses produce a service or product and then look for customers who will buy it. Marketing includes promotion, selling and delivery of the product or service, and more recently, continued follow-up after the sale with consumer hot-lines, email newsletters, online chat groups, technical support, and so on.

Fifty years ago, when there were two brands of canned fruit at the grocery store, few dietitians in private practice, and one local hospital, decisions were easy. Consumers used what was available or they did without. Today, large grocery stores offer thousands of products. There are several thousand private practice dietitians competing with local weight loss and diabetes programs. In metropolitan areas, newer, specialized hospitals compete with the "old guard" for customers (patients). Things have really changed.

With so many options, it seems like customers should have an easier time finding what they want. That is not always the case because of the clutter in the media and the time it takes to sort through the plethora of products and services. The logical answer is for the consumer to try everything for himself before purchasing, but that would be impractical.

Marketing can help consumers sort through the numerous available products and services:

- Consumers can talk to people who have used the product or service (word-of-mouth, testimonials).
- Consumers can buy goods or services from someone they know personally and trust (e.g.,

at church or Chamber of Commerce [relationship marketing]).
- Consumers can check out advertising and brochures that explain the benefits they will experience by using the product or service (promotion).
- Consumers can read reviews and scan websites on the Internet (e-marketing).
- Consumers can buy the most recognizable product or service (brand).
- Consumers can ask questions of a salesperson or customer service department (sales staff).
- Consumers can refer to newspaper articles or broadcast media interviews to assess or form a positive opinion about the business, businessperson, or its activities (publicity or public relations).
- Consumers can go on a list serve or other interactive site and ask peers what they think about the various options (peer-to-peer).

Marketing is not an exact science. There are no guarantees that you will attract more customers than you can handle by having the right slogan, the most expensive brochure, or the best product in the marketplace. Product life cycle, customer whims, competitors, personalities, and competitive positioning of your product or service make marketing more a game of strategy and timing. These variables and others can make or break a new product or service in the marketplace.

The grasp of marketing by businesses has made life easier for the consumer—products are customized (better function, colors, and sizes); there are no-hassle returns; delivery with tracking is faster and guaranteed; and products and packaging are more eco-friendly. The bar has been raised so that it is very obvious when a business does not keep up with its competitors or an employee is rude or inattentive. When this happens, we notice and report it, or we do not come back. Customer satisfaction has become one of the most important parts of new employee training.

Marketing teaches us to look at our product or service from the buyer's perspective, not our own. As dietetic professionals with science backgrounds, we too often assume that customers come to our healthy restaurant for the nutritional value of the fresh food when in fact it is the location near the bay and the fancy desserts. We could be advertising the wrong things if we do not ask and change our perspective to that of the buyer. They come for the view and desserts but they eat our healthy food while they are there—maybe it is not what we planned but it works.

There are lots of similar services to what we sell in food service, clinical counseling, and consulting, but we are not just competing against those services. If you are a nutrition therapist specializing in gastrointestinal disorders, you are competing against the free information on the Internet and anything else the customer might do or buy instead, including the option of doing nothing. In real estate sales, people say you must sell the sunshine coming through the kitchen window and how it makes the customer feel. There are lots of similar houses. What makes this one different? We need to learn how to sell the benefits and sunshine to our customers.

MARKETING TERMS TO KNOW

Customers and potential customers purchase your product or service. They can be described and compared to other individuals; they can be grouped and categorized according to their preferences and dislikes, income, age, buying habits, and so on.

Demographics are observable measurements of a population's characteristics such as age, gender, income, or occupation (2).

The term **psychographics** refers to psychological, sociological, and anthropological aspects of a person's lifestyle and personality used to identify similarities such as preferences in music, movies, fashion, leisure activities, websites, and whether he or she follows the buying habits of some group (2).

Consumption communities, new with the growth of the Internet, are thousands of online groups whose members share opinions about products and services they have tried. There can be pressure to buy things that meet the groups' approval. (2)

Target markets are the primary or potential customers for a product or service. Smart marketers channel marketing efforts and resources to specific market segments or niches that have the highest payoff potential.

Services are intangible products like food service management, nutrition therapy, a massage, computer programming, teaching, consulting in a long-term care facility, and so on. With a service, there is not a physical product that a customer can see, feel, experience, or assess ahead of time, so surrogates that represent the service are used to market it, such as the friendly manner of the person providing the service, referrals from respected people, attractive place where the service is delivered, professional delivery, high quality brochure or business card, and so on.

Products are anything offered in the marketplace to be exchanged for something of value, such as money, time, or commitment. Examples of tangible products are books, food, software, teaching aids like food models and charts, and food service equipment. When a product is tangible, its appearance is important. It must look high quality enough to meet or exceed customers' expectations.

Marketing strategies are a well-thought-out series of tactics or decisions that businesses an organizations use to concentrate their limited resources on the greatest opportunities to increase sales and achieve a sustainable competitive advantage (3–4). A marketing plan contains a set of specific actions required to successfully implement marketing strategies, the fundamental underpinning of a plan (5). Marketing strategies should be dynamic and interactive (6).

The **marketing mix** is commonly referred to as the four P's of marketing (Product, Price, Promotion, and Place) (7); plus three more when marketing a service (People, Process, and Physical evidence); and three specific to the Internet (Personalization, Participation, and Peer-to-Peer) (8). They help people understand the fairly controllable universal elements used in making decisions about marketing strategies and objectives. These terms will be described later in this chapter.

The **perceived value** is the worth that a customer is willing to pay in time and money for your product or service. If the perceived value is not as high as the price, the customer will not buy it. Even if the price is reasonable, but there is poor service, too long of a wait, or too much hassle to get something, the customer will just say, "It is not worth it to me." The goal is to have the perceived value exceed expectations.

EVP (Extra-value proposition or **Value-added)** are extra services accompanying a product or service that are so attractive to consumers that they develop a favorable mindset about the product and remain loyal. You can easily recognize the EVPs used today in the food industry: toll free consumer phone lines, product recipe booklets, free employee training videos with major kitchen equipment purchases, and so on.

Market research is the gathering of factual information about consumer preferences for products or services to establish the extent and location of the market for the product, or to analyze the product in comparison to an alternative or the competition. Primary market research is the research you conduct yourself through private conversations, telephone interviews, and surveys. Secondary market research consists of statistics and information collected by someone else, such as the government, Chamber of Commerce, business organizations, and trade or university groups. To be assured that you have thoroughly researched your concept, use both primary and secondary research.

SWOT analysis is an acronym that stands for strengths, weaknesses, opportunities, and threats; it is a situational-analysis technique often used in market research to help determine your marketing goals. More discussion follows below.

A **market niche** or **segment** is a clearly defined subgroup of customers or potential customers with common characteristics relevant to the marketing of a product (e.g., duel-career couples or 50 to 70 years old with expendable income of more than $60,000 per year). The marketing message would be created to target that subgroup instead of the masses.

Integrated marketing is a holistic approach to all components of the marketing mix that seek to do whatever is necessary to identify, contact, activate, and cultivate individual customers and increase market sales and market share (9). All marketing functions use a common client database so that one hand knows what the other is doing concerning messages and contacts with the clients. Databases provide a useful means to store and retrieve this feedback. By examining this data, you can assess how you are doing and whether customers are satisfied while also doing more promotion that reaches the consumers best.

Individualized marketing is any integrated program of sales communications directly from the advertiser to selected members of the public by any means of direct contact (letters, emails, brochures, telephone, computer disks, advertiser-sponsored events, and so on). The most successful companies are ones that continually carry on dialogues with their target market. In other words, success is built on continuous market research and relationship-building activities (9).

Social marketing is the design, implementation, and control of marketing programs calculated to influence the acceptability of social ideas (such as "eat more fruits and vegetables" or "stop smoking"); social marketing focuses on changing personal or social behavior for the benefit of the person and the public.

Promotion is persuasive communication aimed at target users. Promotion can include everything from billboards, TV and radio ads, sponsorship of a fun run and neon lights to more subtle public relations, pitch letters, proposals, direct-response mailing, monogrammed shirts for employees, and a logo on letterhead.

Advertising is a paid promotional strategy that draws attention to a product, service, or company to elicit a response (a purchase or inquiry).

Brand is a name, term, design, symbol, or other feature that distinguishes products and services from competitive offerings (10). They are created to give an economic advantage over the competition through better name recognition. Brands often have clearly defined personalities or images that are created by product advertising, packaging, branding, and other marketing strategies (11). Today, it is common to see the term extended to people and businesses. A brand image may be developed by attributing a "personality" to or associating an "image" with a product or service, and the personality or image is "branded" into the consciousness of consumers. A good example is how businessmen become free-spirited road warriors when they ride their Harley-Davidson cycles with logos proudly displayed.

Broadcast media is electronic media that deliver messages to mass audiences (e.g., television and radio).

Direct-response is promotion through any method (direct mail, email, phone call, interview, and so on) that is designed to generate direct, measurable action from the recipient.

A **pitch letter** is a letter used to suggest a story idea to a print reporter or program director at a radio or television station, using you as the subject or as an expert source.

A **press release** is the fundamental tool of public relations. It is a brief news release used to generate press coverage for an event, person, product, service or company.

Public relations is a promotional strategy that provides low-cost or no cost publicity; its usual goal is to obtain news coverage, but it can also be to create goodwill (through free services, charitable work, and the like).

A **query letter** is a letter sent to publishers, websites, newspapers, magazines, and other media suggesting a possible story or idea for a book that you want to write for them.

LOWER THE RISK WITH A MARKETING PLAN

There are no magic formulas in business, but you can improve your chances for success by doing your homework, critically assessing all the variables, and then putting your plans in writing. Creating a written marketing plan will force you to anticipate needs and problems, plan your strategies, evaluate the competition, and forecast your financial income and expenses. The process is dynamic. You make the best decisions you can as you begin, but you adapt and adjust along the way to keep on track to your goals (see Chapter 15 for details on how to write a marketing plan).

OVERVIEW OF THE MARKETING PLAN PROCESS

Assume you work for a hospital and want to start an in-house, non-diet, health-at-every-size program for hospital employees that is also open to the public. How would you go about it? The following will give an overview of the systematic creation of the program and its marketing.

Enlist Organizational Support

Five to six months before you want to start the program, write a proposal explaining the project and what you hope to accomplish with it (see Chapter 30). You are seeking preliminary support to see if there is any interest in the idea. At this time, you should offer to develop the business and marketing plans for the venture if the proposal is accepted. Management will use the plans to evaluate the idea and allocate funds for the start-up, or they will request more clarification. They can also turn the project down, but your organized presentation and plans will surely leave a good lasting impression. Remember that weight-loss groups are best started in the fall and after the New Year. Start enough time ahead to allow sufficient time for planning, program development, approval, and marketing.

Write Your Mission Statement

Your mission statement is a short statement of the philosophy and fundamental nature of a business; it sets your course. It helps you decide what your goals should be so you can keep your allocation of resources focused. For this example, your mission statement could be "To provide client-centered, non-diet, health-at-every-size program to the employees of Memorial and people of Centerville through the Clinical Nutrition Office at Memorial Hospital."

Identify Your Major Product and Target Market

Describe your program. In a couple of sentences, succinctly market the project. You might start with some background on the long-term success rate of non-diet, health-at-every-size programs, describe the fitness component and how it is designed to overcome exercise resistance. Then, describe the unique features of this program that will attract people to it.

Now answer: Who will buy it? Describe your target market. Consider age, gender, income, educational level, profession, and the newest parameters that experts use—lifestyle and buying habits. The more you know about your target market, the more you can custom fit your program and marketing to its needs. Also, you will want to market the benefits of your program from the clients' point of view, so you must know your customers' perspective.

Describe your target market's general history with weight-loss programs and obesity. Are obesity, eating disorders, fitness programs, wellness, and disease prevention major or minor concerns to your market? Who cooks the food at home? How often do they eat out? Who does the grocery shopping?

Consider what other items or services you might sell to members of the groups, such as a grocery store tour, a gourmet cooking series, cookbooks, a fitness component, and so on. Some of these items (or free babysitting during the group session) might also be included in the program as value-added extras to increase the perceived value and beat the competition. It is easier and cheaper to sell something to a satisfied customer than it is to find another customer.

Conduct Market Research

This step will help you find out if your idea for a non-diet, health-at-every-size program is a good one.

1. Evaluate the Trends

Look at market trends both locally and nationally to see what is happening in weight loss and to your target market (for example, women 30 to 55 years old diagnosed as overweight with at least one other risk factor such as diabetes, hyperlipidemia, or hypertension). You may feel this step is not too important, but you would be wrong. Even well-financed, national programs are trying to assess where the market will go and what will sell in the future. Are your potential customers looking for a "new" diet? Do they prefer a healthy lifestyle change that does not mention diet, or are they using over-the-counter meal replacements or diet drugs? It is crucial to know for your marketing.

2. General Situational Analysis

What are the general characteristics of the market where you want to start your program? Do most of the women in your area work? What is the economic climate? What does your target market spend its money on? Is adolescent obesity an even bigger problem in your area with fewer competing programs? Talk discretely to potential customers and trusted referral agents. Ask open-ended questions that encourage the person to think through the issue and give his opinions.

3. Conduct a SWOT Analysis

A SWOT analysis (Fig. 3.1) is a realistic, honest examination of your internal strengths and weaknesses, and your external opportunities and threats. In other words, what do you or your department do well that could make this project successful? Your project should use your staffs' strengths to your best advantage. What weaknesses will you delegate, subcontract, or work around? Weaknesses that could sabotage the project must be dealt with or overcome (e.g., no staff with group therapy or non-diet counseling experience). Another weakness would be having only a tiny room in the hospital basement available for the class at the preferred time you want to hold it.

What opportunities and threats are in your environment or marketplace? One opportunity would be the opening of a fitness center that could refer clients or allow your participants to use the facility for a reduced fee. Another opportunity would be a new insurance carrier in the area that recognizes

the value of avoiding obesity in the prevention of disease—its policy holders could be referred to your program. Threats could be increased competition—another local hospital expanding its weight-loss program or a local psychologist approaching the same medical community for weight-loss referrals—or negative publicity on the media from a new long-term study on the futility of weight loss effort.

4. Competitive Analysis

Go deeper in your analysis. Identify your competition, its locations, its products or services, and any advantages or disadvantages it can have. The purpose is to find niches or weaknesses in the competition that will enable you to position your program as different or better. When entering the marketplace, it is important to determine if you are the leader or the follower. A *leader* usually owns the largest share of the market, has the greatest name recognition with its target market, and sets the standards of service. A *follower* looks for and tries to capitalize on the leader's weaknesses. For example, if the leader is a large commercial weight-loss chain that requires customers to buy only its food, your program could say, "Are you tired of cooking a separate meal for yourself? Learn how to eat healthy at a fraction of the cost!" (See Chapter 8 for more information on how to evaluate your competition).

5. Plot Your Product on the Product Life Cycle Curve

Through your evaluation, you will be able to determine which stage the market is in and what kind of market your product is entering. The stages of the product life cycle were discussed in Chapter 2. Most people would call the weight-loss market mature (stage three) with some segments, like extreme fad diet programs, in stage four. Non-diet, health-at-every-size programs are in stage one or two—the competition is not stiff, but the concept is not in prime time yet—which means you will have to educate consumers and decision makers with your 2-minute presentation on the research and testimonials on non-diet, health-at-every-size programs. Explain how the fitness program will offer lessons in beginning tai chi, Celtic dancing, and synchronized swimming.

6. Develop Your Strategic Assumptions

Strategic assumptions are statements about what you expect the market to do. For example, based on your research, your strategic assumptions can be: (a) the local market hit a slump in attendance at traditional weight-loss programs in 2003 and is now recovering to near levels reported in 1997;

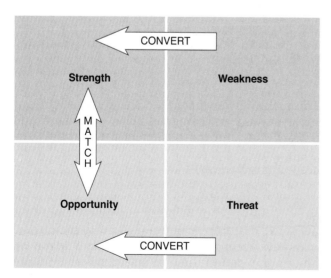

FIGURE 3.1 ■ The four-cell SWOT matrix. (Adapted from Piercy NF. *Market-Led Strategic Change.* Burlington, MA: Butterworth-Heinemann Ltd; 1992:371. Used with permission.)

(b) indications show that the industry has fewer competitors, and the target market is feeling negative about dieting and skeptical of expensive, quick weight-loss programs; and (c) show the statistics and costs of bariatric surgery. By deciding what the strategic assumptions are for your business area, you can better anticipate what will sell and how to sell it. You should review your assumptions yearly to see if they must be altered or if new ones must be added.

Set Your Goals and Objectives

Define what you want to achieve, given the mission statement you wrote. Make goals and objectives as succinct and measurable as possible. Write specific objectives that will help you reach your goals, including profit and marketing (see Chapter 15 for more details on writing goals).

Determine Major Strategies

Now is the time to determine the specifics of your marketing strategies or marketing mix, also known as the four P's of marketing: Product, Price, Promotion, and Place (7). Because marketing a service is different from marketing a product, three additional P's should be considered when marketing a service: People, Process, and Physical evidence. The Internet has created additional marketing strategies in the past few years that will no doubt change the way people market, and three of the most applicable strategies to dietetics are: Personalization, Participation, and Peer-to-Peer (8). The descriptions of these terms follow here.

1. Product

You know the program you want to sell, but take a few minutes to describe its competitive positioning in the marketplace: What is its market niche? What benefits will the consumer get? How is the program unique? What unique aspects will really appeal to the target audience? When you market a service, never forget that you, personally, are part of the total package. That means your personal presentation, communication, interpersonal interaction, and appearance are important to the success of the program. There are many chapters and case studies in this book that deal with these issues.

2. Price

What you charge helps create the image of your program. The assumption of a price-quality relationship is one of the most pervasive market beliefs (12). What are your pricing strategies? (See Chapter 11.)

3. Place

You need to give thought to how you distribute your product or service—where customers buy your product or attend your group classes. This variable could be particularly important if the room is poorly lit, drafty, or difficult to find. If parking is expensive or inconvenient, it can affect your program's success. The keys are to make your products and services as convenient and pleasurable for consumers as possible.

4. Promotion

Specifically explain how you plan to promote your weight loss program. Think of as many ways as you can to spread the name and story of your program: send press releases requesting interviews to local newspapers and radio stations; buy space for ongoing ads in local newspapers; write a brochure and cover letter to send in a direct mail campaign to referring physicians and fitness centers; get free giveaways with the program name or logo to offer attendees, such as mugs, T-shirts, sweat bands, gym bags, or pens. To encourage sign-ups in the hospital, consider paycheck stuffers, articles in employee newsletters, brochures in nursing stations and employee lounges, and signs on bulletin boards. To make the system work smoothly, ensure that the phone number used in promotional materials is staffed every day during normal business hours by someone who knows how to answer the phone professionally and take care of customers and their needs (see Chapter 13 for more ideas on promotion).

5. People

When providing a service, people and interpersonal relationships are inseparable from the service itself in the consumer's eyes. Any person who represents your product or service must be hired carefully, trained thoroughly, and properly motivated to do a good job.

6. Process

This is the delivery of the service (and everything it involves, such as being on time, courteous, and professional) and the quality of the output (thorough, timely, attention to detail, and met or exceeded expectations).

7. Physical Evidence

Since a service cannot be experienced before it is delivered, customers can feel hesitant to try it; there may be a feeling that too much risk is involved. This is the perfect time to use physical evidence that makes the service more tangible, such as letters of reference, testimonials, case studies of successful intervention, and even attractive promotional materials that give the appearance of apparent success.

8. Personalization
Another strategy in the marketing mix since the advent of the Internet is personalization or customization of products and services (8). Dell offers an online service that allows customers to create their own computer from among component options. Amazon.com suggests new complementary products to former purchases each time the customer logs in.

9. Participation
This strategy, which is made possible by the Internet, allows the customer to become involved in the marketing, branding, and advertising of products and services (e.g., recent customer-produced TV advertisements) (8). This concept is laying the foundation for disruptive change through democratization of information (8).

10. Peer-to-Peer
Instead of the passive audiences of the past, there are now thousands of "consumptive communities" or "social computing" websites where brands are debated and debunked or affirmed outside the control of advertisers. This will likely be the most disruptive force in the future of marketing (8).

BOX 3.1 | *Marketing in the Real World*

Once a person knows the theory of marketing and has written and executed a few marketing plans, he or she will start to change how marketing is executed. Very quickly when a new marketing challenge presents itself, marketers will assess the range of options, their knowledge of the customer and his preferences, and the available resources. It does not take long to narrow down the options because there are so many constraints.

Real-life marketing primarily revolves around the application of a great deal of common sense, dealing with a limited number of factors in an environment of imperfect information and limited resources, complicated by uncertainty and tight timetables (13). For most of their time, marketing managers use intuition and experience to analyze and handle the complex and unique situations being faced (13).

GLOBAL PERSPECTIVE: ISRAEL

Yaakov Levinson, MS, Nutritionist

The full potential for nutrition and dietetics in Israel is only just beginning to be recognized. We share the usual health problems, seen in the United States and other developed countries, such as cardiac disease, obesity, diabetes, and cancer, which indicate that nutrition is a critical component in total health care. We have a developing market economy with our citizens striving enthusiastically to achieve Western-style living, including all of its positive and negative implications. The potential market for nutrition services is therefore vast but largely untapped.

National Health Insurance

Every Israeli citizen pays into the National Health Insurance Fund, according to their income, and thereby becomes eligible to join one of the four health services, "Kupat Cholim," literally translated as a "sick fund." They provide basic health services, medical care, hospitalizations, etc. Additional supplementary health insurance for broader coverage is optional. The nice thing is that everyone is covered for basic medical care, Jewish and Arab citizens alike.

Dietitians in Israel

We have two schools of dietetics that offer a bachelor's degree in nutrition, 50 to 60 students per school. Forty percent of our dietitians have master's degrees, and less than 10% have PhDs. Our Ministry of Health has a Department of Nutrition. We also have a dietetic association (ATID), which focuses mainly on sponsoring educational opportunities and employment development. The association includes approximately 1,000 of the 1,400 total dietitians in Israel. The membership is predominantly female, except for 10 males. There are approximately 35 Arab dietitians, mostly working in the north of Israel, who studied in Israeli schools.

To date, about a third of the dietitians work in hospitals, a third are employed by Kupat Cholim in one of the various health funds, and a few work in supervisory capacities in the health ministry. Some dietitians work for businesses, generally one of the pharmaceutical or food companies. A handful of private practitioners are forging their way through unplotted territory. Dietitians are interviewed on the radio and are used in advertisements to promote products. Newspaper interviews and columns are common. *continued*

continued

Diversity in the Population

The Jewish people have been living in almost every nation in the world. Because of this background, we witness today an Israeli society that combines the lifestyles and eating habits of virtually all parts of the world. Our citizens have come from all continents and have recently included massive immigrations from Russia and Ethiopia. It is in relation to this historical and international backdrop that Israeli dietitians face both an immense challenge and an exclusive opportunity for innovation and interesting professional development.

There is, however, a growing consciousness about nutrition in Israel that is quite exciting. Nutrition labeling on food products has gained popularity and is becoming mandatory. Health consciousness, in general, has been increasing, and people are seeking more natural alternatives to health care. In short, the field of nutrition in Israel is wide open for dynamic, well-trained, nutrition professionals willing to take ground-breaking responsibility for raising public and professional awareness and for developing their own new markets.

ABOUT THE AUTHOR

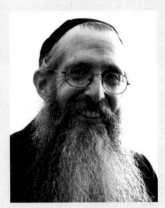

Yaakov Levinson received a BA in biology from Hamilton College (Clinton, NY), an MS in clinical nutrition from Case Western Reserve University (Cleveland, OH), and he worked as a clinical nutritionist at Memorial Hospital (Albany, NY). In Israel, beginning in 1978, he has worked as a nutrition instructor at Zefat School of Nursing, Head Dietitian and Internship Supervisor at Zefat Hospital, as well as other hospitals, and as a private practitioner, clinical dietitian, and long-term care consultant. Levinson has recently had published two breakthrough studies in prestigious medical journals in the United States on a nutritional formula he designed and used successfully with geriatric patients. He presented original research at the International Congress of Dietetics in the Philippines and Scotland.

Develop Action Plans and Assign Responsibilities

In this step, you break down the actions in this chapter into specific activities and arrange them on a timetable showing dates, resources required, budget allocation, deadlines, and so on. Assign responsibilities if someone other than yourself, such as a graphic artist, printer, or publicist, is contributing to the project. Do not assume anything. Stay on top of the project because whatever happens will reflect on you.

Establish a Financial Reporting System and Measure Results

These topics are handled very completely in Chapter 15.

SUMMARY

A marketing plan, just like a business plan, acts as a feasibility study. You become intimately involved with the numbers and marketing decisions that must be made as you create it. Therefore, it reduces the failure rate of projects and businesses. Now you are ready to return for final approval of your project and go forward with a lot more wisdom and confidence . . . and much less risk.

REFERENCES

1. King, K. *The Competitive Edge*, 2nd Ed. Chicago, IL: The American Dietetic Association; 1996.
2. Solomon, MR. *Consumer Behavior: Buying, Having and Being*, 6th Ed. Upper Saddle River, NJ: Pearson Prentice Hall; 2004.
3. UK government businesslink. Marketing strategy guide. Available at: http://www.businesslink.gov.UK/bdotg/action/layer?topicId=1073900352. Accessed December 15, 2007.
4. Marketing strategy. Australian Administration Small Business Guide. Available at: http://www.smallbiz.nsw.gov.au/smallbusiness/Managing+a+Business/Marketing+and+Sales/. Accessed December 15, 2007.
5. Marketing basics. Marketing strategy based on market needs, targets, and goals. Available at: http://www.pages perso-orange.fr/pgreenfinch/mkting/mkting3.htm. Accessed December 15, 2007.
6. Marketing Strategy. Available at: http://en.wikipedia.org/wiki/Marketing_strategy. Accessed December 15, 2007.
7. McCarthy J. *Basic Marketing: A managerial approach*, 13th Ed. Homewood, IL: Irwin; 2001.
8. Mootee I. *High Intensity Marketing*. SA Press; 2001.

9. Rapp S, Collins T. *The Great Marketing Turnaround: The Age of the Individual—and How to Profit From It.* New York: Plume; 1992.

10. American Marketing Association: Dictionary. Available at: http://www.marketingpower.com/mg-dictionary.php?SearchFor=brand&Searched=1. Accessed December 15, 2007.

11. The Chartered Institute of Marketing: Glossary. Available at: http://www.cim.co.uk/KnowledgeHub/Marketing Glossary/GlossaryHome.aspx. Accessed December 15, 2007.

12. Hjorth-Andersen C. Price as a risk indicator. *Journal of Consumer Policy.* 1987;10:267–281.

13. Coarse Marketing. Available at: http://en.wikipedia.org/wiki/Marketing_strategy. Accessed December 15, 2007.

4

MARKETING YOU

Evelyn Tribole, MS, RD, and Kathy King, RD, LD

It's never too soon to write "marketing myself" into your job description (1).

Growing a career is much like growing any business, and the tools used for business growth, especially marketing, can help you get where you want to be. Marketing has become an essential element in the success of any product or person. It is not the exclusive domain of entrepreneurial dietitians anymore since the average person will change jobs eight times within a lifetime (2).

You need to be able to communicate what value you add and what you have to contribute, whether it is to your clients, employer, peers, or community. Competence alone does not lead to professional success (3). Imagine that an author writes a stunning and elegant book; unless others know about it, there is little chance of it making the bestseller list.

CHOOSING YOUR CAREER DIRECTION

Successful careers usually do not just happen to people. Satisfying career growth requires active planning. You need to assess where you are, what you love, what you are good at, what you do not do well or do not like, and the trends that affect where you want to go. (See Boxes 4.1 and 4.2.)

CREATE A PERSONAL VISION AND CAREER PLAN

On any tablet of paper or word processor, write:

- Your personal vision of where you want to go professionally. Where would you like to see yourself professionally in 1, 5, or 10 years? For example, you may want to be a nutrition com-munications executive in a public relations firm, or a personal chef, or an owner of a chain of nutrition clinics in grocery stores, or a nutrition therapist in private practice, or a media spokesperson for food companies, or a food commodities expert, or a top clinical nutrition manager in a teaching hospital.

- Identify the philosophies and values that will guide your major career decisions. For example, "I want to promote natural foods and the vegetarian way of eating. I want to teach people about the environment and the benefits of eating locally and using sustainable agriculture."

- Your career plan will help you clarify your career direction and focus your energy. List your five top skills. Describe your ideal work setting. List five new skills or new knowledge areas that you will need for your dream job.

- Next, identify at least 10 tasks or responsibilities that you really enjoy doing and 10 tasks that you dislike. Keep in mind the process of doing these tasks, not just the outcome. The key to productivity and career satisfaction is to do what you love to do. For example, there is a difference between enjoying the process of writing and enjoying the sight of your name in the byline of an article. If you do not enjoy the process of writing, the glamour of the byline wears off very quickly. Think about it: Do you get great satisfaction helping people who are ill or do you like prevention more? Do you like working with numbers in an office or preparing organic foods in a restaurant? Do you like calculating a feeding more or interacting with people? Does counseling a person who whines

BOX 4.1   *You, Inc.*

WORDS OF WISDOM ON MARKETING YOURSELF:

- Make your brand (who you are) authentic and honest—be yourself.
- 90% of success is just showing up on time! Be prepared and ready 10 to 15 minutes early.
- Do what you love and the pleasure and passion will follow.
- Admit a weakness, confess mistakes, remember names, and keep secrets.
- Exceed expectations and deliver early.
- Praise often; flatter never.
- Keys to successful relationships: reliability, predictability, comfort, and confidence.
- Call back promptly—it shows you think the person is important.
- Listen actively and often—others will find you captivating.
- The future belongs to the communicators—speak and write clearly and simply. In a study on credentials, jurors consistently placed their faith in the person who communicated best, not the one with the most letters after his name.
- Clarity inspires trust and makes you appear the expert.
- Advance one strong argument; people today are overwhelmed with too much information—let them ask for more.
- Precede important comments with a pregnant pause to indicate that what follows is critical.
- Invest in yourself—educate yourself with new ideas, buy at least one great suit, pair of shoes, and briefcase, and spend money where it counts.
- People will avoid you if you gossip or always say critical things—they know they are next on your list.
- Just stay with it—adjust and adapt until it works.

(Adapted from *You, Inc.: The Art of Selling Yourself* by Harry Beckwith and Christine Clifford Beckwith, New York: Warner Business Books; 2007.)

BOX 4.2   *Pursue Your Passions*

Barbara Williams, MS, RD, former Executive Dietitian, ARA Health Care Nutrition Services

As the business climate changes and corporations right-size to save on overhead, some dietetics professionals will be challenged to keep their jobs. No longer are businesses feeling obligated to carry employees who just make do. The person and position must be essential or both will go with the next budget cut.

Nutrition is one of the hottest topics in the public arena today, and new educational programs and job opportunities are flourishing as never before. There is no excuse for remaining in a job that does not excite you or where you have nothing to offer.

If our profession is to grow and continue to flourish, each of us must have a strong sense of commitment to hold dietetics to a higher standard. Take the time to visualize what impact you have. Ask yourself what aspect of dietetics you feel passionate about. Do you feel enough passion that you are willing to pursue solutions, no matter what? Are you visionary enough to see trends and directions in the environment that, if pursued, would greatly enhance yourself and the dietetic profession? Have you thought about the additional skills you will need to take on new responsibilities or upgrade and continue to hold your current position?

Dietetic practitioners must avoid letting others do the things they should be doing. Why not actively become involved in seeking clinical privileges that allow you to determine patients' diets as well as provide total care for monitoring patients nutritionally? If we can be easily replaced by a nurse, a floppy disk, or a person with less training, it may be that our job description needs to be updated and upgraded to a higher level of skills.

Edna Langholz, a past ADA president and Copher Award recipient, stated in her election statement, "Unless we strive for the very best in ourselves, we will never know how good we could have been." So, what are we waiting for?

TABLE 4.1.	ARE YOU IN LOVE WITH THE IMAGE OR THE PROCESS?	
Career Path	**Image**	**Reality: The Process**
Private counseling practice	Independent, successful, lots of clients	1. Do you enjoy the process of counseling? 2. Do you enjoy counseling over and over again each day? (Billable hours are usually hours counseling.) 3. Do you enjoy administrative work?
Nutrition writer for magazine, newspaper, or public relations company	National recognition, creative, authoritative	1. Do you enjoy writing? 2. Do you enjoy tracking down information, researching, and interviewing people? 3. Do you enjoy and work well under deadline pressure?
Corporate executive	Manage projects and people, high levels of respect and responsibility	1. Do you enjoy being responsible for projects and people? 2. Do you enjoy being a team player, or do you get frustrated by red tape and bureaucratic delays?
Entrepreneur	Create and manage diverse projects or a business, risk taker, autonomous	1. Do you enjoy taking risks? 2. Are you good at follow-up? 3. Can you picture yourself preparing project proposals for which you may not get paid or rewarded? 4. Can you handle down times without panic?

and compulsively overeats run you up the wall or is it a challenge?

Table 4.1 can help you understand the difference between process and image. It is devastating to arrive at your career goal only to discover you do not like it!

BUILD YOUR SKILLS

Based on your skills assessment, look at the five new skills you will need and identify the steps you need to take to get those skills.

BOARD OF ADVISORS

To help you decide the best career steps for you, consider developing your own personal board of advisers, a move that could be the single most important career strategy, according to career consultant Jack Falvey. Ideally, this team would consist of five or six people who are willing to provide advice, leads, ideas, and a career overview from a perspective you could not make on your own. Team members might include a favorite mentor, a businessperson skilled in the work you presently do, a practitioner who does what you want to do, your banker or accountant, a trusted dietitian friend, and a business or career adviser.

THE POWER OF SPEECH

Giving a presentation is an effective way to demonstrate your abilities, increase your credibility, and become known as an expert in your field. Hone your speaking skills by speaking locally and speaking often. Work on your content, diction, style, and quality of delivery, jokes or stories, and any audiovisuals. (Word of note: contrary to popular thought, Harry Beckwith, a marketing expert and speaker with 30 years of experience, thinks using audiovisuals like PowerPoint draws away from the effectiveness of the speech and, according to some studies, it does not increase what people remember [4].) Just in case you feel scared of public speaking, you are not alone. In some surveys, people rank it first among their fears, ahead of dying and snakes (4).

When speaking in your local area for only a small fee or no fee, there will come a time of

MINICASE

I had already published a few national magazine articles and one book when I decided to shift my career path to focus on writing. I consulted four writers with whom I had ongoing relationships (from being interviewed for their food and nutrition stories) and posed some key questions: Should I pursue a degree in journalism? Would it make a difference? I was surprised to learn that three of the four writers already thought I had the advantage of being an expert, a dietitian. They thought such expertise, when combined with my published articles and book, demonstrated my ability to write and follow through with assignments. My informal advisory group (three of the four) did not think a journalism degree was necessary, but encouraged me to attend local journalism and writing workshops and classes. Their advice proved to be not only prudent, but (dozens of articles later) time saving.

—Evelyn

deminishing returns, when a decision needs to be made about the value of fees versus more exposure. Offering pro bono work in the beginning as a community service and to become better known make sense, but after a while, speaking for so little pay is not cost effective. Also, group planners do not always try harder to attract a large audience when the speaker can be bought with a chicken salad lunch. Establish a speaking fee that makes it worth your time to get out on a cold night. When you want to increase your professional visibility and your speaking is at a higher level, try marketing yourself to your local, state, and national dietetic program planners—usually a year in advance of the meeting. That will give time for negotiations, preparation and practice. See Chapter 25 for more details on speaking.

One cautionary note: People who speak at conferences for the sole purpose of selling their product or service can sometimes turn off their audiences. Give value and mention your book or product without a hard sell. (See Box 4.3.)

BOX 4.3   *How to Make More Dough in Dietetics*

Joanne Lichten, PhD, RD

Do you feel that you are earning what you are worth? No? You are not alone. Utilizing SurveyMonkey.com, I conducted a 10-question online salary satisfaction survey (June to July 2006) of 552 registered dietitians employed in the field of dietetics. From 2006 to 2007, I sought out "financially successful" registered dietitians who are currently working in the field of dietetics and earned more than $75,000 in 2005. The survey contained a list of 66 different things relating to their education, experiences, and traits. Then from this list, they were instructed to list the top three that related to their "financial" success. Below are the top 10:

1. Passion
"Passion" received 50% more votes than the second ranked item. You cannot make good money by simply going into a field that pays well. If it is not something you love to do, you will never financially succeed at it. One respondent wrote, "If you do not like your job—find something else to do. With a dietetics career you can do almost anything."

2. Communication/People Skills
Are you thinking about getting another degree or certification? Remember that while degrees and certifications might get you in the door for the first job, you will need great communication skills to keep your job, get promoted, and to move on to the next great-paying job.

3. Strategic Thinker
Instead of thinking about what you want to do right now, begin with the "end in mind." Where do you want to be in 10 years? Then look for the jobs that will give you the skills you will need.

4. Vision
Vision is about thinking beyond the way we do things now. Oftentimes, to be financially successful, you have to pave your own path. Instead of trying to duplicate what others are successful doing, find a way to showcase your unique skills and talent!

5. Positive, Can-Do, Optimistic Attitude
Over and over again, I heard from financially successful dietitians that too many dietitians whine (instead of taking proactive steps) about their roles, their responsibilities, and their salary. One of the respondents said bluntly, "So many people do not get it. Attitude will take you farther than skills." How is your attitude?

6. Willing to Work Outside of Your Comfort Zone
Many of the respondents said, "Yes, I can do that!" even if they never have before. Financially successful dietitians never shy away from challenges. When you believe in yourself, you feel confident that you will always succeed.

7. Self-Confidence
Do not feel like you have enough self-confidence to accept work outside of your comfort zone? One participant recommended, "Fake it 'til you make it." She was not suggesting that you lie about your expertise, but rather to give yourself the credit for what you DO know and, if the request is just a mild stretch from what you already do, then feel confident that you can research and practice the rest.

8. Willingness to Take Calculated Risks
There are often risks involved in higher paying jobs. Are you willing to relocate? Work longer hours? Negotiate a contract based on results rather than a salary? Learn new skills, including those outside of the traditional dietetics field? Another risk might be in accepting less money now, in exchange for learning valuable skills that will pay off later.

9. Networking and Creating Strategic Alliances
We all know the importance of networking. But, take some of those relationships to the next level of building strategic alliances. How can you help each other financially?

10. Self-Starter/Self-Motivated
Do not wait for opportunities to come your way. Volunteer for challenging responsibilities that will help to build your resume. Start your own business. Or write your own job description at an established company.

If you are disappointed by earnings that are lower than you feel you deserve, do not give up on dietetics! It **IS** possible to make good money in every dietetics industry if you keep in mind these essential skills.

Dr. Jo has appeared on more than 300 TV and radio shows and has spoken to more than 1,000 companies and conventions. Dr. Jo is the author of *Dining Lean* and *How to Stay Healthy & Fit on the Road*. For more information, visit http://www.drjo.com.

THE POWER OF THE PEN

While writing may not always be monetarily rewarding, you can reap dividends from the personal exposure. Always negotiate the space for a biography note, a brief one-sentence or two-sentence description of who you are and what you do, such as, "Jane Doe is a registered dietitian and health coach in Bigtown, USA. She specializes in lifestyle changes for heart disease and obesity. See http://www.janedoe-rd.com." Most publications offer this opportunity, especially if you are not getting paid (see Chapters 26, 27, 37, and 39). Consider these readily available writing opportunities for career exposure:

- Corporate wellness and hospital newsletters
- Professional newsletters and magazines, such as *ADA Times*, *DPG* newsletters, and *Today's Dietitian*
- Menus that provide space for nutrition tips
- Weekly newspapers
- Trade journals and magazines for the public

BUILD CAREER EQUITY AND CREDIBILITY

Be prepared to pay your professional dues and build equity in your career. You may build some of your most lasting and important relationships when working on committees to host a fun run for the Heart Association or an awards banquet at work. Do not take on projects, however, that make you resent the lack of pay or underpayment; you are not likely to be fully committed, and both you and the organization will lose. Also, take care not to overextend yourself and take on too many projects. While promising career growth, accepting too many projects could stretch you too thin and interfere with your ability to shine.

Credibility is a valuable asset that makes you a desirable employee or consultant. You do not earn credibility overnight; it is a slow investment process. Four key components of professional credibility are honesty, responsiveness, consistency, and forethought. Here are some steps to solidify and enhance your credibility:

- Be accessible. Having a cell phone or voice-mail allows people to reach you.
- Be responsive. Try to return phone calls within 24 hours. Be an active listener.
- Be a resource. If you cannot help, know names of a few competent colleagues.
- Be gracious. Do not forget important details, such as thank you notes for referrals or special efforts by colleagues. Remember to acknowledge the contributions of others. Share the glory.
- Be sensitive to other people's time constraints.
- Be careful when following up on a referral or lead; take care not to use someone's name without first obtaining permission.

PREPARE TO MARKET YOURSELF

Another key to success is to be prepared for marketing opportunities that come your way. Collecting materials for a professional portfolio is one way to keep ready. Samples of projects, clips of articles about you, evaluations from speaking engagements, and letters of recommendation can enhance your professional presence. Of course, you should have an updated resume that is accurate and concise, and a business card. You might also have a Rolodex card, brochure, and brief biography, depending on what kind of work you do. Be careful not to overwhelm people with too much information. Pick and choose carefully from among the options to customize your final presentation according to the position or project you are seeking. Portfolio folders are an easy way to present information without a lot of clutter. Be sure to tuck your business card inside.

For speaking and media work, videotapes of presentations or television appearances will showcase your abilities. If you are seeking writing opportunities, be sure to include samples of your work, whether it is a newsletter, book, newspaper column, or magazine article.

BECOMING KNOWN PROFESSIONALLY AND PUBLICLY

You do not need to become a household name to everyone in your organization, profession, or community to be successful. Focus on promoting your personal assets (based on career goals);

> **MINICASE**
>
> A successful dietitian in a major metropolitan city decided that she wanted to make a career change away from counseling patients and instead to consult restaurants, in which she had little experience. She thought her first step in personal marketing was to become visible, so she began giving a lot of community-based talks. These talks were doing little to get her closer to her actual target, the local restaurant industry.
>
> Her best chance for visibility was to explore opportunities with her existing restaurant contacts. Through one contact, she was able to land a semi-regular nutrition column in a regional restaurant trade journal. This offered her visibility to her potential target customers while keeping her abreast of restaurant trends. She also joined local restaurant organizations to increase her visibility.

choose target markets in which it is important for you to be known—be visible to the right people.

MARKETING TO YOUR CLIENTS

Your best marketing strategies for clients are to keep them satisfied and maintain a good relationship. It is that simple. A satisfied customer will tell a few friends and colleagues, and a dissatisfied customer will tell 20 people.

How do you attract customers in the first place? In private practice, introduce yourself to physicians, clinic managers, head nurses, home health agencies, assisted living managers, hospital social workers, and inpatient and outpatient dietitians. Become known to the referral agents. Send thank you cards for any referrals and send follow-up reports to all referring physicians. Take really good referring physicians to lunch occasionally and bring a holiday basket of healthy foods to offices for the physician(s) and staff—these are your "A" accounts. Your "B" accounts refer less frequently and might receive a holiday card and cookies (or whatever). The goal is to help these accounts step up to being "A" accounts. You might do this through staff in-services over a brown bag lunch or catered sub sandwiches. There are offices where the head nurse and secretary suggest your service to patients more than the physician. Show your respect and appreciation and it will be reciprocated.

Other dietitians have marketed themselves directly to the public through:

- placing small ads in local newspapers;
- having a website;
- speaking to church and other groups;
- using brochures in beauty shops, spas, and fitness centers;
- giving grocery tours; and
- appearing on the local media.

You can keep in touch with your customers through email, a newsletter, a handwritten card, a phone call, Blackberry, or fax. With the new technology coming out, keeping in contact should not be a problem. To set your mind at ease about follow-up contact with clients, ask them during your counseling sessions how they want to stay in touch or if they want to initiate the contact.

BOX 4.4   *Marketing Yourself as a Consultant*

Mona Boyd Browne, RD, Owner, Nutrition Communication Services, New York, NY

It is easy. Just remember service, service, service . . . and quality! Marketing yourself and your services is essential to obtain repeat business from corporate clients in today's marketplace. Use these simple techniques to keep clients coming back for more.

Eye Appeal is Buy Appeal
Image is more than what you see in the mirror; a good image makes people want to enlist your services. All clients want to feel that their consultant is the cream of the crop, the most sought after, the most qualified, and the most successful. A "dress for success" image says to clients, "This consultant is just what we need."

Quality of Work = Your Reputation
The consultant who consistently produces high-quality work and delivers on time is highly valued. The chance to do something bigger and better often arises because of the reputation you have earned for doing a smaller job well. Build your reputation on each project by being creative, dependable, and credible. Arrive for meetings on time (10 to 15 minutes early), be prepared, ask intelligent questions, and provide timely follow-up.

It is in the Extra
Go the extra mile for your clients. Consistently point out opportunities for future projects, clip and mail relevant research articles, send prompt follow-up, and remember appropriate personal dates, anniversaries, and holidays. It is the little things that make a client remember you and your services.

Motto: Go for the Three Es!
A consultant who is excited, enthusiastic, and eager can create job opportunities through hard work and innovation. Work together with your clients for a better bottom line!

MINICASE

When I started my private practice in 1972, I volunteered to the incoming Colorado Dietetic Association president, who asked me to be the Community Nutrition Chair, in charge of National Nutrition Week. I decided that job meant contacting radio and TV stations with our message. Because of that little bit of experience, a registered dietitian suggested me for a TV spot on "Blinky's Fun Club," which lasted over 4 years; another registered dietitian asked me to do a TV interview at the last moment, and the weekly guest spot "Noon-Day Nutritionist" on NBC TV was born. Gail Becker, a registered dietitian, was a guest on our program in 1979 and we met; later, she offered me my first *paid* media spokesperson work. All this grew out of that initial media experience from my volunteer position. After about 3 years in private practice, half of my consultant jobs and speaking engagements (mostly unpaid in the beginning) came from referrals from my peers. I could not afford expensive advertising, so I invested my time and effort.

—**Kathy**

MARKETING TO YOUR PEERS

Peer contacts, especially outside your current employment, can be a valuable asset that is often overlooked. Getting to know peers who are engaged in the type of work you wish to do is a great way to begin carving your niche.

MARKETING TO YOUR CURRENT EMPLOYER

You cannot assume that just because you are holding a job, your career will automatically move ahead. Personal marketing within your own organization is important for your growth. Consider:

- joining cross-department committees;
- writing a column for your company or hospital newsletter;
- taking a member of another department out to lunch. (One hospital-based outpatient dietitian began to take physicians out to lunch; it built a personal network, and her referrals increased.)
- giving presentations to other departments on a nutrition topic of interest;
- identifying the movers and shakers in your company and seeking them out as mentors;
- recruiting your boss to help align your career-development plans with the company's strategic plan.

JOIN AND PARTICIPATE IN PROFESSIONAL GROUPS

Joining a professional group, such as the Chamber of Commerce, Lions Club, Rotary, or a local dietetic association, is a great way to meet people. Too often, however, an individual joins a group and nothing happens. The key to benefiting from organizations is to become an *active* participant. Consider joining committees that you have a real interest in and that can show off or develop your skills. Specialty practice groups, such as the Dietetic Practice Groups of American Dietetic Association, are a good way to meet peers with similar interests. Participating in committee work or taking a leadership role in a national group will also increase your visibility in that area of interest.

Committee work is not a substitute for one-on-one meetings. Your time and money might be better spent if you invest in just a few organizations and save the rest for networking. Take a special contact to lunch to help solidify your business relationship (see Chapter 9 on Networking).

🌐 GLOBAL PERSPECTIVE: JAPAN

Reiko Hashimoto, RD, Managing Director, Reiko Hashimoto Diet Consultations

Japanese Dietitians at a Glance

Presently there are 57,557 dietitians and registered dietitians with membership in the Japan Dietetic Association (JDA). Because of the general economic slowdown and the sluggish growth in areas where dietitians generally work, the number of newly-admitted dietitians has remained low—about 10% of the entire membership.

By industry sector, membership is divided as follows:

- Hospital: 36.4%
- Welfare: 23.3%
- Community health: 17.1%
- School/health education: 9.2%
- Government: 6.5%
- Research and Development (R&D): 4.2%
- Industrial food services: 3.5%

In terms of age composition, over 70% of our members are below the age of 50. Their age breakdown is: 22.8% in their 20s, 26.8% in their 30s, and 21.1% in their 40s.

Changes Affecting Dietitians

Japan is graying at an unprecedented rate with the proportion of the elderly population expected to exceed 26% by 2015. The number of the elderly relying on nursing care services provided through the long-term care insurance system has increased sharply with expenditures almost doubling between 2000 and 2005, jumping from JPY3.6 trillion in 2000 to JPY6.8 trillion in 2005. The rise in medical costs knows no bounds, reaching JPY32 trillion in 2004 and straining Japan's medical insurance finance.

With child obesity and lifestyle diseases a serious societal problem, there is a greater social need and associated responsibility that is expected from dietitians.

Issues

In light of the changing environment, the JDA conducted an industry study and concluded the following

continued

continued

with respect to meeting the need to improve registered dietitians' social standing and developing new businesses in Japan.

1. Employment trends: while new hiring is predominantly in the industrial food services, welfare, and hospital sectors, hiring by hospitals has decreased significantly. Hiring in the educational sector remains flat; and hiring in R&D and government sectors is showing continuing decline.
2. Shift to private sector: except for the welfare sector, employment is shifting **away** from the public sector (hospitals, schools/health education, R&D, and government) and toward the private sector (industrial food services).
3. Expansion to new business areas: As government attempts to reduce medical cost, there is a growing need for expert and effective nutrition services focusing on at-home care (instead of hospitalization) and prevention/self-care. For dietitians, this means honing necessary skills to advance into more consumer-friendly or client-friendly services instead of the more traditional job of working in school/hospital cafeteria.
4. Consignment work: With outsourcing of cafeteria services becoming more prevalent in corporations and hospitals as well as in the welfare sector, a more flexible employment system of consulting and temporary staffing is needed.

In order to respond to these changing market demands and to improve dietitians' social status, it will be pivotal to nurture dietitians who have the requisite skills to provide expert nutritional care and who can remain competitive in the job market. To this end, the JDA has instituted a 5-year continuing education program consisting of mandatory 60 credit sessions. Many educational institutions are revamping their curriculum and have begun to offer practical courses in food service management, business management, marketing, communication, and presentation skills in addition to the core courses on nutrition.

Future

Today, Japanese dietitians are faced with the same predicament that U.S. dietitians experienced 30 years ago. The system and know-how accumulated over the past 3 decades by U.S. institutions, through which dietitians have been given recognition as an established expert profession, is of interest to many in the Japanese dietetic industry. Conversely, Japan is an attractive market to those who can satisfy such need.

ABOUT THE AUTHOR

Reiko Hashimoto is the Founder of the Reiko Hashimoto Diet Consultations (http://www.rh-diet.com), which was established in 2000 with the aim of providing nutritional consultation services to those interested in a healthy dietary lifestyle. Currently she serves as a nutritional adviser to professional soccer and rugby teams, and advises major food companies for conceptual development of new products. She organizes overseas tours geared to dietetic professionals. Ms. Hashimoto has also translated several books on nutrition into Japanese, including *The Entrepreneurial Nutritionist* by Kathy King and *Nancy Clark's Sports Nutrition Guidebook* by Nancy Clark.

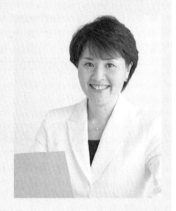

SUMMARY

Marketing yourself can be a very active endeavor. The most successful dietetic practitioners market well and they do it often. They do not wait for opportunity to come knocking; they make it happen. The timeline is usually feast or famine—overload followed by relative periods of quiet. But, as you can see, the quality of your output markets you better than all the brochures and fruit baskets in the world.

REFERENCES

1. McDermott LC. Marketing Yourself as "Me, Inc." *Training Development Journal.* 1992;(September):77.
2. Bolles R. *What Color Is Your Parachute! 2008 A Practical Manual for Job-hunters and career-changers.* Berkeley, CA: Ten Speed Press; 2008.
3. Benton DA. *Lions Don't Need to Roar.* New York: Warner Books; 1993.
4. Beckwith H, Beckwith C. *You, Inc.* New York: Warner Business Books; 2007.

5

MARKETING A SERVICE

Kathy King RD, LD, and Denice Ferko-Adams, RD

Eighty percent of Americans work in service occupations like medicine, teaching, consulting, insurance, and so on (1). Service employment is expected to continue to grow as more women enter the workforce, thus increasing the need for child care, house cleaning services, lawn care, and other time-saving service-fill needs (2). Families have used more financial services, travel, entertainment, and personal care. Businesses use more consultants, equipment leasing, advertising firms, and so on (2).

Marketing a service is all about establishing relationships. Customers buy from people they like and trust, or those who have the qualities or appearance of reliability, consistency, and predictability. They like to buy from people who are confident, personable, and respectful.

A service is intangible; it cannot be physically possessed, looked at, or tested for quality in advance of purchase or use, as a product can. Your challenge when selling a service is to make it seem interesting, high quality, as tangible as possible, and worth every cent to consumers before they buy it.

Providers of professional health services often spend their time researching and providing technically or clinically superior content, but most customers cannot tell the difference (3). Customers want a good quality service from a respected source.

Every day we see nutrition programming with technically correct information and costly audiovisuals that do not attract enough customers to cover the rent. Often, the reasons are (a) inadequate or ineffective marketing—not reaching the target market with the right message—or (b) past poor service.

One overall marketing goal for service providers is to build an image and presence in the minds of their target market. Providers of nutrition services want their target customers to think of them first whenever they want the specific nutrition services the provider offers. Another marketing goal is to create a distinction between your services and your competitors'. (See Box 5.1, Selling What You Can't See.)

In this chapter, we will explore four primary areas of service marketing: (a) identifying a marketing niche, (b) using market signals or messages to build your presence, (c) the value of branding, and (d) developing a market network. See Table 5.1, Dimensions of Service Quality.

IDENTIFYING YOUR NICHE

Identifying and understanding your market niche—that narrow segment of the total market that shares similar needs and desires—is essential. Who are you really selling to? Is it physicians or their patients? Is it the food-service director or the personnel director? Is it all dietitians or just those interested in alternative medicine? Every service has a niche, a market segment that will buy your service more than any other.

It is important to recognize that you cannot be everything to everyone. Determine what services you perform better than your competitors. You may have expertise or particularly enjoy working with certain nutrition problems or with a certain age group, gender, economic group, literacy level, and so on. How are your services unique and different? When you create a service, it is often a mixture of what you like to do and what your market research tells you someone will buy. The process is dynamic. Trial and error with clients will influence what you offer.

What type of relationship do you have with your customers? When you buy a product, such as a pair of shoes, you rarely develop a deep relationship with the sales clerk. However, when customers desire nutrition counseling, they want to know and trust you. Your customers are present for the delivery of the service, and they help determine

BOX 5.1 | *Selling What You Cannot See*

WORDS OF WISDOM FROM A MARKETING EXPERT WITH 30 YEARS OF EXPERIENCE:

■ A small business or service can launch itself faster by convincingly communicating its specialty and how it is different than by using any other single marketing tool.

■ Relationships with clients are more crucial to success than price, brand, quality, or your talent.

■ Even if your service is the best in your market, packaging and image are still important.

■ The challenge in selling a service is to create a perceived value that is higher than the price.

■ Good marketing cannot make up for a service business' unremarkable execution.

■ The fastest, cheapest, and best way to market your service is through your employees.

■ Passionately executed ideas usually win over brilliant, passionless ones.

■ People tend to choose to buy what they hear most about or what seems most familiar.

■ People want to avoid making a bad choice; they seldom seek the superior choice.

■ Focusing on one marketing message instead of multiple ones is a fundamental principle of marketing.

(From *Selling the Invisible* (3) and *The Invisible Touch* (4) by Harry Beckwith, New York: Warner Business Books.)

---

the outcome of the counseling session. For your own consideration, write a description of the typical customer you presently attract to your business. Then write what customers typically say they like or dislike about your services. You can find this feedback in notes, letters, follow-up evaluations, or interviews. Analyzing such information helps you to understand your niche.

MARKET SIGNALS

The term marketing signal first appeared in an article by A. M. Spence in 1974 (5). He described it to mean the observable attributes (like surrogates, attractive office space, brochure, proposal binder, business card, etc.) that help customers draw conclusions about something they cannot see or have incomplete knowledge of. In other words, setting a high fee for your service is a signal to customers that your service is higher quality—and they will expect it to be so. A more expensive brochure or advertising campaign signals that you are successful, presumably because you offer good services.

Signals are used by competitors to let each other know their intentions or capabilities. If you are an industry leader in child nutrition and you make strong statements in the media against marketing poor-quality foods on TV to children under the age of 8 years, you signal to others where you stand.

Unfortunately, consumers' use of signals to make decisions can sometimes be exploited by sellers. For example, customers usually want to buy soft bread because they believe softness signals freshness. Sellers responded by adding chemicals to bread to keep it soft longer instead of working harder to ensure that fresh bread is always available (6).

The use of signaling has increased over the past decade. The reasons are many: product complexity and service content are increasing, the service sector is expanding, media clutter is increasing, shopping time is growing scarce, and technology is rapidly changing. Therefore, the necessity of transmitting attractive signals is growing. In general, the more complex and intangible a product is, the more crucial it becomes to pay attention to the signals that are sent (7). Because advertising time is so short and expensive, websites are being used to better explain what the consumer will receive from a provider: surgeons are explaining their procedures, communication companies describe what they do for clients in more detail—people want to know what to expect. This is why there are scrapbooks of thank you notes and photos of smiling happy babies in the OB-GYN office lobby.

USING SIGNALS TO MARKET SERVICES

Marketing a service usually requires a combination of many different approaches. This section focuses on using signals to market a service. Herbig and Milewicz describe four marketing characteristics: intangibility, perishability, inseparability, and heterogeneity (6). This is a brief review of those signals, with applications and personal examples of marketing the services of a registered dietitian. See Table 5.2, Service Characteristics and Marketing Challenges.

INTANGIBILITY

It is difficult to examine a service without first experiencing it while simultaneously consuming it. This intangible quality makes it important for sellers to signal the tangible aspects of their services. If you have your own office for nutrition

TABLE 5.1. DIMENSIONS OF SERVICE QUALITY

Dimension	Evaluation Criteria	Examples
Tangibles: Physical evidence of the service	Look of the physical facilities Look of the service personnel Handouts, tools or equipment used to provide the service	Safe, clean and professional-looking dietitian's office Clean and neatly attired professional Quality of food in a restaurant Handouts used in a MNT consult
Reliability: Consistency and dependability in performing the service	Performing services when promised Availability for questions in between visits	Appointment time not usually changed Using science-based information Meeting deadlines Arriving on time
Responsiveness: Willingness or readiness of employees or RD/DTR to provide the service	Returning customer phone calls Providing prompt service Handling urgent requests	Forwarding messages with urgency Listening and meeting client's needs Concern for patient's time
Assurance: Knowledge/competence of professional and ability to convey trust and confidence	Knowledge and skills of RD/DTR Company name and reputation Personal characteristics of RD/DTR	Highly trained sports dietitian Known and respected service provider Dietitian's bedside manner
Empathy: Caring and individual attention provided by RD/DTR	Listening to customer needs Caring about customers' interests Providing personalized attention	RD/DTR listening to and trying to understand a patient's needs RD counseling a heart patient

(From: Pride WM, Ferrell OC. *Marketing Concepts and Strategies*, 12th Ed. New York: Houghton Mifflin; 2003. Sources: Berry LL, Parasuraman A. *Marketing Services: Competing through Quality*. New York: Free Press; 1991; Zeithaml VA, Parasuraman A, Berry LL. *Delivering Quality Service: Balancing Customer Perceptions and Expectations*. New York: Free Press; 1990; Parasuraman A, Berry L, Zeithaml VA. An Empirical Examination of Relationships in an Extended Service Quality Model, Marketing Science Institute Working Paper Series, Report no. 90–122. Cambridge, MA: Marketing Science Institute; 1990:29.)

TABLE 5.2. SERVICES AND MARKETING

Service Characteristics	Resulting Marketing Challenges
Intangibility (e.g., nutrition counseling and consulting)	■ Difficult for customer to evaluate without seeing ■ Customer does not take physical possession; cannot hold it ■ Difficult to advertise and display; what do you put in ad? ■ Difficult to set and justify prices; difficult to compare with others ■ Customer leaves with knowledge and feelings but little is tangible ■ Service process is usually not protectable by patents
Inseparability of production and consumption	■ Service provide cannot mass-produce services; most nutrition services are person-to-person ■ Customer must participate in production and can affect outcome; if the patient does not participate, the counseling will be limited ■ Other consumers may affect service outcomes; they arrive late and cut into time for next client
Perishability	■ Services cannot be stored; they are delivered in person ■ Very difficult to balance supply and demand; many months are feast or famine ■ Unused capacity is lost forever; if someone skips an appointment ■ Demand may be very time or season sensitive; people want weight loss after the first of the year but not over the holidays
Heterogeneity	■ Service quality is difficult to control; you have good and bad days, and so does the customer ■ Difficult to standardize service delivery; different people do things differently, even when they are trained the same
Client-based relationships	■ Success depends on satisfying and keeping customers over the long-term ■ Generating repeat business is challenging ■ Relationship marketing becomes critical
Customer contact	■ Service provides are critical to delivery ■ Requires high level of service employee training and motivation ■ Changing a high-contact service into a low-contact service to achieve lower costs without reducing customer satisfaction; is there some way to make the service less labor-intensive?

(From: Pride WM, Ferrell OC. *Marketing Concepts and Strategies*, 12th Ed. New York: Houghton Mifflin; 2003. Sources: Hoffman KD, Bateson JEG. *Essentials of Services Marketing*. Ft. Worth, TX: Dryden Press; 1997:25–38; Zeithaml VA, Parasuraman A, Berry LL. *Delivering Quality Service: Balancing Customer Perceptions and Expectations*. New York: Free Press; 1990; Berry LL, Parasuraman A. *Marketing Services: Competing through Quality*. New York: Free Press; 1991:5.)

counseling, decorate it to appeal to the type of customers you desire. A dietitian who works with obese adults needs large, not-too-soft seating, while the office of a pediatric dietitian needs small chairs and colorful diversions. The way you dress, speak, and present your comments at a meeting to discuss a wellness program with a Fortune 200 company sends many signals about your competency and level of success. Another tangible signal is the quality of your teaching materials, which essentially serve as calling cards for your other services. Identify the many tangible components of your business and signal your customers clearly. In other words, take time to develop the image you want to portray.

PERISHABILITY

Perishability means that you cannot stockpile or sample services in advance. This means that matching seasonal demand (or lack of demand) with your capacity is difficult. You cannot store your excess services the way you would store an inventory of self-published books in your basement or extra cookies in your freezer. How do you handle the periods when your phone rings constantly and other times when it is silent for weeks? When business is booming, it can be great, up to the point where staff gets tired and quality of services decline. This can push customers away.

You will never recover the time and money lost when a client does not show up for a counseling session. However, you can do something to prevent these pitfalls: during off-seasons, by creating more demand, and during peak seasons, by signaling customers that your business is sensitive to their needs. You can:

- create pricing strategies for low times to bring in more people, such as bring a spouse or friend for half price;
- develop an appointment and reminder system so people are reminded of their appointments;
- broaden your service capabilities to include new items or services—sell more to each customer;
- during peak times, such as the New Year's resolution months or pre-summer swimsuit season, hire part-time dietitians to handle increased demand;
- upgrade your reservation systems to improve scheduling; and
- improve responsiveness to consumer calls.

Make clients feel as if they are your number one business interest by showing it!

INSEPARABILITY

Simultaneous production and consumption is called inseparability. Do you both deliver your service and market it? Such inseparability makes it difficult for your business to grow because to provide service, you must always be present. Possible solutions are to teach group sessions, to focus on large-group corporate programs, or to hire dietetic technicians to perform some of the office or assessment functions of a counseling session. Professional services are people-oriented, and inseparability creates the problem of consumers only wanting you as the provider. However, another alternative is to hire reputable, well-trained, conscientious dietitians to assume some of your responsibilities. Slowly assimilate them into your practice: announce their arrival and specific areas of expertise, and introduce them to your clients. Help your clients accept them as capable of providing services similar to yours.

Inseparability from your clients can also cause problems. Much of your success as a counselor or consultant depends on the cooperation and commitment of your clients. Unsuccessful clients can reflect on your services, even when you did all you could.

You can signal your commitment to your clients in many different ways, such as a ready smile, a friendly handshake, and positive body language. You can signal "humanness" by telling a joke or chatting about families and hobbies prior to the consultation. Pictures on your walls or desk and special artwork or antique furniture show your interests. You should hang awards or diplomas on your walls to signal "business" or success (3).

HETEROGENEITY

Lack of consistency, or heterogeneity, means you do not give each client the same quality of service. Standardizing business procedures is very important, whether you are working with consumers, physicians, or companies, because individuals will interact and compare notes on your services.

Service providers need standardized quality-control procedures. Follow-up will set your business apart from the competition. For example, after you finish coordinating and implementing a cafeteria program, use response cards, interviews, and surveys to evaluate customer satisfaction. Provide a written report to let your corporate client know the level of customer satisfaction achieved through your program. For individual counseling, have a third party call to check on customer satisfaction or use a short survey on a return-postage-paid postcard. This attention to detail signals that you care about your clients' satisfaction. Even customers who suggest improvements are more likely to retry your services because of your evaluation efforts.

CHARACTERISTICS OF PROFESSIONAL SERVICES

Certain characteristics help distinguish professional services from all other entities: specialized knowledge, licensing or registration requirements, and technical competency. In addition, services are usually provided by small businesses. These characteristics also give signals to customers.

SPECIALIZED KNOWLEDGE

Specialized knowledge sets dietitians apart from other culinary graduates, health providers, and the lay public. It can also be a limiting factor in that consumers do not know the full scope of our professional abilities and may think of us only as working on hospital floors or in dorm cafeterias. A dietitian's specialized knowledge of diabetes management or weight control can both attract new clients and turn people away, depending on whether they want such services.

Possessing similar work experience to what the consumer is looking for is a highly desirable quality. For example, if you need surgery for a sports injury, you are likely to choose an experienced surgeon who is skilled in your type of injury. Similarly, your clients want to know your success record, and they will ask around. You can help yourself by building a credible reputation in the local community, the media, business networks, and your health professional circle for delivering reliable and effective services.

The need to have experience to obtain clients is not only a problem for new practitioners, but also for professionals who try to change their areas of expertise. In the ranks of professional service providers, being a newcomer is not always favorable. (See the case study that follows by Maye Musk.)

CREDENTIALS/LICENSING REQUIREMENTS

Being a registered dietitian signals consumers that you have met a certain level of professional standards. Place framed certificates and licenses in your office or customer waiting area. If you also have state licensure or other professional achievements, such as a master of science in exercise physiology, then your perceived credibility and level of proficiency will increase. If you work cooperatively with other licensed counselors and health professionals,

be sure to promote this to your customers. To further boost your image, everyone involved with your business must exude professionalism. Customers form opinions as a result of everything they encounter in the process of receiving your service. This includes how the telephone is answered, how the person is greeted on arrival, and even how they are invoiced. Be professional!

TECHNICAL COMPETENCY

Why are your services better than those of less-educated competitors? If consumers do not understand the technical aspects of the nutrition services you provide, then they probably do not feel they need you. An inability to understand the technical aspects forces buyers to focus on the more qualitative components of your services. To counteract this, you must educate clients at multiple levels about your services. Effectively communicate the specific characteristics and advantages that give you a competitive edge!

SMALL BUSINESS ENTITIES

Most professional service businesses are considered small entities. The size of a business can send signals to customers. Large companies may signal that they are more stable, successful, and prestigious. However, smaller companies signal personalized service and better rapport.

Most clients like to meet and assess the person from whom they will receive professional services. For that reason, it is very hard for someone else to market your services for you. Some of the most successful dietitians are ones who learned to market themselves early in their careers. Professionals who improve their selling skills and actively market themselves usually surpass their competition. In fact, evaluating how competitors signal consumers can help you plan your marketing strategy more effectively.

BUILDING A MARKETING NETWORK

One difficult aspect of marketing a service is adapting to continuous changes in population and trends. As a business leader, you need to develop a network that not only promotes your services, but also keeps you informed of changing needs within your niche. Here are five ways to keep involved and be aware of changes that affect your business:

■ Know your local newspaper and radio and television stations. As long as people continue to eat, food and nutrition will always be popular topics in the media.

- Interact with local business leaders.
- Expand your network to other professional groups. If your niche is cardiovascular health, become involved with professional organizations for nurses and exercise physiologists.

- Do not forget past satisfied customers.
- Be involved in your own professional group. By becoming involved, you will gain valuable insight into how other practitioners reach their target mark.

BOX 5.2 | ***Starting Over: A Service Business in a New Location***

Maye Musk, RD

As I have started my own business in seven cities and three countries, let me share some marketing insights with you.

You have built up your private practice. Business is going well. Your clients and the physicians in your area are happy with you and keep a steady stream of referrals coming in. The local media call you for TV, radio, and newspaper interviews. Spokesperson work is sporadic but regular. Life is good.

Then you have to move, for whatever reason, and you have to start over. You know what success feels like and look forward to continuing this feeling in your new city. You expect your name and reputation have traveled so well that minimal marketing is necessary. Unfortunately, this does not happen when you have your own business. A move means going from "celebrity" to "nobody" in a few hours. However, do not fear, help is near.

YOUR FIRST YEAR IN A NEW LOCATION

Before leaving your area, contact dietitians in your new city. Go to http://www.eatright.org to find your state and regional dietetic associations and local members of your dietetic practice groups (DPGs). Members of the Nutrition Entrepreneurs (NE) DPG will understand your needs the best. Call or email them about opportunities, challenges, locations, media or spokesperson opportunities, and fees. The NE listserv is a wonderful way to get good advice, although you cannot discuss fees due to legal issues. Update your location on your website (which you really need to have).

Private practice: If you do not have savings or someone supporting you, start part-time as you will need a steady stream of income. Colleagues can help you find a day job. Start counseling in the evenings and Saturdays. Fix up a home office or find a health club that will not charge you rent, but you will need to pay a percentage of your fees to the club. If you start your practice by paying rent, you can drain your finances quickly.

Consulting, speaking, and spokesperson work: Send change of addresses to former clients. Find new clients on the Internet. With new clients, success is obtained through marketing yourself, continuous contact with the target market, and persistence. When you hear that it takes seven tries to make a contact; that is certainly close.

Media work: Find the TV and radio stations, newspaper and magazine offices in your area. Send the health producers or editors your articles and demo-reels, or refer them to your website, which should contain your articles and videos.

Consulting, speaking, spokesperson, and media work can be done from your home.

Marketing

For all entrepreneurial activities:

- Print cards and stationary as soon as you have settled in.
- Update your website and add interesting articles.
- Join the state and local dietetic associations, and the Nutrition Entrepreneurs DPG (volunteer on one of their committees). Start a mini-NE group in your area. You will be surprised at how willing colleagues are to share their experiences, failures, and successes.
- Attend functions, social or business-related, and then network.
- Start a database of key people (doctors, potential clients, colleagues, public relations [PR] firms, media, and other movers and shakers in the area).
- Keep busy (writing, phoning, emailing, faxing to potential contacts).
- Write articles for DPG newsletters so colleagues think of you in your new location.
- Give free talks at Rotary clubs, the Chamber of Commerce, health fairs, churches, libraries, and other community groups.

For private practice, send letters introducing your practice to doctors, chiropractors, fitness centers, massage therapists, and psychologists in your area. Visit doctors' offices, talk to their staff, and leave a handout for their patients.

Introduce yourself to PR companies for spokesperson work. Send a change of address to past clients or introduction letters to the local media, PR agencies, and food companies.

Image

Change your image to suit your city. At first, I did not understand how important that step is. When I moved from San Francisco to New York, I was told I looked Californian. This was not good. You need to dress

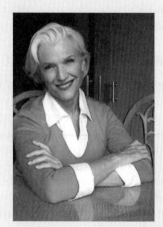

continued

continued

to suit your city, and as sophisticated as your clients. I asked a stylist friend of mine to shop with me and bought her lunch for payment. Now I wear a lot of black! This would not work if I moved to Miami.

Adapt to Fit Local Cultures

Learn about the different cultures in your city. In San Diego, know Mexican foods; in Miami, know Cuban foods; in New York, know foods from all the countries in the world! This is not as difficult as it seems. During a dietary history, you will see what different cultures eat, and use that information to plan their meals to suit their lifestyle.

- Use the Internet and read whatever you can on the client's culture.

- Expand your horizons with different cultural foods and food practices.

- Do not apologize because you do not understand their culture's eating habits. Explain this is new to you and you will learn from them, and adapt their foods to a healthy meal plan. When I moved from Johannesburg, South Africa, to Toronto, Canada, I had a client threaten to walk out of a counseling session because she had binged on Oreos, and I did not know what an Oreo was. She felt I was ignorant.

- Do not fear taking on a client from a different culture; you can learn a lot and help them as well. Often, they do not have someone from their own culture who is available.

- When moving to a new country, learn the spelling, metric blood values, and local foods quickly. Taking the country's dietetic registration exams will get you started. Send transcripts of your degrees and internships direct from the college or institution to the new country's registration department.

First Year Initial Results

Private practice: You have done all your marketing correctly and sent a mailing to physicians. No one responds to your nice letter. Do not despair. Send out letters again. You will slowly receive a few calls from patients of doctors. Unfortunately, they will say, "Do you take insurance?" "No, that is not what I had in mind. I need a prescription for diet pills." "Thanks, but I cannot afford your fees." "I will get back to you." This leaves you depressed, desperate, and wondering if you have made the right decision. You have, it just takes longer than you think.

Keep on sending out letters and meeting people. Soon, bookings start coming in. If some clients start and then quit, do not take it personally. It happened to you in your former practice, but you were too busy to notice.

Consulting, speaking, or media work: This is where you have to be the right person at the right time. Even though you are doing all the right marketing, these clients may not have a project for you, or you may not be right for their current projects. Keep on networking with colleagues, who are your best referral source. If you are not right for a job, you may know colleagues who are. For example: an African American for a lactose-free food; a young mother for a breakfast cereal; or a Spanish-speaking dietitian for a popular Mexican food. When PR or food companies know you are a good source of referrals, they will keep you in mind when you fit the right project.

SECOND YEAR

Private practice: You are becoming a little more established, not as successful as you would like to be, but receiving a little name recognition. Upgrade your office or rent an office, budgeting for the slow months— January, December, and the summer. Increase counseling fees.

- Speaking: Charge for your talks.

- Spokesperson work: Keep in contact with potential clients.

- Consulting: Become more active in your local dietetics association and DPG groups.

- Media: Continue to send press releases and write articles for local newspapers. Update your demo-reel.

THIRD YEAR

By now your business should be ticking over nicely. You are not inundated, but you are surviving and even saving. Money and the work are coming out of the woodwork.

- Invest in an office. Make it look warm and friendly, not clinical. Increase counseling fees. Increase fees for talks.

- Write a book.

- Become the president of your state dietetic association.

- Become a director for Nutrition Entrepreneurs.

- Moderate at local dietetic and ADA meetings.

- Be a role model and mentor for your colleagues.

- Dress and act like a successful professional.

I wish I could tell you it takes 3 months to go from "starting from scratch" to being "rich and famous," but I have not found the formula. When I do, you will know about it. In the meantime, enjoy your move and your new business!

🌐 GLOBAL PERSPECTIVE: HONG KONG

Susan Chung, MS, RD

Hong Kong has approximately 250 to 300 dietitians. It does not currently have its own dietetic registration system. There are two ways to become a practicing dietitian in Hong Kong:

- Dietetic education at Hong Kong University SPACE Institute (co-organized with the University of Ulster, UK) offers a Postgraduate Diploma (MSc) in Human Nutrition and Dietetics. This program consists of a year of academic study and a full-time, 28-week clinical placement in local hospitals.
- Dietetic education overseas to obtain a degree in Nutrition or Dietetics and be recognized as registered or accredited by one of the following boards:
  a. Commission on Dietetic Registration, American Dietetic Association
  b. State Registered Dietitian of Health Professions Council, UK
  c. Registered Dietitian of Provincial Registration, Canada
  d. Accredited Practicing Dietitians, Dietitians Association of Australia

Job Market

Dietitians work in a variety of work settings in Hong Kong:
- in a clinical setting, usually in a hospital, providing medical nutrition therapy to patients with diabetes, hypertension, gout, etc.;
- in community settings where they advise people on optimal nutrition for disease prevention and health promotion;
- in food service where they plan, supervise, and manage the operation; and
- in sports nutrition, health screening, dietetic research, teaching at the universities, commercial food companies, and so on.

Marketing Projects

Over the years, many dietitians individually, or as representatives of the Hong Kong Dietitians Association (HKDA) or Hong Kong Nutrition Association (HKNA), have been involved in various community programs used to promote healthy eating to the public. Recently, both HKDA and HKNA were members of a task force work group promoting healthy eating in restaurants throughout Hong Kong: EatSmart@restaurant.hk.

For more information go to:

HK Nutrition Association: http://www.hkna.org.hk/en/default.asp?page=home

HK Dietitian Association: http://www.hkda.com.hk/

ABOUT THE AUTHOR

Susan Chung, MS, RD is the Sports Nutritionist for the Hong Kong Sports Institute, and part-time nutrition lecturer at the Chinese University of Hong Kong and Hong Kong University. She is a registered dietitian (British Columbia, Canada), registered Chinese medicine practitioner (Hong Kong), and has obtained a Master of Health Science (Human Nutrition) in Australia. Ms. Chung's work at the Sports Institute includes counseling, monitoring athletes' food intake, developing educational materials, and conducting applied nutrition research. Recent published research: *Nutritional Profile of Hong Kong Adolescent Athletes* and *Dietary Intake of Hong Kong Male Road Cyclists During a Multistage Event.*

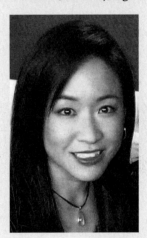

SUMMARY

Marketing a service is a continuous process. To be more successful, take the time to define your services, identify your niche, send the right signals, and build your network. Make your messages clear with only one focus. Tell customers what you can do for them.

REFERENCES

1. Herschol NC, Carraher SM, Buckley MR. Measuring Service Orientation with Biodata. *Journal of Managerial Issues* 2000;(Spring):109–120.

2. Pride WM, Ferrell OC. *Marketing: Concepts and Strategies,* 12th Ed. New York: Houghton Mifflin; 2003.

3. Beckwith H. *Selling the Invisible.* New York: Warner Books; 2001.

4. Beckwith H. *The Invisible Touch.* New York: Warner Books; 2003.

5. Spence AM. *Market Signaling: Information Structure of Job Markets and Related Phenomena.* Cambridge, MA: Harvard University Press; 1974.

6. Herbig F, Milewicz J. Market signaling in the professional services. *Journal of Professional Services Marketing* 1993; 8:2.

7. Bloom PN, Reve T. The role of strategic information transmission in a bargaining model. *Economic Journal* 1990;98: 50–57.

6

MARKETING A PRODUCT

Kathy King, RD, LD

Volumes are written on the different strategies for marketing a product. Obviously, you market broccoli differently than you market a book. But it is not so obvious that you market a new natural sports drink differently than you market Gatorade. The pricing, packaging, distribution, marketing strategies, and advertising mix will be different because the natural sports drink is intended to appeal to a different target market.

The revenue from a product is sometimes called passive income because once the product is manufactured; you do not have to be there to make the sale. But anyone who has tried to sell homemade cookies while they are still fresh, or pack and transport glass jars of gourmet fruit jam, or negotiate with a bookstore to sell a new cookbook, or market a software program by direct mail will tell you that you cannot be passive if you want to be successful. It takes everything you have to make it all work.

If you look at the financial success stories in the dietetic profession, you will see that selling a product is a promising way to make money. Using the same philosophy, a clinical department can develop and sell gluten-free cooking videotapes and a hospital food service can add catering, contract bulk feeding, or off-hours wholesale pastry production. But, unlike selling a service, selling a product often requires a larger financial investment and, some believe, higher risk.

FIVE KEYS TO SUCCESSFUL PRODUCT MARKETING

Five very important keys to success in marketing a product are:

THE CHARACTERISTICS OF THE PRODUCT

Do not introduce a new, expensive product unless it has proprietary (patented, copyrighted, trademarked) competitive advantages (1). If it is not unique, do not spend your time and money on it. If there is no barrier to a competitor entering the market with a product that is just as good as or better than yours, you will quickly be competing on price. You could have a marketing success, but you will have a business failure if you cannot sell it at a profit (1).

THE TIMING IN THE MARKETPLACE

If your target market is not ready for your product, it usually will not sell well. With our fast-paced communication and lifestyles, it may not be long before the market is ready, or it may take years. For example, until the popcorn market matured, Orville Redenbacher was unable to attract enough interest in his high-priced, high-quality popcorn.

In 1977, when I tried to sell a natural sport drink product to Coca-Cola of New York, the new products manager said, "I do not know if 'natural' is where the market is going. If we are first in the market with a natural drink, it will cost us millions of dollars to educate the public, and then everyone else will come along and say, 'me too.'" Timing can make or break a product. That is why it is so important to watch nutrition and health trends when you want to be one of the first in the market to take advantage of them.

THE COMPETITIVE POSITIONING OF THE PRODUCT

Look at and evaluate the competition to your product. Then decide how you will make your product more attractive to potential buyers. You may choose a different niche of buyers than the strongest competitors pursue, or you may decide to change the message. If there is a strong, well-financed leader in the market, as the follower, you must capitalize on what you can do better and different. You might change the packaging or name to appeal to a more elite group. Or you might decide that you will keep your overhead very low, change the packaging to lively colors, reduce the price slightly, and go for volume sales in the youth market. (Check out the discussion on positioning and marketing strategies in Chapter 8: Competition.)

Whatever your strategy, make your advertising, image, and messages unique and appealing to your target market. If you cannot attract attention and solicit the intended response, it does not matter if the product is wonderful.

BRANDS

As mentioned in Chapter 3, a brand is the personality or image of a product or service that is "branded" into the consumers' consciousness. (Think: Apple computers, Target's bull's eye logo, Starbucks, Nike, Betty Crocker, and so on.) Brands affect selling through (2–4):

- increasing word-of-mouth marketing;

- converting more inquiries into sales; and

- taking less time and expense to sell because they are trusted.

Consumers choose brand names in 13 out of 14 sales; brands account for 93 percent of products purchased in the U.S. (2). A brand is one of the most valuable elements in an advertising theme. (3)

THE MARKETING MIX (4 Ps) YOU CHOOSE FOR THE PRODUCT

Product

As mentioned earlier, your *product* should have proprietary competitive advantages that will keep your competitors from copying it exactly. You can patent the function or design; copyright any written booklets, artwork, or music score; and trademark the name or logo.

There are exceptions, such as A&W Root Beer, which is not patented. It owns the majority of the root beer market because of its good taste and people-pleasing frosty mug. Sometimes being first pays off. Another business strategy used years ago by the first commercial manufacturer of granola was to hit the market making a big splash and lots of money, and then sell out to a big cereal company before being put out of business by Kellogg or Quaker Oats.

Many markets today are so saturated with new products that very few will actually make it big. Consider hiring a university entrepreneurial department to assess the market potential for your product. Check with your state universities, government libraries, and invention groups for referrals.

Place, Location, or Distribution

Place, location, or distribution will be another major hurdle in selling your product. Distribution-related factors should be thoroughly checked out before you manufacture your product because you do not want it to be the wrong size to fit on a typical retail shelf, or in a carton to ship by UPS, and the like. If your buyers want your children's drink in a plastic bottle to avoid breakage, you want to know that before you have a warehouse full of product packed in glass.

You may think that it would be great to sell your gizmo in big discount stores, but suppliers say that the Wal-Mart chain requires that you have 2 million gizmos in inventory. And you must be willing to take every piece back if customers return them for any reason. Moreover, you will usually negotiate away most of your profit to make such a big sale in the first place. In the grocery industry, budgets for new cereals must include $5 million more than they did 5 years ago to cover the slotting fees grocery stores charge food manufacturers for shelf space. So distribution can be tricky and expensive.

Price

Price is important in creating the perceived value of a product in customers' minds. Price is not much of an issue if the function, design, and physical packaging or persons involved (as in a video) meet or exceed the customers' expectations. Price will be a barrier to sales if expectations are not met. Usually, the price of a product is higher when it is first introduced on the market (before competitors hit and under-price it), so you recoup some of your initial investment. (See Chapter 11 for more information on pricing strategies.)

Promotion

Promotion lets the target market know what the product is, what it does, how wonderful it is, how it fits their needs, and where to get it. A product should have a distinctive brand name and a short, easy-to-remember slogan or subtitle that quickly explains important information to the consumer. The right colors in packaging or product design can easily distinguish a product from its competition and be a strong marketing tool.

As mentioned in this book many times, advertising is changing to include more direct contact and individualized marketing. Direct mail, web shopping carts, TV home shopping, catalogs, cable TV, and trade shows that promote closer contact with customers and their needs are growing in popularity. Developing and selling a product to the dietetic market is not as risky as selling to the public because we know our needs better. However, potential sales volume is greatly reduced. (See Chapter 13 for detailed information on promotion.)

THE FUNDING MUST BE ADEQUATE

Enough must be allocated to manufacturing and promoting your product or you should not spend your time and energy producing it. You will face many expenses, such as product inventory, legal and accounting fees, engineering designs, models and molds, import fees (on products or components made overseas), telephone and office expenses, transportation of inventory, warehousing, packaging, labels, advertising copy or taped commercials, air time, and so on.

John Luther and Jim McManus, marketing consultants from Westport, Connecticut, offer two additional suggestions (1):

- Do not bet the ranch. Always hold some personal or business assets in reserve.
- Test market your product by getting into business. There is nothing theoretical about it. Just do focus groups in at least two geographic regions to get a reality check that you are on target. The old thinking was that if you test marketed a product in a "representative" city, like Denver, and consumers liked it, it would sell nationwide. That did not prove to be true. (See Chapter 38 for details on how to create and use focus groups.)

BUNDLING AND UNBUNDLING

Bundling and unbundling can be successful marketing strategies, especially when you sell several lower-cost items. For example, if you have a $9.95 weight-loss tape and a new low-fat cookbook that retails for $12.95, you could offer them both for $19.95 (the price of all great deals)! That is bundling, or grouping products together. Unbundling is just the opposite.

PRODUCT FAILURE

Although there is no way of actually knowing how many new products are created each year, it has been estimated by consulting firms, statistical bureaus, and trade publications that at least one

---

CASE STUDY 6.1

COMPUTRITION, INC. SOFTWARE COMPANY

Ellyn Luros-Elson believes in luck. But she does not wait for it. She creates it. Fresh out of a dietetics internship at Wadsworth VA Medical Center in Los Angeles, Ellyn launched her first company and opened a new frontier for dietitians in long-term care consulting. A decade later, she saw the need for a better way to analyze the nutrient content of recipes and menus and patient/resident nutrient intake. Partnering with three colleagues, Ellyn created Computrition, Inc., a software solution provider. Over the next 30 years, that company grew into a multi-million dollar international enterprise employing 65 people, many of whom are dietitians. "Frankly, I started Computrition because I hated doing nutritional analysis," Ellyn admits. "If I hated doing it, surely other dietitians did, too. Turns out, I was right."

Just like marketing ventures that "go by the book," the company determined a need and then filled that need. They positioned their products to the owners and CEOs of businesses and to requirements of the end-users, the foodservice director and dietitians. The company has grown from a collection of nutritional analysis tools to the world's leading suite of software products for foodservice operations and diet office management.

Ellyn has always had a clearly defined mission for Computrition, that is, to provide the highest quality products and services with an emphasis on customer service, employee fulfillment, and profitability. This mission does not change. Rather, it is the company's energy, creativity, and innovation that respond to the changing environment. "It's critical to have a goal," Ellyn explains. "And it is equally important to be open to new ideas about how to reach that goal."

Over the past 3 decades, Computrition has solidified its competitive edge not only by understanding its target market and offering the products its customers need, but also by supplying leadership, expertise, and resources that move the hospitality industry forward. "We have a responsibility to give back to the industry that has been so good to us," Ellyn says. "And as dietitians, I believe we have a responsibility to give back to the profession as well. Helping others achieve their goals can be one of life's greatest rewards."

---

in three fail and some report an estimated product failure rate at 80% to 90% with only half of all pioneer products (first in the market) surviving (4). Besides lack of funding, there are other reasons why products fail: customers not seeing the need for it, ineffective branding or wrong message, poor technical or design, poor timing, overestimation of the market size, ineffective promotion, and insufficient distribution (4).

INTERESTING READING

Two very interesting books on product marketing are *How To Create Your Own Fad and Make a Million Dollars*, by Ken Hakuta (5), and *Toyland: The High-Stakes Game of the Toy Industry*, by Stern and Schoenhaus (6). Both books are available used on Amazon.com but are out of print. Although these two books talk about the toy industry, the manufacturing trials, competition, retail problems, and the like, are often similar to those in other markets.

A third book that offers very entertaining reading is *The Rejects*, by Nathan Aaseng (7). It explores the difficulties and negative feedback that inventors of well-known, highly successful products or services had to endure to make their ideas successful.

CASE STUDY 6.2

NEW CAREER AVENUE—MARKETING A FOOD PRODUCT

Manette Richardson, RD, Director of Nutrition Services, Eggland's Best Eggs

In 1991, I was faced with looking for a new job. My position as the director of a hospital-based weight management program had been eliminated. I was weighing my options when I responded to a job posting in the local paper looking for a candidate with cholesterol education experience. The recruiter scheduled me to interview with Heartland's Best (now Eggland's Best), a new food marketing company. I knew working for this company would potentially launch me into a new career path, which meant there were challenges ahead, but that sounded fun.

The initial challenge was to get my foot in the door. During the interview, it was mentioned that the company would need to conduct further clinical trials using their product. They would need the services of a registered dietitian (RD) who would assist the research RD at the medical center. Two months later I was called and offered the opportunity to work in the clinical trials. Thus began my career at Eggland's Best eggs 17 years ago.

The best way to describe my role (that grew into a permanent position) of the Director of Nutrition Services comes from what I learned when I attended an American Wine and Food Workshop "Taste Meets Health." I had to evaluate my pantry to see what ingredients I had in inventory (skills, education, experiences, etc.) and determine what new ingredients I would need (marketing, sales, PR). I had to learn how to blend the business, my personal needs, and family because my job required that I travel approximately 50 days per year.

As a RD with 15 years of experience, I had the basics necessary for this job. I also knew that, as an active member of my local and state dietetic associations, I had a wealth of resources available to me. But I had to learn how to market myself to the company as well as market the company and its products. I had to learn about the egg business, marketing, sales, and public relations. I loved to cook, so recipes were not a problem, but handling a media interview while I cooked was a new skill I had to master, and cooking for 100 to 2,000 people per day in a booth made me learn more about sanitation, personnel management, food logistics, budgeting, multi-tasking, and trade show marketing. I have written cookbooks, pamphlets, customer education flyers, and participated in numerous executive planning meetings for new marketing ideas.

It was important to build my credibility with the company executives. Over the years, they saw how the company benefited from having a staff RD who was involved with the state and American Dietetic Association. As they worked with me in our booth at state dietetic meetings, and as we discussed sponsorship opportunities at dietetic meetings to highlight our eggs, they saw the value of having someone with credentials taking their scientific and marketing messages to the public and food professionals.

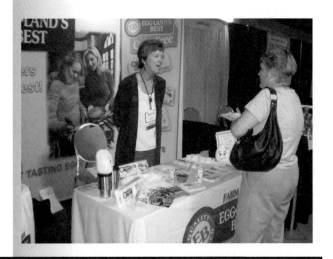

🌐 GLOBAL PERSPECTIVE: PHILIPPINES

Sanirose Orbeta, MS, RD, FADA

Dietitians in the Philippines have educational experience that is comparable to the United States. To practice, dietitians must successfully graduate with a baccalaureate degree in foods and nutrition, take a dietetic internship, and pass a two-day exam administered by the Philippine Professional Regulation Commission, a governing agency. Continuing education is required, and licensure is mandatory to practice. In 1993, reciprocity was established between the Commission on Dietetic Registration and the Philippine Professional Regulation Commission that allows dietitians trained and educated in either country the opportunity to take the other's registration exam without returning to school or taking an internship or other supervised segment.

At this time, our Philippine dietetic profession (like other health fields) is losing many of its potential students to the nursing profession. Due to the world-wide nurse shortage, nurses are in demand and they are able to easily land jobs here and abroad.

Dietitians are typically employed in hospitals and other health care agencies, like public health. Others work for school food services, industry, restaurants, on-board shipping food services, weight loss centers, in teaching or research, and private practice.

Our Newest Project

The Commission on Higher Education, which formulates rules, standards, and policies for Nutrition and Dietetic educators and practitioners in the Philippines, has initiated and approved a *Harmonized Curriculum* to be used in all schools offering nutrition.

The *Harmonized Curriculum* prepares the dietitian for a well-rounded, integrated approach in all the facets of nutrition and dietetic practice. This new form of the discipline will cut across the fields of clinical dietetics, public health, food service, education, and research. This academic milestone allows fluidity in future career paths in keeping with contemporary wellness and lifestyle needs. Such an approach addresses the demand for global competitiveness, allowing our graduates more working opportunities here and abroad.

ABOUT THE AUTHOR

Sanirose Singson Orbeta, MS, RD, FADA, is the founder of the first private Nutrition Therapy and Diet Clinic in the Philippines, and she is the first sports nutritionist in the Philippines and currently Head of the Sports Nutrition Unit, Philippine Center for Sports Medicine. She is also Sports Nutrition Consultant to the Philippine Olympic Committee. Mrs. Orbeta is currently the vice president of the Philippine Association for the Study of Overweight and Obesity, which studies the overweight population in the country, and acts as the delegate to the European Obesity Organization.

Mrs. Orbeta is a busy clinical private practitioner, sports nutrition lecturer, and a corporate nutrition presenter to big corporations in Manila, Southeast Asia, and the Pacific, seeing personal clients in Hong Kong, Taiwan, and Malaysia. She is a columnist for *Health and Wellness*, *Food Magazine*, and *Living Nutrition*.

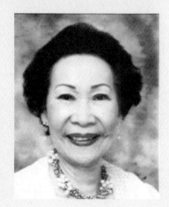

To organize a venture to sell a product, you should always research and write a business and a marketing plan (see Chapter 15). These plans will help you organize and check the feasibility of your venture.

SUMMARY

Developing a new product is fun and exciting. Trying to get it into the stores, catalogs, grocery stores, the Home Shopping Network, and the like is time-consuming, challenging, and expensive. It can be frustrating because investors and banks want to see the product first and see the results of a test market on target consumers. Most high-tech manufacturers will not do an electronic prototype for less than $50,000 to $100,000 for one or two samples. Food products cost less, but packaging, trademarks, etc., start to quickly add up. Videos, books, audio recordings, soaps, foods, and CDs are usually more reasonable to produce—costing $5,000 to $25,000, but you must add test marketing, packaging, distribution, shipping, and so on. After learning a little more about marketing a product, it makes you appreciate the effort it takes to have that item so readily available. (See case study on Manette Richardson and Eggland's Best Eggs.)

REFERENCES

1. Richman T. How to grow a product-based business. *Inc.* April 1990.

2. Beckwith H. *Selling the Invisible*. New York: Warner Books; 2003.

3. Kotler P, Pfoertsch W, Michi I. *B2B Brand Management*. Berlin, Germany: Springer; 2006.

4. Pride WM, Ferrell OC. *Marketing: Concepts and Strategies*, 12th Ed. New York: Houghton Mifflin; 2003.

5. Hakuta K. *How To Create Your Own Fad and Make a Million Dollars*. New York: Avon Books; 1989.

6. Stern S, Schoenhaus T. *Toyland: The High-Stakes Game of the Toy Industry*. Chicago, IL: Contemporary Books; 1991.

7. Aaseng N. *The Rejects*. Minneapolis, MN: Lerner Publications; 1989.

CUSTOMER SERVICE

Kathy King, RD, LD

In the early 1990s, at an American Dietetic Association (ADA) Futures Conference in Chicago, one of the speakers made the statement that U.S. businesses had discovered the customer and were now consumer-oriented, but there were two dinosaurs left in the United States—education and health care—that still believed the world revolved around educators and health professionals. He stated that in the next 10 to 20 years we would see huge changes in these two hold-outs and discovering customer service would lead the way. From a private practitioner's point of view, we learned from day one that customer service is the reason you have a business and will remain in business—customer service was our highest priority.

In 2002, ADA's House of Delegates recognized customer service as a core value of the profession and charged a committee to research it and bring it to the membership (1,2). Although lagging behind business and industry, health care is experiencing a paradigm shift from facility-centered care to a customer-focused culture and from purely clinical outcomes to incorporating customer satisfaction outcomes (3).

WHAT GOOD CUSTOMER SERVICE MEANS

Top quality customer service exceeds your customers' expectations and sets you apart from your competitors. To be effective, it must be consistently good in every part of your business—from when the customer first contacts you through each step of the way when delivering a product or service, and even after they leave (4). On careful evaluation, you can see there are opportunities where improved care of the customer could make his or her hospital stay, school lunch, nutrition consultation, or culinary experience more enjoyable or effective.

Where does customer service fit in with the other variables a business has to consider? A Genesys Telecommunications Labs 2007 poll of adults found the biggest influences on their loyalty to a company were 48% customer service, 37% product or service quality, 13% price, and 2% brand name or reputation (5). Now that puts things in perspective!

Dietetic professionals must improve customer service because (1):

- increased customer satisfaction drives the demand for dietetics services,
- increased demand for dietetics services drives reimbursement and salary increases,
- demand for dietetics services also increases recognition by our constituents, and
- increased demand for our services potentially means more work, better pay, and more job satisfaction.

WHAT WE KNOW ABOUT CUSTOMERS (4,6–10)

THE GOOD NEWS:

- Customers can't always tell which service is a superior service, but they know if it's good and whether they liked and respected the provider. That's where they will return.
- Customers can tell intuitively if they are being treated with respect and they expect it.
- Customers will pay up to 10% more for the same thing if they get top service.
- Word-of-mouth communication is the most effective form of promotion and it is controlled by you.
- The most important time with a customer is the first 4 minutes (greeting and getting to

know them) and the last 2 minutes (how you leave them).

- When customers get top service, they tell 9 to 12 people.
- Customers expect accuracy, timeliness, reliability, and availability.
- Once a long-term relationship is developed, a customer will tell an average of five new people about it every year.
- By retaining 5% of the customers you normally lose, you can increase profits 25% or more; it helps to create an aggressive plan to prevent losses and regain lost customers.

THE BAD NEWS:

- It costs five to six times more to get a new customer than to keep an existing one.
- Six out of ten customers who have a bad experience will never tell you.
- Research shows that on average a customer will tell 5 to 6 people about you when pleased with service and 8 to 10 when they are unhappy with it.
- When service is really bad, 91% of customers never go back and they tell 18 people who each tell five more people.

WHO ARE YOUR CUSTOMERS?

In order to serve your customers better, you must know who they are and where to find them. Ask yourself the following questions (5):

- How would you describe your most valuable customers?
- Where are your best customers in relation to your business location?
- What attracted them to you initially?
- What do they value?
- How long have they been your customers?
- What do they think about you and why?
- Are there any customers who actually cost you money? (They monopolize your time or excessively return items.)

WHAT DO YOUR CUSTOMERS NEED OR WANT?

In health care, patients are often very scared and sometimes in pain; it is a needy time. They are also sick of having to endure excuses, blame, and generally cold and unfeeling treatment from health care providers (10). Dietetic professionals have the enviable job of providing the one pleasure patients

and the public look forward to several times each day. What can we do to make that happen? Ask!

There's no point providing services that are not valued by your customers (4). That is a waste of time and resources!

Use a quick phone call, email or written survey, or online SurveyMonkey to find out your customers' wants and needs. You might also include an evaluation in with orders; print it on a self-addressed postcard. You can ask a few open-ended questions or use a scale (1–5 with 5 being the highest). Some suggestions include (4,6,7):

- Regularly ask your customers how well they like your business services.
- Phone, email, or mail a postcard to patients or clients a week or two after the sale to see if they are satisfied or if there are areas that need improvement.
- Keep a list of all suggestions and complaints to identify any patterns and the cause of the dissatisfaction.
- If there is a complaint, apologize immediately (no matter who was at fault) and offer to take care of it. Call back to tell the customer what was done about the issue and thank them for bringing it to your attention.

IDENTIFY YOUR KEY CUSTOMER SERVICE INTERACTIONS

Each step along the way in an interaction with a customer should be analyzed for ways to make it better. Typical situations include (4,6):

- answering the initial phone call or email to ask questions or get product information;
- responding to call-backs or missed contact opportunities;
- taking customer orders for products or providing service;
- scheduling follow-up and completing any referrals to other health practitioners;
- billing or collection of fees;
- follow-up visits or after-sale communication; and
- dealing with any complaints.

MAKE YOURSELF MORE VALUABLE— HOW THE BEST COMPANIES DO IT

The perceived value of a service or product is intertwined with customer service, not just the quality of the purchased product or delivery of the service by the professional. For that reason, all personnel involved must be carefully hired and trained. Also, all stages of contact with the customer must be scrutinized and improved if necessary.

Here are suggestions for making yourself valuable to your target market (1,3,4,6,7):

- The best businesses are guided by values, not slogans.
- Hire strong employees, train and treat them well, and empower them to make most customer service decisions.
- Make it very easy for customers to do business with you—have good phone coverage, a website, email, and toll free number if you have a large regional selling area. Deliver with minimal hassle.
- Respond immediately whether by phone or email—make customers feel appreciated.
- Offer helpful suggestions; let customers know how to use the portfolio system better or how to save money using a different one of your products, refer them to another professional who can serve their special needs better, and so on.
- Act like you enjoy being of service. Have a helpful, upbeat attitude, and listen well.
- Be honest about your timelines and what you can deliver.
- Remember a customer's name and use it in all conversations. Review the chart and any notes you made during the last visit before seeing the patient or client.
- Adapt your product or service to the customer's needs or wants. Offer convenient times and location, offer reasonable prices consistent with your image and experience, consider bundling revisits to offer a reduced price in return for prepayment, use your survey results to hone which tactics and strategies to include in your service, and so on.
- Attend to small details. Handwrite the thank you notes and notify customers of delayed deliveries.
- Pay attention to appearance—of you, your surroundings, and your promotion materials and advertising.
- Put processes in place that will allow you to know when problems arise, before they are out of hand.
- Take full responsibility for your products and services. Make sure you stand behind them, and if something goes wrong, take action to fix them.
- Differentiate your products and services by offering something valuable that your competitors do not offer.

TRAINING EMPLOYEES

The most successful businesses create a service-oriented culture that supports their employees, keeping them happy, productive, and consumer-oriented. Good employees support each other and have an understanding that the customer may not always be right, but the customer always comes first. When things go wrong or they were fine but the customer perceives them as wrong, the challenge is to make the experience with your company end on a positive note.

Brainstorm with your employees to try to match what you offer with what customers want (6). Slim down your procedures so there is less to go wrong and whatever you do, do it well (6). Reward and recognize good employees in order to help retain them, thus reducing turnover.

Don't assume that an employee will know how to answer the phone as you want or interact with customers as you would do. Design a training program to bring them up to your standards and then offer coaching, hands-on training, and actual practice while they learn the job. Have them know the answers to all frequently asked questions (FAQs); in fact, you can help relieve customer service personnel of the repetitive questions by posting FAQs on your web site and in your company brochure.

When communicating, it is important to use a warm tone of voice, be respectful, courteous, use friendly body language, good communication skills, and excellent telephone etiquette (5).

USING EMAIL IN CUSTOMER SERVICE

There are some rules to follow when using email to correspond with customers (6):

- Respond quickly, and if you need more time to formulate the answer, tell the customer.
- Let customers know approximate times when you check emails so they don't get so frustrated when you don't answer immediately.
- Don't use emails to deliver bad news—set up an in-person appointment; don't put anything into writing that you don't want to live with—consider if it could be used against you at a later date.
- Keep messages short, and send only necessary messages.
- Break the message into paragraphs or bullets for easy reading.
- Don't use all caps—it's considered shouting.
- Always proofread all your messages.

HANDLING AN ANGRY CUSTOMER

If a customer gets angry, even when you try to help solve the problem, what can you do? Stay calm. Let the person vent. Be professional and ask about the details of the problem. Don't blame anyone, but say the problem will be resolved and you are very sorry it happened.

EXTRA TOUCHES THAT REALLY WORK

- Throw in something special to your best customers when they make a purchase. Give a discount on their next purchase, send an overstocked cookbook home with them after a consultation, etc.
- Send something to your best referral agents. Give flowers to referring physicians' offices in the spring or a deli platter or gift basket at the holidays for their office.
- Send an online newsletter to customers.
- Use a database to remember significant dates and buying habits of individual customers. Use the information to personalize your services, promotion campaigns, and giveaways.

 GLOBAL PERSPECTIVE: UNITED KINGDOM

Paula Hunt, BSc, RD

There are approximately 6,000 dietitians in the United Kingdom (UK), and the vast majority of them are women and members of the British Dietetic Association (BDA).

Anyone claiming to be a dietitian must have an approved qualification and be registered with the regulatory Health Professions Council (HPC), which commits the registrant to certain professional standards and Continuing Professional Development (CPD).

Of the BDA members who are practicing, the most recent data show about 70% work for the National Health Service (NHS). The NHS has increased its number of dietitians by 76% since 2000. The NHS is funded by the government, and everyone is entitled to good quality health care through this system. A small proportion of people opt to buy additional private health care through insurance companies.

Changes in Dietetics

Dietetics in the UK is becoming increasingly diverse and more highly specialized. There is growth in community-based NHS work with an emphasis on health promotion. Much of this work is being done by dietitians working with general practitioners and the wider multidisciplinary primary health care team. There is also an increase in opportunities for dietitians to work outside the traditional NHS role, in industry, or in a freelance or consultancy capacity. Dietetics is becoming more business-oriented and client-centered, with an increased emphasis on evidence-based practice, needs assessment, and evaluation/audit of practice.

Strategic Plan

In 2005, the BDA developed a 3-year strategic plan to focus the work of the Council, Standing Committees, and staff as they carry out the BDA's work in advancing the science and practice of dietetics, providing trade union support to dietitians, and educating the wider public in nutrition and health issues. The BDA supports members' CPD commitments by offering courses and activities at its Centre for Education and Development that count towards learning hours, and by encouraging members to carry out research to improve dietetic practice and to publish their findings.

Externally, the creation of the post of Food and Health Policy Officer is aimed at giving the BDA a voice in the development of health policy at a national level. The National Public Relations Officer has grown into a full-time role to increase the Association's media exposure, an objective which has been further helped with the BDA Media Hotline, which is staffed by media-trained dietitians. The BDA has also created the role of Sponsorship Officer to develop links with commercial organizations and other partners in the health sector. This includes the Association's Food First project, an annual campaign that targets healthy eating messages at different sections of society.

The Future

Health policy has been given to each of the UK's four constituent counties and dietitians in each will work with other health care professions to achieve their relevant objectives. Health policy in England is driven by a white paper called Choosing Health.

continued

continued

At the same time, the Food Standards Agency, an independent government department set up in 2000, sets nutritional health targets and food nutrient standards for publicly procured food (for hospitals, schools, prisons, etc.) across the four counties.

A major theme from all the bodies setting health targets in the UK is the problem of obesity, particularly among children. A report in 2006 found that the UK was the fattest country in Europe, and there are major policy initiatives underway attempting to address the obesity crisis.

ABOUT THE AUTHOR

Paula Hunt, BSc, RD, works as an Independent Nutrition Consultant in England. She is perhaps best known for her work as an advisor to Weight Watchers UK and her expertise in health behavior change and motivational interviewing.

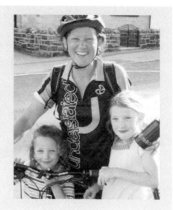

SUMMARY

Treat customers like you were treated in the best customer service experience of your life. Think about it! What experience so far in your life impressed you the most? What can you learn from it? As a dietetic professional, what food-related interaction can you have with a customer? Several private practitioners share beverages and healthy foods with their clients during consultations. In surveys, their clients identified this practice as their favorite.

REFERENCES

1. ADA Customer Service Tool Kit. Available at: http://eatright.org/cps/rde/xchg/ada/hs.xsl/governance_127_ENU_HTML.htm. Accessed February 22, 2008.
2. Laramee SH. Customer satisfaction advances the dietetics profession. *J Am Diet Assoc.* 2004;104:1519.
3. Finley D, Diekman C, Dorner B, Lofley DK. Putting the WOW!" in dietetics. *J Am Diet Assoc.* 2005;105:1149–1151.
4. Customer Service. *NSW We Mean Business.* Available at: http://www.smallbiz.nsw.gov.au/NR/rdonlyres/92E17D53-197A-4BBD-8B16-885B46294FFA/0/CustomerService.pdf. Accessed February 8, 2008.
5. Customer service plays big role in consumer loyalty. *USA Today*, May 30, 2007.
6. Win with Great Customer Service. Chicago, IL: Socrates Know How Made E-Z; 2004.
7. Beckwith H. *Selling the Invisible.* New York: Warner Business Books; 2002.
8. Is Your Customer Service Impacting Your Bottom Line? Irving, TX: Lowe's Talk of the Trade; September 1999.
9. Press I. *Patient Satisfaction.* Health Administration Press; 2002.
10. McClusky KW. Customer service in health care—Dietetics Professionals can take the lead. *J Am Diet Assoc* 2003;103:1282–1284.

8

EVALUATING YOUR COMPETITION

Mindy G. Hermann, MBA, RD

A dietitian had a successful private practice at the city headquarters of a major corporation. Suddenly, budget cutbacks forced him out of a steady position. What should he do—open an office near his home in a densely populated suburban area, or set up shop in a high-rent, upscale business district one hour from home? Renting office space in the suburbs is less expensive; rents in the business district are very high. Several dietitians have private practices near his home; only one dietitian serves the business district. After evaluating his competition in each location, the dietitian decided to sublease office space in the business district. His practice is booming.

The dietitian immediately improved his chances for business success by taking the pulse of the competitive environment. He determined that the suburban market, while attractive, would be too difficult to break into because it was so saturated with well-established dietetic consultants. On the other hand, the business district offered far more opportunity, even though start-up costs were higher. By jumping into a wide-open market, the dietitian not only avoided the competition, but also achieved a competitive advantage over other professionals who might decide to compete with him at a later point in time.

COMPETITION—WHY WORRY?

Good marketing practices require constant assessment of the competition. It is essential to know who you are up against in the competitive market, how their businesses are similar to or different from yours, and which consumer needs you fill that your competition does not. In every nutrition market—food service, counseling, consulting, writing, educating—successful dietitians and companies have developed distinct advantages over their competitors by meeting specific customer needs. Those who do not fill a unique need or maintain their competitive edge are at high risk for failure. The dynamic nature of the marketplace also requires constant surveillance of the competition to enable you to change and adapt your practice based on what your competitors do.

FINDING THE COMPETITION

Competition includes not only those businesses that are exactly like yours, but also those that are similar in one or more of three areas: products or services, customer base (target market), or geography. The grid in Table 8.1 illustrates the ways in which a dietitian who specializes in high school food service could define her competition. The better you define your own business, target markets, products, and services, the easier you will find it to define and identify your competition.

Keep in mind that your competition extends beyond other dietetics professionals. Physicians, chiropractors, non-registered-dietitian nutritionists, food service management companies, practitioners of alternative therapies, and even health food stores may be competing with you for the same clinical clients. All eating establishments within a certain radius may compete with your corporate cafeteria for employees or with your campus dorm dining room for students.

The next step is to get as much information as possible about competitors who appear to fit the product or service, target market, and geographic profiles of your business. For a general but incomplete list of potential competitors, start with the Yellow Pages. However, the limitations of the Yellow Pages are that they give little or no specific information and can be time-consuming to use. Instead, for a clinical business, speak to as many

TABLE 8.1. COMPETITION GRID

Major Players	Product or Service	Customer Base	Geography
Close competitors	Sack lunches	Students at Central High	Stores and fast food within 1-mile radius
	7-11 fast food Vending snacks McDonalds		
Broad competitors	All restaurants, fast food, vending, home cooking	All teenagers	In the same county

local health professionals as possible—physicians, nurses, physical and occupational therapists, and pharmacists—to get a feel for who the major players are and how saturated the market is.

Market research can help identify unmet customer needs, such as nutrition services that competing practitioners currently do not offer or catered foods that clients like but no one offers. Consider developing a brief market research questionnaire to distribute to members of your target market or referral sources.

One of the best ways to get information on the competition is to network, network, network. Talk to friends, neighbors, and local merchants to learn about private practitioners in your area—who they are, how well-known they are, and what they do. Talk to colleagues in dietetic practice groups. Telephone contacts and potential clients in public relations, advertising, food-service management, nursing-home management, home care, or other fields related to your area of business. Each call should generate the name of at least one additional person to call.

Bonnie Taub-Dix, a nutrition consultant with private practice in the New York City area, attributes her success to networking. After each new client appointment, she sent letters to both the referring physician and the primary physician, whom she did not know. Her mailing to the primary physician included a nutrition report on the client, along with a letter of introduction, a resume, and a business card. Every letter was followed up with a phone call. Taub-Dix used this type of networking to introduce herself to potential sources of new clients and to keep her name prominent in the physicians' minds for future referrals.

Identify at least one dietetics professional who has firm roots in the professional community, is not a direct competitor, and can be trusted. Ask in confidence about the scope of business, professional reputation, and image of each potential competitor. Ask this dietitian to please keep your business plans private to prevent competitors from knowing your ideas.

Dietetic practice groups are another good source of information on competitors. Look at the Internet, newsletters, and directories for names of both contact persons and potential competitors. Contact one or more prominent practice group members for additional information on who is doing what type of business. Information on competitors can be documented in a log book or on a computer. Include information on type of business, target market, approximate size (big, medium, small), strengths and weaknesses (for example, well-connected in food industry [strength] or not available for evening counseling [weakness]). Finally, add an assessment of perceived threat, that is, how much your competitor's business overlaps yours. You can then use this information to define and modify your own business.

FITTING INTO THE COMPETITIVE ENVIRONMENT—POSITIONING

Armed with a comprehensive profile of your competitors, you can now structure and market your business, or position your products and services competitively, to fill unmet consumer needs better than anyone else.

First, decide how broad to make your product or service line. A nutrition consultant, for example, could offer a full line of counseling services if no other competitors serve the same geographic market. Consultants in highly competitive markets should look for specific market segments whose needs are not being met (e.g., pregnant women or overweight teens).

Seeking out windows of opportunity where you will encounter little or no competition improves your chance of success. Leni Reed, founder of Supermarket Savvy, spotted a window of opportunity in supermarket tours. Although other dietitians had been conducting supermarket tours for years, none had developed a formal program. Reed turned Supermarket Savvy into a marketable product that included instruction kits for dietitians, slide sets, and a newsletter. She sold her company to Linda McDonald, who expanded it (see Chapter 21). Julie Hagan, a nutrition consultant in Mount Kisco, New York, became an expert in counseling children because few, if any, services were available for children with nutrition-related medical problems.

Use information on your competitors' price structures to set up or fine-tune your own pricing. In a saturated market with an abundance of competition, lowering price may seem the only way to build your business, but use it as your choice of last resort! To grow strong in the marketplace, you and your products or services must have some inherent competitive advantages other than price! If you are the only player in the market, you have the luxury of charging higher prices, as long as clients will pay. Higher prices often, but not always, connote higher quality. Conversely, some markets respond only to lower prices.

Linda Jones, a consulting dietitian in Sandy Hook, Connecticut, worked for one of two local fitness centers. The other fitness center attracted a wealthy, older crowd, while the center employing Jones was frequented by young singles. Jones created package deals for pre-paid multiple visits to appeal to her unique market, which reduced the overall cost per visit. To be profitable, it was important that Jones' overhead was low and that a higher volume of sales made up for lower profit on each sale.

Evaluate how you are most likely to succeed and remain profitable: getting into the market first, making your product or service different from the competition (differentiation), or focusing on a market segment that others are unlikely to go after. The first in the market (the leader) has the most time to iron out bugs and build a loyal customer base. Theoretically, the longer you have been in the markets, the more you have learned from your experience; the more you know about your business and market, the better able you are to compete.

Product or service differentiation works well if there is an unfulfilled need or desire in your target market. For example, you could develop an office delivery service for busy businesswomen or men for the evening meal; this is for the person who does not want to go home and cook or eat alone at a restaurant at night. The menu could range from comfort foods to gourmet entrees for small dinner parties.

The final course of action might be to focus on a specific market segment that competitors are unlikely to go into (e.g., a particular immigrant population not fluent in the English language). Dietetic professionals fluent in less widely spoken languages may encounter little if any competition.

KEEPING AHEAD OF THE COMPETITION

Business environments constantly change. Outside factors, such as Diagnose Related Groups (DRGs), growth of the TV Food Network, health care reform, and peaks and valleys in the economy have catalyzed change in the food and nutrition business. Competitors have dropped out, new products and services have entered the market, businesses have folded, and other businesses have merged. The goal of any business is to remain competitive in spite of shifting forces in the marketplace. Businesses usually fall into one of four competitive categories: market leader, challenger, follower, or niche marketer. Marketing strategies change to better fit the competitive positioning.

MARKET LEADER

If you are the biggest in the market, you are the market leader. When the target market needs a particular product, they think of the leader first. This can make the leader very powerful in setting the standards by which products and services are measured. But on the downside, lack of competition may make leaders lazy and complacent. Market leaders continually must fight off competitors and keep costs under control. It is expensive to be the market leader because keeping competitors away usually means cutting price, increasing advertising, or adding promotions. Market leaders are forced by competitive pressures to introduce new products and services, improve existing products and services, set appropriate prices, and strengthen weaknesses.

CHALLENGER OR RUNNER-UP

The number two spot in the market is held by the challenger, or runner-up. Challengers often try to go head-to-head and overtake the market leader, even though it is expensive and difficult to do. One strategy is to offer the same services or products as the market leader does, but at a lower price, with a different flair, or with a different distribution channel. For example, the market leader in nutrient analyses may offer 15-nutrient computerized diet analyses for $30 per diet; the challenger charges the same for the same analysis but offers a 24-hour turnaround time.

GLOBAL PERSPECTIVE: LEBANON

Najat Yahia, PhD, RD

Evolution of Nutrition and Dietetics

In Lebanon, the evolution of nutrition and dietetics started in 2003 when three private Lebanese universities, namely Kaslik, Notre Dame, and Saint Joseph, joined the American University of Beirut in offering this curriculum. Currently, in all universities, the academic requirements are based on the standards of the American Dietetic Association.

Dietetic students must successfully complete 3 years of courses, a supervised practical training of not less than 6 months in a Lebanese hospital setting, and pass a national exam. The 3-year program includes courses in biology, chemistry, biochemistry, sociology, psychology, and several core nutrition courses. A Bachelor degree in Nutrition and Dietetics prepares students for employment or advanced study in one of several professions in the broad areas of food, nutrition, and dietetics.

Government Policy

In 2005, the Lebanese government issued a nutrition law to enforce academic standards, establish proper qualifications for nutrition and dietetics, and insure high standards of performance in the profession. According to the Lebanese Nutrition Law, Lebanese graduates cannot practice dietetics unless they are registered and licensed by the Ministry of Health. To date, 115 dietitians are registered and licensed. However, there are more than 500 Lebanese graduates that can undergo registration.

Career Market

In Lebanon, clinical nutritionists and dietitians work closely with other health professionals in hospitals, nursing homes, outpatient clinics, public health agencies, corporate health, or food processing industries. Administrative dietitians direct food service planning, purchasing, production, and service of meals in medical centers, restaurants, and schools. Holders of graduate degrees in nutrition work in colleges, technical schools, and universities. They teach future doctors, nurses, dietitians, and other health professionals the science of nutrition and foods. They also conduct research experiments to solve critical nutrition questions and provide dietary recommendation to the public. Currently, an increasing number of dietitians are completing other kinds of graduate degrees such as Master of Public Health and Master of Health Administration/Business Administration. Similarly, others are completing PhD degrees, which are not offered in Lebanon.

Lebanese Associations

In Lebanon, there are many non-government associations that deal with food, nutrition, and dietetics issues. The Lebanese Association for Nutrition & Food Science was founded by the American University of Beirut, and the Lebanese Association for Nutrition and Dietetics (LAND) was founded by Notre Dame University and Lebanese American University. Their aim is to provide scientifically based nutrition information to the country. Membership to any association is voluntary. Dietetic licensure and registration is under the jurisdiction of the Ministry of Health.

Future Market Trends

As rapid advances in medicine increase the dietitian's role as a member of the health care team, dietetics in Lebanon is becoming increasingly popular in health promotion and the well-being of the Lebanese population. Nutritionists and dietitians are in demand in community health. They are becoming a common sight in the media and are more widely available in private health clubs. All hospitals in Lebanon have at least one dietitian. Dietitians are developing important relationships with food manufactures, food service companies, and industries specializing in marketing and food development. Future growth for dietitians appears to lie in community health and private practice. Some Lebanese dietitians have affiliation with international organizations such as the British Dietetic Association, the American Overseas Association Dietetic Association, and the American Dietetics Association.

ABOUT THE AUTHOR

Najat Yahia, PhD, RD is registered and licensed by the Ministry of Health, Lebanon, and is an ADA member. Dr. Yahia is employed as an assistant professor of Nutrition at Notre Dame University (NDU), where she was the founder and implementer of the Nutrition and Dietetics major at NDU and initiator of the program at other Lebanese universities. She 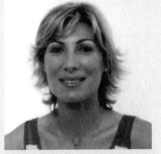 participated in the preparation of Lebanese Nutrition Law. Dr. Yahia graduated from American University of Beirut with a BS degree in Medical Laboratory Technology (MLT), an MS in Nutrition and Dietetics, and a PhD in Clinical Nutrition from King's College, London. She has a certificate in weight management from the ADA and is serving as the National Coordinator for Research for the International Diabetes Outcome Study (IDOS), supported by the ADA, in Lebanon. She has a private practice for weight management and she has been a speaker on nutrition issues in many local radio and TV shows.

FOLLOWERS

Followers are providers of products and services who are not positioned to become market leaders. As a follower, your strategy is different. A follower tries to capitalize on the leader's weaknesses or satisfy needs in the target market that the leader overlooks, albeit not for long, if the strategy is successful. Many followers are comfortable with the size and scope of their businesses; for example, a freelance magazine writer with small children at home who decides to accept only one article assignment a month, or a media spokesperson who limits traveling to two weeks per month. The follower's main challenge is to keep business at a steady level.

NICHE BUSINESSES

Niche businesses are so specialized that they are not in conflict with the market leader. The owners of such businesses are faced with the challenge of finding a niche that is profitable, has growth potential, and is not in direct competition with the market leader. For example, you consult to food services that are ready to convert from full-service cafeterias to salad and sandwich preparation only.

SUMMARY

The competition can be a valuable source of information on which factors lead to business success. Carefully evaluate your competition—what they are doing right, what they did wrong, what made them succeed. Use that information to modify and build your own business. Remember that a one-time look at the competition is never enough; follow your competitors throughout the life cycle of your business.

BIBLIOGRAPHY

Corey ER. *Marketing Strategy: An Overview*. Boston: Harvard Business School Case Services; 1978.

Kotler P, Keller KL. *Marketing Management*, 12th Ed. Englewood Cliffs, NJ: Prentice Hall; 2006.

Pride WM, Ferrell OC. *Marketing: Concepts and Strategies*, 12th Ed. New York: Houghton Mifflin; 2003.

BUSINESS SKILLS AND MARKETING PLAN

MARKETING THROUGH NETWORKING

9

Sharon O'Melia Howard, MS, RD, CDE, FADA, LDN

Why do dietetic professionals need to network? We may be trained to be nutrition experts, but we have a lot to learn about the real world of business as intrapreneurs and entrepreneurs. Networking can enable you to:

- meet people with new resources and perspectives;
- share your expertise and knowledge;
- boost your business, get referrals, and find new opportunities or careers;
- find a job or assistance with career management;
- improve your professional image in your field or community;
- find qualified business advisers, employees, and mentors;
- learn new business and problem-solving skills; and
- reduce feelings of isolation and gain emotional support.

Communication channels become less formal as jobs become less secure and opportunities are more entrepreneurial. Networks for the purpose of job searches become crucial. Many consultants report that 70% to 80% of their jobs come through networking rather than from sending out resumes and answering ads.

Networking is fun, potentially profitable, and effective!

WHO SHOULD BE IN YOUR NETWORK?

Your network can move in many directions, like a spider's web or the spoke of a wheel with you at the hub. Select your directions carefully and evaluate your steps as you go, because you have only so much time and energy. Develop networks where you can make a contribution and realize long-term benefits for your business.

You already have many people and contacts in your network: friends, family, their friends and colleagues, community and religious groups, dietetic associations, clients, physicians, employers, co-workers, cultural and hobby groups, neighbors, local and national business or political organizations. Join committees—the program committee allows you to make connections with people of interest as you solicit speakers. You can find networking groups in the Yellow Pages. A resource in a business library, *American Society of Executives Directory*, lists over 20,000 organizations!

HOW DO YOU NETWORK?

1. *Write your personal and professional goals.* As you clarify these on paper, you will find it easier to select the directions to pursue (See Chapter 4).
2. *Get an attitude.* Develop a positive attitude to make the effort to get to know others. Networking should become a habit. You never know where or when a business opportunity may arise.
3. *Have a plan.* Based on your time and energy, decide how many networking opportunities you can attend or create each month. Attend local and national meetings to meet people as well as to hear speakers. Call an acquaintance for lunch.
4. *Improve interpersonal skills.* Set a goal for each large function you attend. Collect 10 business cards and give out 10 of yours. Be sure to greet people openly and be able to describe what you do in 20 words (see #7 below). As you elicit information from another person, think about what you do to benefit him or her. Be resourceful and genuinely interested. A person who networks well is confident, enthusiastic, and caring.

BOX 9.1	*Networking Groups (not industry specific)*

- National Association of Female Executives: http://www.nafe.com
- American Business Women's Association: http://www.abwahq.org
- BusinessNetworkInternational (BNI): http://www.bni.com
- Leads Club: http://www.leadsclub.com
- Le Tip International, Inc.: http://www.letip.com

BOX 9.3	*Service Groups*

- Lions Club
- Rotary Club
- Chambers of Commerce
- The League of Women Voters
- Political groups
- Charities
- PTAs
- Church groups

5. *Know networking etiquette.* Know how to dress, shake hands firmly but comfortably, have good eye contact, smile, and be friendly. Make a good first impression. Just as you would use a marketing or PR firm for your business image, consider an image consultant to help. Know proper manners in social situations, such as introductions. If meals are involved, know your meal etiquette.

6. *Make good conversation.* Be ready with conversation "starters" to get past that first awkward moment. People like to talk about themselves. Be an effective listener by following up with pertinent comments or questions. "What has brought you to this event?" "What do you do?" "What do you like best about your job?" "I need some help with finding (an accountant, a good steak restaurant, or other people in my business)." "Could you give me (referrals, directions, or introductions)?" Listen more than you talk.

7. *Practice your "elevator speech."* In less than 30 seconds, you can make an impact with a summary of what you want the listener to know about you and your business. Give your name, business, and what you can do for others. Do not drone on about yourself, but learn to be

comfortable with self-promotion. Women tend to downplay their accomplishments and credentials. If no one knows about your *successes*, you will not be noticed. Prepare a biography that highlights your achievements and experience. Send press releases announcing your business, news, and successes.

> Sample elevator speech:
> "Hi, I am Sue Smith; my business is Calci-Cookies. I make getting more calcium in your diet a lot more fun than a pill."

8. *Be visible.* Offer a course at your local community college on your special expertise or interest. You could extend a free consult to the participants. Host a Chamber of Commerce meeting. Write articles in your subject area for newsletters, trade journals, and local newspapers. Volunteer to be a speaker at your networking group. Become a media resource; you will get called as the authority and get quoted.

9. *Follow up your contacts.* Send an informal, friendly letter to all your new business card contacts within 3 days. Mention ideas that might be interesting to pursue. If you have a reason to meet, suggest it, and call within 2 weeks to schedule it. Enclose any materials or

BOX 9.2	*Industry-Specific Groups*

Following are examples of groups formed around a specific profession or industry; they may provide information, education, certification, or regulation:

- American Dietetics Association
- Society for Nutrition Education
- Trade Associations (e.g., Dietary Managers Association: http://www.dmaonline.org)
- Use Google to search for trade associations http://www.google.com/intl/en/options/. Browse by topics.

BOX 9.4	*Special Interest Groups*

- Book clubs
- Health or Wellness clubs
- Hobby groups: autos, stamping, trains, etc
- Game clubs: bridge, tennis, bowling, chess
- Sports clubs: biking, basketball, football
- Fraternities and Sororities
- Alumni groups
- Business or executive networking groups

articles that may be of interest to the person. Keep a file of the business cards, arranged either by event, state, country, or alphabet.

10. *Build relationships.* Be genuinely interested and helpful. You will be remembered by the person if you are able to "do a favor" by providing them with valuable information they are looking for or by introducing them to a good contact, restaurant, or car repair shop! You will stand out in his mind after the event, and you will feel more connected. People naturally want to "return the favor"—what you give can very well come back to you.

11. *Persevere.* People do not always remember casual acquaintances. It often takes several meetings before someone will remember you. Salespeople know that 82% of their sales are made after the fifth call. You may need to attend five events or meetings before you reap benefits from your efforts. Be visible, be a good listener, and be yourself.

12. *Say thank you.* Send short notes to let others know you appreciate their efforts. One very successful businesswoman told me that in 5 years not one woman has thanked her for leads and special favors, but men have reciprocated with business leads and helpful feedback. Women need to see the benefit in helping other women in their businesses and careers. Men have been doing this very well for some time.

CASE STUDY 9.1

COMBINING NUTRITION AND A PASSION FOR COSMETICS

Tendai Kaisa, MS, RD, LDN, Philadelphia, PA

I am a Registered Dietitian with a Post-Masters Certificate in Nutrition Marketing and I am also a licensed esthetician (makeup artist) with my own company called Nutri-Beaute. For 15 years, I worked as a dietitian in clinical, community, wellness, and health promotion settings. I have always had an interest in cosmetics, especially makeup. Makeup artistry was a fun hobby. As a dietitian, people always asked me if there were any foods that promoted healthy skin or if certain foods caused acne or other skin breakouts. I had also noticed over the years that healthy, unblemished skin needed little or no makeup. After a few years of hearing these questions, I decided to get a better understanding of skin care and treatment. My main focus was to learn to create a healthy "canvas" for makeup application.

With that in mind, 11 years ago, I became a makeup artist, and then a licensed esthetician. Upon completion of my training, I began working for cosmetics companies at promotional events, in retail sales, and at day and wellness spas.

There is an increased consumer interest in health and beauty reflected by the emergence of "cosmeceuticals," as well as natural cosmetics and beauty aids. Pick up any women's magazine and you will find articles or advertisements about beauty benefits of good nutrition. According to Jennifer Haid, in *Wellness & Vanity*, consumers are looking for beauty products that provide health benefits (1). *Nutraceuticals World* trade magazine developed, Beauty I/O, a magazine devoted to beauty with features on the food and nutrition and the beauty link (2). In 2006, *Forbes* magazine reported that the cosmetic industry was a growing industry with global sales of $230 billion (3). This is great news for dietitians interested in the beauty industry. The options are endless.

CAREER OPTIONS FOR DIETITIANS

A dietetics degree provides a good physical science and nutrition background, which allows an esthetician a better understanding of appropriate products and treatment to recommend. Esthetician job options for dietitians with cosmetology training include:

- Work in or owning a Day, Destination, or Wellness Spa, providing nutrition counseling for health and wellness (which is key in promoting healthy skin), providing "beauty" treatments, conducting workshops and developing education materials.
- Assist in product development, marketing, promotion, and consumer education for cosmetics companies. The latest industry trend is interest in the role of nutrition in promoting healthy skin and anti-aging remedy.

BEAUTY TRAINING

MAKEUP ARTISTRY

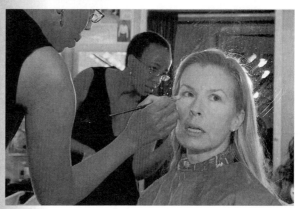

continued

continued

Education/training varies, depending on your areas of interest and career goals. Makeup artistry programs offer training from basic beauty makeup to advanced courses in special effects makeup for television and film. Cosmetics companies also offer makeup artistry training. Although the training is specific to that cosmetic company's product line, the general application techniques taught are transferable to other cosmetic lines. Regulations vary from state to state, but in general, a makeup artist does not require a license for routine makeup application. The exception is if you work in a salon, spa, or other settings where you may be required to provide services that require formal training as an esthetician, such as hair removal (waxing), eye brow tinting, etc. If you are working in an area where these services are not required, such as retail, a license may not be required.

ESTHETICIAN

Education/training is offered at state accredited schools. The Esthetics (skin care) curriculum includes theory and hands-on practical training. The curriculum covers biology, chemistry, and physiology of skin; general nutrition; and ingredients in cosmetics. This is valuable information when advising clients on appropriate products for their specific skin type. The number of required hours of training varies from state to state, but a license is required to practice. State board examinations include testing on theory and practical competence.

DIETETICS

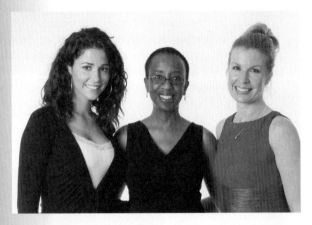

My education and training provided a wonderful foundation for my interest in beauty:

- Biology, chemistry, physiology, and nutrition courses provided better understanding of skin health. As an esthetician, I better understand the importance of diet on overall health and how it reflects in your skin's health (e.g., the importance of adequate fluid intake for hydration. I believe that healthy skin begins with "nourishing your beauty inside out."
- Counseling skills developed as a dietitian are an advantage in conducting skincare and treatment assessments as well as educating my clients about skincare and nutrition at home.
- Education background is also beneficial for facilitating workshops, and developing education materials.
- Healthy skin requires a wellness approach, which includes a healthy diet, exercise, stress management (minimize those lines), a good amount of sleep (prevent those dark circles in the morning), and sun protection (to protect from the damaging effects of the sun), all of which are not easily attainable without the means to effectively communicate your message.
- A marketing background is an essential tool for developing creative ways to make nutrition relevant to different segments.

I am very excited that this is a great time to be a dietitian especially if you have an interest in the beauty industry.

Copyright T. Kaisa

1. Haid J. Wellness & Vanity: Where Health and Beauty Meet. *Nutraceuticals World, Beauty I/O.* Available at: http://www.nutraceuticalsworld.com/beautyio/200709/wellness-vanity-where-health-and-beauty-meet. Accessed November, 2007.
2. Nutraceuticals World, *Beauty I/O* Available at: http://www.nutraceuticalsworld.com/beautyio/200709. Accessed November, 2007.
3. Momma Heliodor. World's Best-Selling Makeup. Available at: http://www.forbes.com/2006/02/08/best-selling-cosmetics. Accessed November, 2007.

A PERSONAL EXAMPLE

As a dietitian in private practice, I often feel isolated from other professionals because most of my days are spent in one-on-one contact with clients. To illustrate how networking works and the potential it can offer you, let me share this personal example.

A client of mine mentioned she was the editor of a newsletter for a local organization for businesswomen called Women's Referral Network. The group meets monthly to network over lunch and listen to a speaker on a topic of interest to women in business. This struck me as a great opportunity to learn how other women solve business problems, increase my professional visibility outside of dietetics, and maybe even make new friends!

I was introduced to the group by my client. I quickly became involved with the program committee and accepted the opportunity to speak about nutrition and women's health at one of the luncheons, which was attended by 150 women. From my networking at the luncheons and my speech, I attracted new private clients, found a new office to sublease, hired a firm to do my mailings, obtained a part-time secretary, and was asked to work with the caterer to provide light, low-fat meals for our meetings.

More opportunities followed. I met an enterprising woman at one luncheon who was starting a news magazine for women entrepreneurs. As we chatted, I mentioned that I occasionally wrote for local newspapers and would love the opportunity to write for her. Not long after that she offered me a regular column in her magazine. Her business grew substantially, and she now offers business seminars. Because of my column, I receive complementary registration for her wonderful programs, where I meet dynamic businesspeople in the Philadelphia area. As a result of their advice and examples, I have improved my business practices.

My involvement in the business world landed me a job teaching entrepreneurship to dietitians in a graduate school. My magazine editor friend, and now mentor, benefits from having my students attend her seminars and subscribe to her magazine. This story has no ending; it is exciting to know that being open and willing to participate can bring many unpredictable benefits in return.

SUMMARY

The business world where we work is relationship-based. To get ahead, you must have a web of relationships inside our profession as well as with key players outside of dietetics and nutrition. Just as other people give our private lives fun, depth, and meaning, so too will networking and building professional relationships. Most good jobs come from knowing someone.

NEGOTIATING AGREEMENTS

10

Felicia Busch, MPH, RD, and Julie Mattson Ostrow, MS, RD

Your ability to negotiate may be key to the success or failure of your business or department. In today's business climate, negotiations can and should be conducted so that both parties win. The ultimate goal in the negotiation process is to reach an agreement that is satisfying to all. For many, the idea of negotiating a contract with a potential client may seem intimidating. Actually, it is a skill often used in our daily lives. We negotiate chores with our families, project assignments with coworkers, and entertainment schedules with friends. Entrepreneurial and intrapreneurial dietitians need to develop and practice their negotiation skills to attain the appropriate compensation for their work.

EIGHT STEPS TO EFFECTIVE NEGOTIATIONS

To enhance your effectiveness in negotiating, try this eight-step approach.

STEP 1: PREPARE

Learn all that you can about the other side or company and key contacts before any sales efforts are begun. Read the business section of the newspaper, community business papers and magazines, and research in the library. Find out who your competitors are and how to differentiate your services from what they offer. Determine what has to be done and develop alternatives. Focus on the value that you can bring.

STEP 2: DISCUSS

During the discussion, listen. Listening is a skill you may need to work on because it is often easy to talk too much. Not only is talking too much unprofessional, but it could also lead to making too many concessions.

STEP 3: SIGNAL

Signaling is a method of moving negotiations forward by testing the other side's willingness to modify their position. Asking a potential client to consider a particular option or feature of your service is a signal. For example, you might ask, "If enough employees sign up for the weight-loss class to fill two groups, can we schedule two groups?"

STEP 4: PROPOSE

Once your signal is read, it is time to discuss the proposition. Offer a position that has some room for compromise. It might be advantageous to offer several levels of service instead of a fixed proposal. Consider asking for more than you will settle for so you will have items or fees to bargain away. For example, you might say, "We can offer your corporation a group weight-loss program, a healthy lifestyle seminar, individual nutrition consultations for employees with heart disease and diabetes, and healthy food selections for your vending machines and cafeteria. Our most comprehensive plan offers all four services."

STEP 5: RESPOND

Now is the time for you to respond to any new objections. Carefully consider any concession that the other side may offer as an opportunity for compromise. Determine what they really want and what you require in return. Consider options that may be new to the discussion and will better satisfy both parties.

STEP 6: BARGAIN

You may have to bargain to get what you want. Be sure to keep your offer conditional by making comments such as, "If I agree to this, then you agree to . . ."

STEP 7: CLOSE

The key to a final agreement is the close. Restate the final decision so that all parties understand what the proposal is. To bring the other party to closure, consider asking, "What will it take for you to come to an agreement?" or "How soon can we start if we agree today?" or "So if you get . . . and I get . . ., do we have an agreement?"

STEP 8: AGREE

The goal of every negotiation should be to agree. When an agreement is reached, write it down before anyone leaves. Before starting the project, make sure the agreement is described in detail in writing and signed off by all parties.

CONTRACTS

Contracts are one of the tools of a successful businessperson. Today's business environment demands that dietitians use clear and meaningful documents to outline their services. Contracts also form the basis for negotiations.

A contract is an agreement that creates an obligation. To be considered legal, a contract must include these basic parts: an offer and acceptance, consideration of who gets what, parties who are capable of entering into a contract, and subject matter or a purpose that is legal.

While some verbal agreements may be legally enforced, written contracts are far more preferable. A written contract may take various forms, ranging from a simple letter of agreement to a detailed formal document drafted by an attorney. A written contract can spell out the terms of your proposed work and help avert misunderstandings. If necessary, a written contract can also be used as evidence in a court of law.

Generally, a letter of agreement is a contract written in simple language that spells out the details of a work proposal. Such agreements may be written on your own company stationery and typically run no longer than three pages. Included at the end of the letter is space for both parties' signatures. See Figure 10.1 for an example of a letter of agreement.

More formal contracts may be required when:

- financial risk is greater,
- intellectual property is involved, or
- you are working with a large corporation, many different people, or over a long period of time (see Fig. 10.2).

Since contracts contain more legal language and include many more details, have an attorney write or review a contract before you sign it. You should never verbally agree to a contract's provisions if you intend to have your attorney review the contract before signing it. Voicing premature agreement can create significant misunderstanding if you later decide to renegotiate something.

1. *Who* is the key decision maker who will authorize work? Who will own the copyright or legal right to your work?
2. *What* exact services are you to perform? What is needed from your client for you to carry out your work in the manner described? What products are included in the agreement? What can you hope to gain from this work in addition to fees?
3. *When* does the work start? When is the expected completion date of the project? Is there a final deadline or a series of deadline dates prior to completion? When will you be paid?
4. *Where* will meetings be held and services performed? Are travel expenses included in the fee or paid as an additional reimbursable expense?
5. *What* are the client's expectations in this agreement? Can you show the client a sample of your work that is similar to what is expected?

FEES

A contract should also spell out the method in which you will be paid. Two of the most commonly used methods are fixed fee (by the project) and cost per hour or day. (For a detailed explanation of how to determine your fees, see Chapter 11.)

Fixed or Project Fee

When charging a fixed fee, you must accurately estimate the number of hours you will spend on the project, plus make allowances for additional expenses you may incur. Most clients like a fixed-fee arrangement because it enables them to budget the entire project up front. Under this method, you assume all the risk if the project goes over the budgeted number of hours, so it is wise to estimate a range of hours to give yourself some leeway. Be sure to ask for separate payment for reimbursable expenses, such as mileage, long-distance phone calls, and supplies purchased on behalf of the project. Your client may want to place a limit on such expenses.

Cost

Under the cost method of payment, you simply charge your hourly or daily rate, which should

AGREEMENT FOR NUTRITION CONSULTING SERVICES

This document shall serve as a Letter of Agreement between Nutrition Consultants, Inc., 1234 Apple, Saint Paul, Minnesota and HealthSystems, Inc., 0000 Avenue South, Minneapolis, Minnesota. The contract period is from October 15, 2009 through October 14, 2009.

Nutrition Consultants, Inc. shall be compensated for services in developing a registered dietitian referral system in the amount of $5,500.00. Reimbursable expenses in addition to the fixed fee shall include long-distance telephone calls, photocopying, postage, fax services, mailing lists, incentive awards, and other incidentals directly related to provision of services.

In addition, Nutrition Consultants, Inc., agrees to seek out promotional opportunities for HealthSystems, Inc., to assist in increasing its client base. These activities will focus on RDs, the local media, and corporations. For this ongoing service, Nutrition Consultants, Inc., will be compensated by a monthly retainer of $1,000.00 for the duration of this agreement.

Requested services outside the scope of this agreement will be billed at the rate of $85.00 per hour. All additional services will require advance authorization from the designated HealthSystems, Inc., representative.

A monthly activity report will be submitted, along with an invoice for direct and other authorized expenses, by the first of each month. Invoices are to be paid by the fifteenth of the month in which they are submitted. Interest in the amount of 8 percent per annum will be added to all late payments.

Nutrition Consultants, Inc., agrees to maintain current registrations, licenses, malpractice insurance, and all other requirements necessary to practice as registered dietitians in the state of Minnesota

Both Nutrition Consultants, Inc., and HealthSystems, Inc., acknowledge that the relationship entered into by this agreement is that of independent parties and not that of employer and employee. Both parties enter into this temporary relationship for the purpose of affecting the provisions of this Letter of Agreement, and do not deem or construe to create a relationship as agents, employees, or representatives of each other.

Either party may terminate this agreement, with or without cause, at any time upon giving the other party sixty (60) days' written notice.

HealthSystems, Inc.   Nutrition Consultants, Inc.

By_____   By_____

Designated Representative   Designated Representative

Date _____   Date _____

FIGURE 10.1. ■ An example letter of agreement.

AGREEMENT BETWEEN
CORPORATE HEALTH CARE CORPORATION
AND
NUTRITION CONSULTANTS. INC.

THIS AGREEMENT, effective January 1, 2009 between Corporate Health-Care Corporation ("CHC") and Nutrition Consultants, Inc. ("NCI").

WHEREAS, CHC is a for-profit corporation organized and operated for the purposes of developing and marketing alternative health care delivery systems and related products and services; and

WHEREAS, CHC desires to arrange for the development and implementation of health-promotion programs and NCI are duly registered dietitians and health educators who desire to develop and implement health-promotion programs for CHC;

THEREFORE, in consideration of the mutual covenants herein contained, the parties hereby agree as follows:

SECTION 1. NUTRITION CONSULTANTS. INC. OBLIGATIONS:
1.01. <u>Food for Health Program.</u> NCI shall develop, implement, and maintain the Food for Health Program for CHC. The Food for Health Program shall consist of, but not be limited to: (a) presentations on good nutrition; (b) the development of guidelines for healthy eating; (c) demonstrations of practical and healthy food preparation: and (d) the development of brochures and other literature on the subject of good nutrition. See Attachment A for details.

1.02. <u>Health-Promotion Program Articles and Publications.</u> NCI shall research, develop, and write health-promotion articles for the magazines, brochures, and other written media published by CHC. NCI shall develop and provide health-related scientific data for the magazines, brochures, and other written media published by CHC. The publication of such articles and scientific data shall be subject to the final approval of CHC.

1.03. <u>Media Placements.</u> NCI shall develop, implement, and coordinate media placements for the promotion of the Food for Health Program and other health-promotion programs developed by NCI or CHC. NCI shall also develop, implement, and coordinate media placements concerning general health information as a public service to local communities. NCI shall obtain final approval on all media placements prior to scheduling a media placement or committing CHC in any manner.

1.04. <u>Liability Insurance.</u> NCI shall procure and maintain, at their sole expense, professional liability insurance with remaining coverage satisfactory to CHC. Upon request by CHC. NCI shall provide evidence of insurance coverage. NCI shall notify CHC, to the attention of the Chief Executive Officer, in writing within ten (10) days of changes in carriers, changes in remaining coverage, or notification to NCI of any claims against, denials of, restriction on, termination of, or changes in NCI professional liability insurance.

1.05. <u>Laws, Regulations, and Licenses.</u> NCI shall maintain all federal, state, and local licenses, permits, and association memberships, without restriction, required to practice as registered dietitians or health educators. NCI shall notify CHC in writing, to the attention of the Chief Executive Officer, within ten (10) days of any suspension, revocation, condition, limitation, qualification, or other restriction on NCI's licenses, permits, and/or association memberships by any state in which NCI is licensed as dietitians, health educators, or other health-care professionals.

SECTION 2. CHC OBLIGATIONS
2.01. <u>Payment for Services.</u> CHC shall reimburse NCI for services rendered under the Agreement ("Contract Fee") an amount equal to thirty-three thousand and six hundred dollars ($33,600) in the contract year January 1, 2009, through December 31, 2009. The contract year thereafter shall be the calendar year from January 1 through December 31. CHC shall pay NCI in monthly payments of two thousand eight hundred ($2,800.00) the first business day of each month beginning with January 1, 2009. made payable to NCI.

2.02. <u>Payment of Out-of-Pocket Expenses.</u> CHC shall reimburse NCI for all reasonable out-of-pocket expenses, including, but not limited to, supplies, subscriptions, educational resources, travel expenses, and mileage that are incurred in connection with the provision of services under this Agreement. Said out-of-pocket expenses shall be limited to $1800.00 per annum for supplies and travel, and to $350.00 per annum for subscriptions and educational resources as determined by the budget. Said out-of-pocket expenses shall not include normal travel and mileage between NCP's place of business and CHC's corporate headquarters.

2.03, <u>Office Space.</u> CHC shall provide adequate work space and support staff to NCI at CHC's corporate headquarters as detailed in Attachment B.

FIGURE 10.2.   ■   An example of a formal contract. *(continued)*

2.04. <u>Copyrights and Trademarks.</u> Any health-promotion data, information, articles, publications, brochures, or programs, and any specific information connected therewith, uniquely developed or implemented by NCI for CHC shall be considered the property of CHC. CHC shall have the rights to all copyrights and trademarks for all uniquely developed health-promotion data, information, articles, publications, and programs, and the specific information connected therewith.

SECTION 3. TERM AND TERMINATION

3.01. <u>Term.</u> The term of this agreement shall commence on January 1, 2009 and shall continue and remain in effect through the remainder of the calendar year 2009, and for each calendar year thereafter until such time as this Agreement is terminated as hereinafter provided.

3.02. <u>Termination.</u> This agreement may be terminated by CHC, with or without cause, or by NCI, with or without cause, upon sixty (60) days written notice to the other party.

SECTION 4. MISCELLANEOUS

4.01. <u>Independent Contractors.</u> The relationship between CHC and NCI is that of independent contractors only and NCI is not an employee or agent of CHC. Nothing contained in this Agreement shall constitute or be construed to be or create a partnership, joint venture, or an association between CHC and NCI, nor shall either party, or its employees, agents, and representatives be considered employees, agents, or representatives of the other party.

4.02. <u>Amendment.</u> Any amendment to this Agreement proposed by CHC at least thirty (30) days prior to the effective date of such amendment is incorporated herein; provided, however, that in the event any change or modification to this Agreement is requested by any State or Federal regulatory authority as a result of a filing of this Agreement with such authority, such change or modification shall be incorporated into this Agreement from the effective date of this Agreement.

4.03. <u>Assignment.</u> CHC shall have the absolute right, in its sole discretion, to assign all or any of its rights or responsibilities hereunder to any corporation that is a subsidiary or affiliate of CHC. In the event of assignment, this Agreement shall be binding upon and inure to the benefit of CHC's successors and assigns. NCI shall not have the right to assign any of their rights without the prior written consent of CHC, which consent shall not be unreasonably withheld.

4.04. <u>No Waiver of Rights.</u> The failure of any party to insist upon the strict observation or performance of any provision of this Agreement or to exercise any right or remedy shall not impair or waive any such right or remedy. Every right and remedy given by this Agreement to the parties may be exercised from time to time and as often as appropriate.

4.05. <u>Entire Agreement.</u> This Agreement is the entire Agreement between the parties. No representations or agreements between the parties, oral or otherwise, has any force or effect.

4.06. <u>Impossibility of Performance.</u> Neither CHC nor NCI shall be deemed to be in default of this Agreement if prevented from performing for reasons beyond its control, including without limitation, governmental laws and regulation, acts of God, wars, and strikes. In such case, the parties shall negotiate in good faith with the goal and intent of preserving this Agreement and the respective rights and obligations of the parties.

4.07. <u>Governing Law.</u> This Agreement shall be construed in accordance with the laws of the state of Minnesota.

IN WITNESS HEREOF, the parties hereto have caused this Agreement to be executed.

CORPORATE HEALTH PLAN CORPORATION   NUTRITION CONSULTANTS, INC.
0000 Eagle Drive   1234 Apple St.
St. Paul, Minnesota XXXXX   St. Paul, Minnesota XXXXX

By_____   By_____

Designated Representative   Designated Representative

Date _____   Date _____

FIGURE 10.2. ■ *(continued)*

CASE STUDY 10.1

MARKETING MNT TO INSURANCE COMPANIES

Barbara Ann F. Hughes, PhD, MPH, RD, LDN, FADA, Raleigh, NC

When B. A. Hughes & Associates was founded in 1991, I marketed directly to physician practices through letters announcing the new business and requesting patient referrals. I also advertised in the local Yellow Pages, contacted managed care organizations, and made many calls to various insurance companies asking to become a provider. One major company, CIGNA Health care, contracted and listed B.A. Hughes & Associates in its database, which was available to all policy holders. I mailed letters to CIGNA physician practices requesting client referrals, and our business picked up with access to this information.

Over the next several years, three more insurance companies agreed to contract with us, but the state's largest company, Blue Cross and Blue Shield of North Carolina (BCBSNC) remained unwilling to contract with registered and licensed dietitians/nutritionists. Meanwhile, the rise in adult and childhood obesity became an epidemic in North Carolina in the late 1990s and early 2000s.

In early 2004, I proposed to a few other private practitioners that a letter be sent to BCBSNC requesting reimbursement to credentialed and contracted dietitian/nutritionists; BCBSNC responded by proposing a date to meet. Three of us met with six company executives. We offered a packet of information about the scope of practice of RD/LDNs in private practice. The meeting opened with the chief medical director announcing the company was committing to reimburse for MNT services, but the planning process and imple-mentation would require at least 18 months. I proposed that there be a research component.

In the fall of 2004, BCBSNC sent its first announcement to recruit RD/LDNs across the state, but only a handful responded. In the spring of 2005, a major presentation was given at the North Carolina Dietetic Association (NCDA) annual meeting in an effort to inform and recruit more RD/LDNs. In early 2006, the American Dietetic Association obtained a small grant from the Commission on Dietetic Registration to permit willing BCBSNC policy holders enrolled in the "healthy lifestyle choices program" to consent to having their data sent electronically to Duke University for research. The flow of referrals to the 30 RD/LDN providers greatly increased. Providers are self-employed or work in hospital and out-patient facilities.

The official name of our study is ADA BCBS MNT Lifestyle Case Management Cost Benefit Analysis. "Most insurance companies provide coverage for nutrition counseling only for diabetes, renal disease and a few pediatric diagnoses. In October 2005, BCBSNC began offering coverage for all individuals including hyperlipidemia, obesity, hypertension, and even those who simply wanted to prevent health problems!! This case study will describe a historic research study that is going on in NC with the ADA Office of Scientific Affairs and Research, the Dietetic Practice Based Research Network, and Blue Cross Blue Shield of North Carolina. Nearly 30 registered and licensed dietitians/nutritionists around the state are part of this historic study which is being watched eagerly by RDs across the country. If the data show that RDs reduce health risks and save money, BCBSNC will continue this benefit and other insurance companies may be willing to add medical nutrition therapy benefits in the future."

The Weight Management Dietetic Practice Group announced that I am its second recipient of its Excellence in Practice Award (perhaps because of this research). This is a recognition for which I am grateful.

---

include overhead for the duration of the project and other expenses. Many clients prefer to limit the total number of hours allowed. You can include a "not to exceed" clause in such cases.

SUMMARY

The purpose of negotiation is to identify, discuss, and reach agreement about the expectations of each party involved in a business situation. The clearer the parties can be in describing their needs and expectations, the more likely they are to reach an agreement that satisfies all. Jim Rose, MS, RD, a for-mer consultant and foodservice director, used to write a list and description or show a sample of what the client would own at the end of their contract, such as a new staffing schedule, a new employee policy manual, or a new patient trayline layout, so there were no miscommunicated expectations.

BIBLIOGRAPHY

Dawson R. *Secrets of Power Negotiating*. Franklin Lakes, NJ: Career Press; 2001.

Donaldson MC. *Fearless Negotiating*. New York: McGraw Hill; 2007.

Harvard Business Essentials Guide to Negotiation. Boston: Harvard Business School Publishing; 2003.

11

SETTING PRICES AND FEES

Elizabeth Hamilton, RD, and Kathy King, LD, RD

Of all the marketing decisions that must be made, the one that likely causes dietetic professionals and other members of the helping professions the most anguish is the setting of prices and fees. How much should you charge? Research has shown that services that differentiate themselves from their competitors through better marketing, building trust, and enhancing the customer experience have better return on equity and capital than services that compete on price (1,2).

Price is the value exchanged for products in a marketing exchange (2). Barter is the oldest form of exchange where products are traded and money is not usually involved. Because most buyers have limited resources, they must choose between the many options and decide if the benefit gained is worth the buying power sacrificed (2).

KNOWING YOUR WORTH

PERCEIVED VALUE

People buy more than products and services. They buy what they perceive the products and services will do for them. In other words, they buy benefits. A weight-loss program does not make them exercise and eat less food, it makes them happier and more attractive. Your challenge is to package your service or product at a price that does not exceed the customer's perceived value of it. Arriving at this figure is a process of trial and error or negotiation.

A low fee is often perceived as indicating lesser quality. A fee that is too high stifles sales. You can tell your prices are too high when more than 25% of your potential customers complain, according to service marketing expert, Harry Beckwith (1). Your reputation, name recognition, years of experience, and expertise all factor into the fee you can charge. Your fee can be higher when the work you do requires more skill and expertise that few people possess. Your fee can be higher, or you can ask for a fee and a royalty, when your product or service is going to be used to generate profit for your client, for example, when you write a script for a video series, create a weight-loss program for a fitness center, or write a cookbook for a food company.

If your product or service does not have any perceived or actual advantage over the competition except for price, a simple price cut by a strong competitor might put you out of business. In other words, you might reconsider going into a business venture if your products or services are not different or better than those of the competition and if a low price is your only advantage. Beckwith warns that bargain-hunting customers that only come to you because you have the lowest price will seldom remain loyal as your business grows because their nature makes them look around for a better bargain (3).

Also keep in mind that customers do not often want to be the first to try an intangible service without a track record; they want to make sure the service is worth the price (3). If the perceived value is good, word-of-mouth advertising will help make the business reputation grow.

It boggles the mind to those of us who are price conscious, but time after time research has shown that human nature makes us value something more if it costs more or it seems more exclusive—within reason of course. Marketers tell stories about how products flew off the shelves when the price and image were raised instead of lowered (1–3).

COMPETITIVE ANALYSIS

A competitive analysis is simply an in-depth look at who your competitors are, what they are selling, and what they are charging. You then use this information to create or adjust your services or products so they are different and better; that is, you competitively position them to have advantages in the marketplace against your competitors. Price is just one factor to use. Other perks could be easy-open packaging, home delivery, child care during group classes, accepting payment by credit card, phone-in ordering, or overnight delivery—depending upon what you sell.

VALUE-ADDED

Another strategy that is popular in business today is value-added—the addition of something to give customers more value for their money. For example, you could offer a free computer diet assessment for new clients, or give a healthy holiday cookbook with each event you cater through the holidays, or a coupon for 10% off the next visit or purchase.

PRICING STRATEGIES

When pricing your services, the two most important considerations are your level of expertise and your years of experience (3). The prices and fees you set need to match your target market's ability to pay and perception of value of the service or product. The image you wish to create (your competitive positioning) and your client's ability to pay will help you decide how much to spend on the quality of your materials, meeting space, packaging, promotion tools, and other overhead.

The six common pricing strategies for services or products are:

1. *Skimming:* charging a very high price to reach a small, elite, and profitable market.
2. *Trading down:* adding a lower-priced, less-prestigious service to an existing elite service; this is a technique used to expand to a less elite or affluent market segment.
3. *Trading up:* introducing an expensive service or product to increase the status of other generally low-priced services and to attract new buyers.
4. *Cost plus:* starting with what it costs to produce the service or product and adding a markup based on a standard policy (commonly used on books and clothing).
5. *Demand-oriented:* setting a price according to an estimate of what the market is willing to pay. (All the strategies use a little of this method.)
6. *Underbidding:* setting a price with a low profit margin in order to be more attractive than competitors. This has been a very common

method among dietitians, but it often means that you work very hard just to break even. Also, consider your image: do you want to position yourself as the least expensive or one of the best? In tight economic times, underbidding can be an appropriate option. (Wal-Mart appears to succeed with this philosophy, but in fact, it has used its world-wide buying power to demand lower wholesale prices from its suppliers; so its volume is high and it still generates profit because goods cost less when its wholesalers move to locations with very poorly paid labor.)

SETTING PRODUCT PRICES

In the manufacturing of goods, estimates vary, but most experts suggest that manufacturing costs should not exceed one-sixth to one-eighth of the suggested retail price. For example, if you think your product will sell best at $40 retail, but you have to sell it through distributors or brokers to reach retailers, you may have to give 10% of the price to the distributor and 40% to the retailer to sell it. That means you have $20 left to pay for:

- the product,
- its packaging,
- insurance,
- transportation and postage,
- marketing (advertising and public relations),
- salaries,
- phone and office,
- your salary, and
- profit.

By knowing your probable expenses and how much consumers are willing to pay (determined through focus groups or competitive analysis), you have a better idea of what price you must manufacture the product for to make it worth your time.

ESTABLISHING PROFESSIONAL FEES

QUOTING FEES

Do not rush into quoting fees. Do your homework first. Ask questions about the job and carefully evaluate what the client wants you to do. Consider any additional costs, such as travel expenses (additional time away from home, added child care), or tight deadlines (you might need to pass on other job opportunities, use the phone and overnight mail more, hire additional help, and pay overtime for secretarial work).

When you have a job opportunity that is new to you, talk to businesspeople in your area, call employment services that place dietitians and technicians, and call practitioners in other parts of the country. Take the time to find out what the going rates are for the kind of work you plan to do. Be sure to compare like services and economic conditions.

If a business calls and wants to know your fees, do not answer immediately unless you know exactly what you want. Say instead, "I need to know more about the job and then I need to work the numbers to see what it will take. Do you have a ballpark amount that you want to offer?" You play a game. You do not want to commit to a low amount when they may be willing to pay you more and they do not want to offer too much in case you may be willing to work for less.

THE COST OF DOING BUSINESS

A salaried person may not give much thought to the cost of doing business. When you have to cover all your business expenses as a consultant, private practitioner, or entrepreneur, however, rent, telephone bills, and health insurance premiums take on new meaning.

You must determine your cost of doing business. To more accurately establish your fees, you need to consider both direct and indirect costs. Direct costs are costs incurred while working with a specific client, such as educational materials, billable research time, travel, special messenger service, faxes, and long distance phone charges. Such costs are usually passed along to the client or patient. Indirect costs are your overhead to run and maintain your business venture (e.g., rent, telephone, secretarial service, computer, furniture, supplies, photocopying, postage, advertising and marketing, legal and accounting services, licenses, insurance, continuing education, professional dues, social security, and taxes).

One way to estimate a range for consultant fees is to determine the hourly pay range of salaried dietetics professionals in your area. It is against the law to discuss fees in a manner that might suggest price fixing. However, calls to Human Resource Departments of several hospitals and clinics or to consultants will probably provide you with usable figures, or buy the most recent national salary research publication from the American Dietetic Association.

To determine where you might place yourself within the range you have found, consider how much experience you have, what the work entails, and what unique expertise you can bring to the table. Then multiply the hourly pay of a similarly qualified and experienced, full-time employee by 2.5 to 3 times to determine your hourly rate as a self-employed professional who must also cover all the business overhead (1).

Example: Assume the salaried worker's pay is $30 per hour. Your rate would be $30 × 2.5 or 3 = $75 to $90 per hour.

You may use $75 to $90 per hour as your first rough estimate because your overhead in a very expensive location could add $50 or more to the equation. Keep those figures in mind as you proceed.

UNIQUE EXPERTISE

If you have unique expertise, notoriety, or you just published a national bestselling book, the ball game totally changes. For example, you may charge $3,000 or more for an hour of speaking if you are a nationally renowned speaker who is known for attracting crowds and making programs successful. As a media spokesperson or media personality, you might charge $2,500 to $10,000 or more if your appearance with the product or program lends credibility and has a reputation for attracting viewers.

BILLABLE HOURS

How much time are you willing to work? As an entrepreneur, you may enthusiastically commit to a 60-hour week. However, those will not be 60 billable hours. Professionals consider they are doing well if they can bill 50% to 75% of their working hours (3). The remainder is spent on paperwork, administration, preparation, travel, and marketing. That brings your 60-hour week down to 30 to 40 billable hours or less (there may be zero income on projects like writing a book for only royalties). How soon will you burn out at that pace? How many weeks per year are you going to work? Remember, there is no paid vacation or sick days when you work for yourself.

IS IT WORTH IT?

You have considered your number of billable hours and your overhead, but now there is something else to consider—your profit. What is going to be left over for you? The low bid that landed you the contract may find you working for less than you had anticipated. Businesspeople hope to make a 20% profit. Use your own figures to check the validity of the original hourly rate you made by extending the formula as follows (1):

1. Billable hours per week × number of working weeks per year = billable hours per year
2. Annual overhead − billable hours per year = hourly costs
3. Hourly costs + hourly pay + 20% profit = hourly rate

You may want to adjust the resulting figures. It may or may not be possible to raise your hourly rate without pricing yourself out of the market. If that is the case, you need to look at how you might lower your costs or increase your number of billable hours.

FEE STRUCTURES

There are six common ways of charging for products or services. Depending on the nature of your business, you may choose to use any number of them.

- *Flat rate.* The same fee is charged for the same service to any client. People use flat rates when selling the same service again and again because they have a good idea of the time and expense involved. Such rates are easy to use for counseling visits, speaking engagements, routine consults, and group classes.
- *Per-hour rate.* If the number of required hours of work is variable or unknown in advance, it is logical to charge only for the hours worked. Such rates are used for subcontracting, long therapy sessions, and consulting projects. To set clients' minds at ease, it is helpful to estimate an approximate time frame or maximum number of hours.
- *Per-head rate.* With this rate, the amount of money you make depends on the number of individuals who participate in an event. This rate is often used for workshops, courses, and speeches to groups when attendees pay at the door. It does involve some risk, but if attendance is good, you can do very well.
- *Project rate.* This rate covers your direct and indirect costs, provides a profit, and leaves some room for unexpected delays or miscalculations in developing something (educational materi-

als, a kitchen plan, a marketing tool, and the like) for a client. Clients like this rate because they know what the final cost will be and because you will usually be expected to absorb any cost overruns (unless the clients created them). To protect yourself from nonpayment, have your agreement in writing and ask for one-third to one-half of the total fee up front.
- *Retainer fee.* This fee is charged, usually monthly, for your availability. Dietitians receive retainers for being on-call consultants to food companies and public relations firms. You could charge a clinic to see patients every Tuesday. No matter how many patients you see, you are paid the same amount, so the clinic takes the risk for inconsistent patient loads, not you. If the patient load is more than you can handle in one day, renegotiate the retainer to include another partial or full day. A retainer should be tied to an amount of time (like 10 hours per month), with any time over that amount billable at an hourly or daily rate. If a commercial client (food company or hospital or pharmaceutical company) wants to state that you are a staff member or consultant, ask for a retainer fee and have your lawyer draw up a letter of agreement on your rights (including the right to review all materials and ads associated with your name) and any liability limitations. Talk to your advisers before signing anything.
- *Contingency fee, commission, or royalty.* Such fees are paid only as money is generated. The product or book must sell, or the recruiter must place a prospect. The risk is high because a lot of time and overhead may be invested without any promise of income. If someone asks that you work on commission, make sure the reward is worth it, either financially or professionally.

CASE STUDY 11.1

SETTING AND CHANGING FEES IN YOUR NUTRITION PRACTICE OR CLINIC

Theresa Wright, MS, RD, LDN, President, Renaissance Nutrition Center, Inc., East Norriton, PA

Setting your fee schedule in private practice is a thorny issue, and critical to your success. Your fees influence other areas of your practice: how many hours you will work, how much you will earn, and ultimately, the fu-

ture of your business. Your attitude as you discuss fees with your clients will affect how they feel about paying you, and will ultimately affect your practice. The purpose of this case study is to discuss how I change my fees. As the owner of a successful nutrition counseling business for the past 18 years, perhaps my mistakes and successes can benefit your business ventures.

The first time I raised fees was really difficult for me. I thought long and hard about the effect of the increase on individual clients. I worried so much

continued

continued

about it that a friend finally asked me to consider the effect on *me* of not raising fees when I really needed the money. I learned that I had to consider myself as well as my clients.

I checked my proposed fees against the fair market value of my services and the reasonable and customary fees in my area. (You can find this out by talking to your patients, listening at meetings, and reading published fee surveys.) What do other nutritionists charge, and what do other related programs cost? Would my fees be competitive with others' fees for similar services? I asked friends and associates how much they would be willing to pay for a service. Many of my referrals come from psychologists and other therapists. I found that a fee two-thirds to three-fourths of what the referring therapist charges, is generally a good benchmark.

I also needed to charge enough to allow time for non-income-producing essential tasks like administration and business development. My clients have become national now, rather than local, so my website (http://www.sanefood.com) has become a critical communication tool. It must be kept updated and that takes time.

This year, my clients have asked me to create audio recordings of my lectures and a cookbook featuring recipes we have developed over the years. I have to balance my needs with what is appropriate for my practice. When I charged minimal fees, I starved myself and my practice. When I charge fair fees, and have the time I need for myself, I can be fully present with my clients and give excellent service.

While I am making fee changes, I consider changes to other policies and fees. What about cancellation notices? Must clients pay at the time of the consultation or will they be billed? Must clients pay in advance for the initial session? Being clear with clients about this and all fee-related matters is essential to avoid misunderstandings, resentments, and lost referrals.

Clients frequently request sliding-scale sessions. They tell me about their financial difficulties and their need for my services. I tried sliding scales in the beginning of my practice, but I had no real way of assessing their income and ability to pay, and I often discovered that the sliding-scale clients could afford vacation trips and other amenities of life that I could never afford. Now, if people cannot afford my standard sessions, I offer them shorter sessions, less frequent sessions, or a group class. I now see my time as my most precious resource, and I guard it more carefully than ever before.

For each new client, I include written payment and cancellation policies within my HIPPAA forms; clients initial a line agreeing to pay for sessions not cancelled 24 hours in advance, as well as other conditions needed for my smooth operation. The day before their appoint-

ments, my secretary calls and confirms their sessions, and makes note of the need to call when canceling. When billing for a no-show, I send the client a copy of their agreement with the bill. I may lose a client over this issue; often they pay the bill and do not return. I have noticed, however, that waiving the fee when a client is not committed does not make the client more committed, it just increases my "no-show" rate.

As you plan fee changes, consider the following:

1. How long has it been since your last fee increase? It is best to maintain the same rate for 1 to 2 years. If you need to raise fees in less than a year, you probably did not plan properly. If you delay a rate increase too long, the amount you have to increase to bring yourself up to the right level may be a shock for your clients. I realize now that if I had increased fees by $5 or $10 per session every year, my clients would be more prepared for it. Better to make small increases every 1 or 2 years than significant increases spaced farther apart.

2. Consider the general economy. In the middle of an economic recession or war may not be a good time to raise fees. If you wait a few months until conditions improve, your fee increase may be better received.

3. Consider timing your rate increases to coincide with the introduction of other programs. New classes, courses, or support groups offer good opportunities to raise rates. You may also coordinate the timing of client sessions with a rate change. For example, if you offer a 1-hour initial visit followed by 20-minute follow-up visits, you may want to change to 1 1/2-hour initial assessments followed by 30-minute follow-ups. (Be careful not to adjust your time so that you continue to charge at your same old rate!) You can present the change so that clients will feel they are getting more for their dollar, and the rate increase will become part of "a package of expanded services to better meet your needs."

4. Write down your decisions. Talk about them with trusted advisers, such as your accountant, lawyer, or other professionals, and listen to their counsel.

5. As you implement the fee structure you have chosen, give your clients adequate written notice. Four to eight weeks is adequate time for most people in your practice to see your notice and discuss it with you. In your notice, indicate why the change is necessary (see Fig. 11.1). Be prepared for comments from clients like, "I do not think I can afford this!" Have some answers ready, like "I am sorry if this is a problem for you." Use your counseling skills to hear and validate your clients' feelings with comments like, "I understand, it is difficult," and "It is really tough to make ends meet these days."

continued

Renaissance Nutrition Center, Inc.
2500 DeKalb Pike (Suite 200) ● *East Norriton, PA 19401*
(610) 275-3699 ● *Fax (610) 275-3799*

Date

To all my clients,

While I am pleased to have maintained my hourly rate for nutrition counseling for the past several years, it has become clear that due to rising costs, I cannot continue to do so. I have given this matter much thought and consideration, and find that I must raise my rates for nutrition counseling to $_____ per initial session and $_____ for each follow-up effective March_____, _____.

My clients' welfare has always been of paramount importance to me, and I trust the importance of our work together is apparent and valuable to you. If you have concerns, or if this fee creates undue hardship for you, please feel free to discuss the matter with me. Thank you for understanding, commitment, and continued effort.

Sincerely,

FIGURE 11.1. ■ Sample letter announcing price increases.

continued

Each time I change my fees, I risk losing some clients. Those who adjust easily and who come regularly are really committed to the work we are doing together. Clients must believe that they are coming to a quality provider and will receive excellent services delivered in a caring and creative atmosphere.

I have written a food plan guide, available for sale to clients and other practitioners, which provides specific guidance about food choices. I offer support groups, as well as scales, books and other items in the office and on the website. These items really help the client stay focused and committed to the work we are doing.

Setting and maintaining a fee structure is a very important part of private practice. My lawyer, one of my most trusted advisers, always says, "Either you are making money or you are having fun, or both. If you are not, change your business till you are!" Take this advice and use it to make sure you get both a livable wage and fun in your practice!

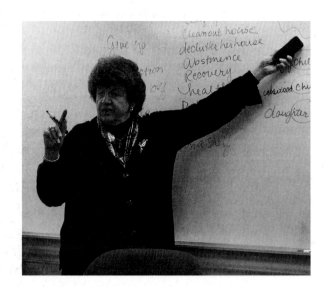

ANNUAL EVALUATION OF FEES

It is necessary to evaluate your fees at least annually. An appropriate time might be when you review annual statements with your accountant or CPA. Determine whether your fees covered your expenses and gave you the profit you had predicted. If not, decide if you can increase your fees without charging more than the market will bear, or if you can, cut your costs. Other possibilities might be to add a new service or trade up into a new target market.

SUMMARY

Remember: when setting fees, they must give customers value that is equal to or higher than expected and not more than they are willing to pay. Prices help create a powerful image and are one of the most potentially effective marketing considerations.

REFERENCES

1. Beckwith H. *Selling the Invisible*. New York: Warner Books; 1997.
2. Pride W, Ferrell O. *Marketing Concepts and Strategies*, 12th Ed. New York: Houghton Mifflin; 2003.
3. Beckwith H. *The Invisible Touch*. New York: Warner Books; 2000.
4. Kelly K. *How to Set Your Fees and Get Them*. New York: Visibility Enterprises; 1989.

BIBLIOGRAPHY

King K. *The Entrepreneurial Nutritionist*, 3rd Ed. Lake Dallas, TX: Helm Publishing; 2003.

MARKETING AND BUSINESS ETHICS

12

Mindy G. Hermann, MBA, RD, and Kathy King, RD, LD

Recent growth in the visibility of and respect for dietitians has opened up tremendous opportunities in the business world. It is no longer unusual for dietitians to work in public relations firms, food companies, Fortune 500 corporations, and entrepreneurial ventures. Additionally, more and more dietitians consult for companies that market nutrition-related products or services. Yet, as these and other nutrition business links continue to strengthen, dietitians will be forced to make more decisions regarding the ethics of their affiliations with business and its use of marketing.

ETHICS DILEMMAS

One school of thought holds that medical and health care fields cannot be both professions and businesses since the morals and economics of the two appear to be incompatible (1). A fundamental moral tenet of health care is to care for the masses. In fact, the mission of The American Dietetic Association (ADA) includes "the promotion of optimal health and nutritional status of the population" (2). However, once financial considerations enter into health care delivery, the public may no longer be able to receive consistent information or levels of care; affordability, rather than quality, may become a major influence on health care decisions.

In marketing a product or service to the public, it is imperative that the dietetic professional represent the facts accurately and fairly. The professional must avoid conflicts of interest, especially of creating the impression that a personal opinion is objective and free from outside influences when in fact there is potential bias. This can occur when a dietetics professional works for or owns a company, or in some other way would benefit from downgrading the competition or promoting a product. It is common today for companies to want to hire dietitians to represent them. The practitioner's credibility can lend support to the claims made by the product's marketing team. The ethical concern arises when the practitioner's credibility is used to bolster an otherwise lacking product or service.

When articles or books are written, credit should be given to the original sources of quotes and information. Copyrighted materials (videos, booklets, educational materials, and so on) should not be reprinted without the copyright holder's (publisher or author) consent.

To assist in ethical decision making, many health care professions, including dietetics, have developed codes of ethics, the principles of which can and should be used to make business decisions.

PERSONAL AND PROFESSIONAL ETHICS

The following are the principles from the "Code of Ethics for the Profession of Dietetics" (3).

ADA ETHICS PRINCIPLES

1. The dietetics practitioner conducts himself/herself with honesty, integrity, and fairness.
2. The dietetics practitioner practices dietetics based on scientific principles and current information.
3. The dietetics practitioner presents substantiated information and interprets controversial information without personal bias, recognizing that legitimate differences of opinion exist.
4. The dietetics practitioner assumes responsibility and accountability for personal competence in practice, continually striving to

increase professional knowledge and skills and to apply them in practice.

5. The dietetics practitioner recognizes and exercises professional judgment within the limits of his/her qualifications and collaborates with others, seeks counsel, or makes referrals as appropriate.

6. The dietetics practitioner provides sufficient information to enable clients and others to make their own informed decisions.

7. The dietetics practitioner protects confidential information and makes full disclosure about any limitations on his/her ability to guarantee full confidentiality.

8. The dietetics practitioner provides professional services with objectivity and with respect for the unique needs and values of individuals.

9. The dietetics practitioner provides professional services in a manner that is sensitive to cultural differences and does not discriminate against others on the basis of race, ethnicity, creed, religion, disability, sex, age, sexual orientation, or national origin.

10. The dietetics practitioner does not engage in sexual harassment in connection with professional practice.

11. The dietetics practitioner provides objective evaluations of performance for employees and coworkers, candidates for employment, students, professional association memberships, awards, or scholarships. The dietetics practitioner makes all reasonable effort to avoid bias in any kind of professional evaluation of others.

12. The dietetics practitioner is alert to situations that might cause a conflict of interest or have the appearance of a conflict. The dietetics practitioner provides full disclosure when a real or potential conflict of interest arises.

13. The dietetics practitioner who wishes to inform the public and colleagues of his/her services does so by using factual information. The dietetics practitioner does not advertise in a false or misleading manner.

14. The dietetics practitioner promotes or endorses products in a manner that is neither false nor misleading.

15. The dietetics practitioner permits the use of his/her name for the purpose of certifying that dietetics services have been rendered only if he/she has provided or supervised the provision of those services.

16. The dietetics practitioner accurately presents professional qualifications and credentials.
    a. The dietetics practitioner uses Commission on Dietetic Registration awarded credentials ("RD" or "Registered Dietitian"; "DTR" or "Dietetic Technician, Registered"; "CSP" or "Certified Specialist in Pediatric Nutrition"; "CSR" or "Certified Specialist in Renal Nutrition"; and "FADA" or "Fellow of The American Dietetic Association") only when the credential is current and authorized by the Commission on Dietetic Registration. The dietetics practitioner provides accurate information and complies with all requirements of the Commission on Dietetic Registration program in which he/she is seeking initial or continued credentials from the Commission on Dietetic Registration.
    b. The dietetics practitioner is subject to disciplinary action for aiding another person in violating any Commission on Dietetic Registration requirements or aiding another person in representing himself/herself as Commission on Dietetic Registration credentialed when he/she is not.

17. The dietetics practitioner withdraws from professional practice under the following circumstances:
    a. The dietetics practitioner has engaged in any substance abuse that could affect his/her practice;
    b. The dietetics practitioner has been adjudged by a court to be mentally incompetent;
    c. The dietetics practitioner has an emotional or mental disability that affects his/her practice in a manner that could harm the client or others.

18. The dietetics practitioner complies with all applicable laws and regulations concerning the profession and is subject to disciplinary action under the following circumstances:
    a. The dietetics practitioner has been convicted of a crime under the laws of the United States which is a felony or a misdemeanor, an essential element of which is dishonesty, and which is related to the practice of the profession.
    b. The dietetics practitioner has been disciplined by a state, and at least one of the grounds for the discipline is the same or substantially equivalent to these principles.
    c. The dietetics practitioner has committed an act of misfeasance or malfeasance which is directly related to the practice of the profession as determined by a court of competent jurisdiction, a licensing board, or an agency of a governmental body.

19. The dietetics practitioner supports and promotes high standards of professional practice. The dietetics practitioner accepts the obligation to protect clients, the public, and the profession by upholding the Code of Ethics for the Profession of Dietetics and by reporting alleged violations of the Code through the defined review process of The American Dietetic Association and its credentialing agency, the Commission on Dietetic Registration.

CAN YOU CONSULT FOR A COMPANY AND REMAIN UNBIASED?

The following hypothetical situation offers one example of how ADA's Code of Ethics can be used to make business decisions about a nutrition product:

Dietitian #1 is approached by Company W to speak at a conference sponsored by Company W and to serve on its medical advisory board. Company W also plans to use Dietitian #1's name in its publications and in a listing on its letterhead of Advisory Board members. Dietitian #1's acceptance of this offer will constitute an implied endorsement of Company W's product (Product W). According to the Code of Ethics, Dietitian #1 should be able to (a) avoid conflict of interest between Product W and her existing work, (b) disclose any implied or explicit endorsement, and (c) remain neutral in her present and future decisions, evaluations, or actions regarding Product W and its competitors. The principles mentioned earlier from the Code of Ethics can help Dietitian #1 to make a sound decision regarding whether or not to affiliate with Company W. If Dietitian #1 decides to work with Company W, she can remain ethical by being totally objective and honest when asked to render a professional opinion on the category of products to which Product W belongs (e.g., predigested enteral formulas or high-fiber cereals), or on specific products. Be careful when you are choosing your alliances because they will reflect on your clinical and professional judgment.

CAN YOU BE A SPOKESPERSON FOR A FOOD COMPANY?

A second scenario involves Company X, the manufacturer of a line of luncheon meats (Product X), some of which are relatively low in fat and others that are quite high in fat. Dietitian #2 is approached to act as Product X's spokesperson, representing Product X to the media and to other dietitians.

Dietitian #2 feels that all aspects of this potential business arrangement adhere to the Code of Ethics. However, he has reservations about promoting luncheon meats to his colleagues, even though he subscribes to the maxim that foods are neither good nor bad.

In making his decision, Dietitian #2 must realize that his reputation will be closely aligned with all of Company X's products unless he clearly promotes only the lower-fat items, which could be the case. Then he must decide whether Product X's message can fit into his personal concept of a healthy diet and take the job, or whether the message is misleading or false and turn down the job. Again, ADA's ethical principles can facilitate Dietitian #2's decision making.

Other health professions are faced with similar challenges to remain ethical once ties with industry have been forged. The ethical standards of pharmacists, for example, are at risk when drug companies pay pharmacists for research or presentations (4). A heightened awareness of ethics is creating an environment in which pharmacists, physicians, and other medical professionals routinely disclose to colleagues their financial relationships with industry. ADA fully supports this practice.

Beginning in January 1992, the *Journal of the American Dietetic Association* required that authors reveal any financial support of research or other work that is related to a journal article's authorship.

CAN YOU BE EMPLOYED, SERVE ON ADA, AND CONSULT FOR A FOOD COMPANY?

Ethical decisions that affect one's employer(s) are more complex. The most important step is to evaluate who one's employers are and what the potential impact of one's business action is on each of them.

Dietitian #3 is a full-time employee of a world-renowned medical center and also serves on several important ADA committees. Company Y, whose products are used by the medical center, invites Dietitian #3 to serve on its Medical Advisory Board, receive financial remuneration for consulting time, and have her name appear in Company Y's publications.

In this case, Dietitian #3 has three "employers" or affiliations: the medical center, ADA, and Company Y. The medical center should be approached first for approval. The use of Dietitian #3's affiliation is valuable to Company Y because it lends credibility to Product Y and suggests product endorsement by the medical center. For this reason,

Dietitian #3's appropriate ethical action is to first ask her employer for approval.

Depending upon the will of the employer's decision makers and their regard for the product, there are three options: (a) use the employer's name, (b) allow the dietitian to consult but not mention the employer, or (c) refuse to allow the dietitian to consult. The dietitian should contact ADA next. ADA spells out standards of behavior not only for employees but also for volunteers, officers, committee and council members, and their immediate families. Its conflict of interest statement prohibits a volunteer from disclosing "information relating to the business of the Association that can be used by another entity that does business or seeks to do business with the Association" (5). Dietitian #3 cannot reveal any information about the inner workings or business plans of ADA to Company Y. Furthermore, any mention by Company Y of Dietitian #3's position in ADA must be cleared by ADA. The primary ethical question pertaining to Company Y is whether Dietitian #3 can work for Company Y while upholding her professional standards and those of the medical center and ADA. The dietitian does that by first gaining permission to work with the company, then by representing her affiliations as agreed with the employer and ADA, and, finally, by keeping the proprietary information of each business separate and confidential.

CAN YOU REMAIN UNBIASED WHEN YOU WRITE?

Dietitian #4 works full-time in a public relations firm and does freelance writing outside the scope of her regular job. A magazine asks Dietitian #4 to write an article on fat-free salad dressings. Dietitian #4's full-time employer represents a salad dressing manufacturer (Company Z). The ethically correct decision is to turn down the magazine assignment because of conflict of interest. It is virtually impossible for Dietitian #4 to write an article without the appearance of bias, given her prior relationship with Company Z and her employer's objective to have Company Z's products mentioned in the media. However, in this case, the dietitian can tell the magazine editor about the apparent conflict and let the editor decide whether to go forward, or she can turn down the assignment without mentioning it.

CLIENT CONSIDERATIONS

As illustrated previously, ADA's Code of Ethics spells out guidelines for ethical decision making as it pertains to clients (3). Unfortunately, these guidelines become harder to uphold as economic considerations cause dietitians to run their practices based as much on finances as on services.

CHILDREN AND FOOD MARKETING

As long as we are talking about ethics, it is a good time to bring up the uncontrolled marketing of food products (the highly processed, high-sugar, high-fat varieties supported by tons of marketing) and consumer goods to young children in America. Why haven't we, as practitioners and parents, and more significantly, the American Dietetic Association, taken a stand on this for the health of American children?

In 2004, American corporations were targeting children with a combined marketing budget of *2.5 times more than in 1992*—a total of $15 billion! That is with a "b." In polls, 90% of parents are becoming increasingly concerned about tactics aimed at their children, making them too materialistic and craving the wrong foods. Today's children spend almost 40 hours per week engaged with media—radio, television, movies, magazines, the Internet, and even at high school with Channel One—most of which is commercially driven. Two-thirds of children between the ages of 2 and 8 have televisions in their bedrooms. They see more than 40,000 commercial per year. Advertising appeals to emotions, not to intellect, and it affects children even more profoundly than it does adults.

In 2007, legislators in the United Kingdom passed legislation to restrict marketing "junk foods" in media programming to children until 9 p.m. The movement was spearheaded by health professionals and educators in England to help combat its rising obesity and eating disorder problems in children. Our epidemics are no less severe. (The source for information in this section is Susan Linn's *Consuming Kids* [6]).

SUMMARY

Dietitians can use ADA's Positions and Code of Ethics to help them make decisions regarding the ethics of their professional business behaviors and practices. Additionally, guidelines and guidance must be culled from one's own standards of conduct and the policies of one's employer. It is helpful to break ethical decision making into at least two steps: (a) determining what one's personal rules of conduct are, and (b) thinking through who will be affected by the decision and how to weigh their interest in it (7).

Dietitians can ask themselves, "What, if any, aspects of this situation might have ethical consequences for me personally, for my superior, for the members of my work group, for my organization, and for society as a whole?" (8).

REFERENCES

1. Agich GJ. Medicine as business and profession. *Theor Med* 1990;11:311–324.
2. The American Dietetic Association. *Bylaws* 1990.
3. Code of ethics for the profession of dietetics. *J Am Diet Assoc*, June 1, 1998.
4. Zilz DA. Interdependence in pharmacy: risks, rewards, and responsibilities. *Am J Hosp Pharm* 1990;47(8):1759–1765.
5. The American Dietetic Association. *Policy and Procedure Manual*. Conflict of interest/general. August 1989.
6. Linn S. *Consuming Kids: Protecting Our Children from the Onslaught of Marketing & Advertising*. New York: Random House; 2005.
7. Cadbury A. Ethical managers make their own rules. *Harvard Business Review* 1987;65:69–73.
8. Rice D, Dreilinger C. Rights and wrongs of ethics training. *Training & Development Journal* 1990;44:103.

PROMOTION: PR, ADVERTISING, WEBSITES, AND OTHER STRATEGIES

13

Kathy King, RD, LD

Promotion is a component of marketing. Marketing encompasses all the planning and strategizing while promotion's purpose is to attract attention. Tooting your own horn is the best way to lead the parade to your doorstep. Promotion includes distributing business cards, creating web pages, advertising in the Yellow Pages, writing newspaper columns, appearing on TV talk shows, and giving speeches to civic groups. Promotion is all the communication used to familiarize others with you and your products or services. It's more important now than ever because of increased competition, clutter in advertising, and the public's growing but limited awareness of what you do outside of the traditional work settings.

PROMOTIONAL STRATEGIES

Some professionals naïvely assume that promotion is not necessary because we possess the right credentials and our products or services are good. We sometimes inadequately budget for promotion not realizing that an excellent program may fail, despite meticulous attention to its development because of insufficient or poor-quality promotion.

Promotion will attract far more clients to our doors than will any form of legislative mandate. The focus of health care is shifting toward health promotion and the well individual, and we dietitians must realize that our services are only one of many nutrition options available to the consumer.

SERVICE BUSINESSES

Because of the nature of our business—health care and service—our products are usually intangible (except, of course, in food service). An intangible product cannot be held, visually evaluated, or tasted like a piece of cake. Weight-loss programs or consul-

tation services cannot be experienced in advance. Therefore, surrogates that represent and promote our services (advertising, testimonials by satisfied clients, business cards, brochures, resumes, proposals, letters of reference, portfolios, and the like) are extremely important, especially to those who have not yet sampled our programs and skills. The provider of an intangible service is inseparable from that service in the minds of most clients, and for that reason, interpersonal relationships between the customer and provider, successful outcomes and feelings of goodwill, and customer service may affect the eventual success of a business or program more than promotion, price, brand, or quality (1). Nevertheless, you need promotion to attract the first customers and to grow the business faster than word-of-mouth marketing alone can do.

We hear so much about benchmarking and following industry standards in business. However, people in very successful service businesses know that every service industry can be dramatically reformed and following industry standards or best practices is an invitation to ordinariness (1). The more innovative the idea, the less market research and surveys will help, you need to seek out a few, trusted individuals who have exceptional insight and love exploring a problem and reaching new conclusions to be your sounding boards on promotion ideas and business design (1). Good marketing will not make up for unremarkable execution, so first make the service exceed expectations and then market it to make it successful.

CREATING A BRAND

A brand is a name, term, sign, symbol, or any other feature that identifies one seller's goods or service as distinct from those of other sellers (2). A brand image may be developed by attributing a "personality" to or associating an "image" with a product or service, whereby the personality or image is "branded" into the consciousness of consumers, like Starbucks or Whole Foods (3). Advertising and other forms of promotion play a major role in creating the brand and managing its use and growth (2,3). A brand is one of the most important elements in an advertising theme and the most precious asset owned by a business. It allows a firm to communicate consistently and efficiently with the market (4). In the past, brands were associated with products and large businesses, but that is no longer the case. Marketing people today also talk about brands for services and individuals—and what contributes to their unique identities.

Are brands really important? According to marketing expert Harry Beckwith, author of *Selling the Invisible* and *Invisible Touch*, customers buy brand name products or services over generics (or unknown names) in 13 out of 14 purchases (5,6)! Customers want familiar names, trusted reputations, and warranted service with good reputations. As time in our schedules shrinks, the importance of brand names increases because consumers do not have the time to compare and they don't want to buy a poor quality, unfamiliar product or go to a Nutrition Therapist they don't know when another is available that has a good reputation according to a trusted health professional, a neighbor, or friend (5).

If one brand makes a person feel good, cared for, even loved, customers will be more loyal. By developing emotional connections with your constituents, you will ensure that people respect you even if they don't agree with everything you do (7). To build your personal brand, illustrate your competence in all you do to show your credibility while you produce results, and then couple this with the four personality traits that contribute to a person's likeability: friendliness, relevance (common interests or needs), empathy, and realness (authenticity) (8). The goal is to inspire loyalty beyond reason (6). Here are five tips to make that happen (6):

1. Inventory your personal brand attributes (both rational and emotional). This website offers a complementary self-assessment: http://www.reachcc.com/360personalprofiler
2. Determine from others how you are currently perceived. Let them validate or refute your personal assessment.
3. Look at your attributes and decide which ones are relevant and important to your target market. Which ones make you distinctive in the market?
4. Use this information to change everything you do—improve every report you write, each email you send, and every telephone conversation you have.

5. Evaluate your results and outcomes. Are you more successful or fulfilled? Is your image more consistent and customers more loyal?

SELF-PROMOTION

One-on-one communication can be your most effective form of promotion. It affords the opportunity to speak, hear, see, and exchange viewpoints face-to-face. With this direct approach, people are more likely to remember your message. You can read the body language and expressions of each listener and then adjust your presentation to maximize its impact.

If you look closely at professionals and businesspeople you consider successful, you will notice they promote themselves well. Self-promotion is a skill that can be learned. It creates greater awareness of you and your expertise, increases professional and personal opportunities, and creates demand for your services.

Some people overlook or ignore opportunities to promote themselves for fear of looking too aggressive or self-serving. In today's competitive and fast-paced marketplace, no one can afford to let opportunities pass by so easily. If you do not distinguish yourself, others will quickly take your place. The most effective ways to promote yourself are:

- Look good and distinctive, and act successful but humble. In conversations, be genuinely interested in what the other person has to say.
- Learn how to "work" a room. Write and practice your 20-second promotional speech and use it to introduce yourself to people in your environment: peers, community leaders, health care professionals, media, and so on. Use a professional handshake, move away from the comfort zone of standing with friends, and get to know people!
- Networking with other individuals in and out of the dietetic profession is an important promotional tool that may change your perspective and offer new professional opportunities. When you start a new job or join a business or professional organization, it is especially crucial that you introduce yourself to peers, supervisors, and executives alike. Offering support and showing eagerness to become involved may increase your personal influence and power (see Chapter 9).
- Become known: write a newspaper article or ongoing column, contribute to journals and magazines in your areas of interest; offer to give short presentations at physicians' offices, Chamber of Commerce meetings, church groups, PTAs, fitness centers, or other appropriate locations.

- Hire someone to create your logo and brand look, and use it on your business cards, letterhead, envelopes, website, email signature, and so on.
- Encourage word-of-mouth promotion by saying, "If you know someone who might need my services, please give them my card" or "I like working with food service operations that are ready to consider a healthier menu. If you know any colleagues who are considering that change, please give me a call or have them call me." Satisfied customers are invaluable walking promoters. Potential clients are often influenced to try a dietitian's service by a satisfied former client who receives no profit or gain from the referral and therefore has high credibility.
- Remember that third-party endorsements carry great weight. Ask referring physicians or past satisfied customers for a letter of reference or quote that can be used in your promotional efforts.
- Keep your personal opinions about people and competitors to yourself or among only close friends. Negative publicity or comments travel as fast or faster than the positive form. Off-the-cuff statements overheard in elevators may be damaging to your professional image.

PLANNING YOUR PROMOTION

When trying to evaluate which forms of promotion to use, review a list of promotional options, such as the one in Figure 13.1, and hypothetically try to fit each form to your product, budget, and audience. Look for ideas that are creative, unique, affordable, and in good taste. Promotion is most successful when designed for multiple exposures of the name, logo, and message to the target market over an extended period.

Advertising and public relations firms will create a promotional campaign for you for a fee. You can expect to pay anywhere from $100 to $300 per hour plus out-of-pocket expenses, materials, and advertising placement costs. If you are seeking the advice of a public relations firm, consult the Internet and your local Yellow Pages, and call colleagues who may have suggestions. There also are individuals who do freelance promotion at a more modest rate. Dietitians who work as employees may have access to in-house public relations or advertising departments that can make a program sparkle if given adequate time, guidance, and budget.

Promotion costs should be seen as part of the investment necessary to create demand for nutrition services. The challenge is to choose wisely so that promotional programs are cost-effective.

Principal Marketing Methods for Small Business

Word-of-Mouth	**Direct Marketing**
Networking	Food sampling
Mentors and Gatekeepers	Coupons or incentives to buy
Volunteerism	Direct mail
Sponsorships	Discount pricing
Business name	Newsletters-print and online
Charitable donations	Circulars and flyers
Referrals	Trade shows and exhibits
Contests and giveaways	Cooking demonstrations
Letterhead and business card	Sales seminars
Product packaging	Direct mail
Point-of-sale display	Bulletin boards and tear pads
Public Relations	**Inventive Advertising**
Writing articles	Classified ads
Letters to the editor	Business directories
News releases	Yellow Page ads
Speeches and seminars	Websites
Publicity	Blogs
Newspaper	Your own radio show
Magazine	Your own TV show
Radio and TV	Online networking
Business & trade publications	Fax
	YouTube
	iPhone

FIGURE 13.1. ■ Principal Marketing Methods for Small Businesses (Adapted from Edwards P, Edwards S, Douglas, E. *Getting Business to Come to You*. New York: Tarcher/Perigee; 1991).

THE PIECES OF THE PROMOTION PUZZLE

There are seven potential pieces of a promotional plan:

1. Public Relations
2. Advertising
3. Internet
4. Direct Mail
5. Trade Shows
6. Personal Promotion
7. Graphic and Print Materials

Each piece is important to the whole because each piece works to reinforce the others. The more pieces you use, the stronger the image you present to your customers, potential customers, and referral agents. But remember that advertising clutter and over-saturation are growing problems that reduce effectiveness of promotion campaigns.

HOW THE PIECES WORK

The pieces work together or separately (3):

- public relations provides low-cost or no-cost publicity about you and your service, product, or company;
- advertising elicits a response from the customer;

- websites provide your customers with the means to read about you and your business twenty-four hours a day and make an immediate purchase;
- direct mail puts a targeted message in front of a specific target market;
- trade shows offer you the opportunity to meet a large number of high-potential new prospects in one setting; and
- personal promotion materials keep you and your message in front of your customers on a daily basis.

Begin your comprehensive promotional plan by looking at the pieces. First, get your personal appearance, 20-second self-promotion statement, and business cards under control; then you might promote yourself as a speaker or consultant. Then do a direct mailing or advertising campaign to tell your target audience more about your department, service, or product and encourage them to take immediate action. Enter a trade show or wellness fair and run an ad inviting attendees to stop by your booth for a free demonstration or gift. Join the Chamber and host a breakfast where you discuss your business or the services provided by your employer.

PUBLIC RELATIONS

Public relations (PR) is an organized effort to promote a favorable image of an individual, an organization, or a product in the marketplace. PR can be internal or external. Internal PR focuses on employees or their families, awards or recognitions, and new product/service updates. External PR is aimed at outside target audiences, such as customers, clients, suppliers, the press, the government (local, state, or federal officials), local business leaders, stockholders, or the local community.

Public relations can involve many different activities that increase exposure by:

- staging major media events;
- producing brochures, newsletters, or other promotional materials;
- sponsoring a community event; or
- offering customer perks to promote goodwill.

Today, most health organizations have an in-house PR staff or hire public relations consultants as needed. Some national companies and associations have a network of spokespersons or media training for its top officers. For example, The American Dietetic Association has trained ambassadors and state media representatives who are interviewed by print and broadcast media on nutrition topics while putting the profession in a good light.

FIVE KEYS TO A SUCCESSFUL PR CAMPAIGN

As you plan, ask yourself the following five keys to a successful PR campaign:

1. *Purpose.* Why are you creating this campaign?
2. *Product.* Are you promoting yourself, your product, or a service?
3. *Plan.* Who are you trying to reach and what do you want them to do or think?
4. *Packaging.* How can you differentiate yourself in a way that will grab attention?
5. *Promotion.* What is the vehicle? A feature story? A blurb? An article?

PUBLICITY

Publicity is planned news, but not paid advertising, so coverage is not guaranteed. You can easily recognize publicity when you see media coverage of a company-sponsored 10K race or a hospital's new mom's class on the evening news.

Your publicity should include an announcement of your coming event or newsworthy story packaged with a good story line or "hook" that will interest the media and its viewers or readers. When planning a special event, you may want to include a local celebrity or consider cosponsorship with a philanthropic organization to improve the possibility of media coverage and attract a larger attendance. You should call and talk directly with the programming editor or media personality to improve your chance of coverage since they receive hundreds of emailed news releases each day. There is no charge for publicity (other than the cost of your time and materials), but since you are not paying, your story may be upstaged by a bigger story and never be used, or it may run without a photo or fanfare on a back page. (For more specific advice on publicity, see Chapter 31.)

PRESS RELEASES

News releases or press releases are the staple of the public relations business. Releases are used by dietitians for many purposes:

- to announce staff changes or the opening of a practice;
- to give details of a special event;
- to announce an upcoming appearance before a local group; or
- to announce the introduction of a new product, the publication of a book, or the release of an association's position paper.

For suggestions on how to write a press release, see Chapter 32.

PRESS KITS

Press kits are used to interest the broadcast and print media in a story on your service, product, book, or speaking engagement (see Chapter 34). The kit may include a variety of items:

- a press release or pitch letter describing the product you wish to publicize (see Chapters 32 and 33);
- a sample of the book or new food product;
- copies of newspaper articles, advertisements, brochures, or critical reviews;
- a resume or short biographical sketch (see Chapter 29);
- sample questions (in kits designed for radio or TV interviews);
- backgrounders describing related studies, endorsements, historical information, and the like;
- 5″ × 7″ black-and-white glossy photos of you or the product.

Press kits should be descriptive, attractive, and to the point. They should provide solid information and explain why the public would be interested in the topic. Although press kits can be very elaborate, with printed covers and numerous photos, they can also be as simple as several of the above items placed in a large pocket folder.

MEDIA INTERVIEWS

Media interviews expose the local area—or sometimes the nation—to a dietitian's views and influence. You can reach more people in five minutes on the radio, TV, or in one newspaper article than you can in 10 years of one-on-one counseling and public speaking combined. Being introduced on a television program or quoted in the newspaper as an expert in nutrition quickly establishes you as a credible professional in the eyes of the public. (See Chapter 14 for more information on gaining media exposure.)

NEWS CONFERENCES

News conferences are called to announce to the media an important event, scientific discovery, product, or the like. Usually, a formal statement is made, followed by a question-and-answer session.

PRESS BRIEFINGS

Press briefings—one-on-one, desk-side interviews or more formal editorial board briefings—are used to provide the media with in-depth background information on a specific subject.

COSPONSORSHIP

Cosponsorship of events and activities has proven to be a very successful promotional method for many ventures because it cuts costs. It also may increase your visibility and extends your reach through exposure to your cosponsor's viewers, readers, members, or fans. When considering potential cosponsors, evaluate what skills, resources, and public image are required to complement what you have to offer. For example, a hospital could cosponsor a city health-promotion campaign with a local newspaper and television station. The media cosponsors could offer publicity and exposure, while the hospital could provide the project development, management, personnel, and help recruit a celebrity.

In any partnership, all participants should contribute to and benefit from the relationship, or problems will arise. A project plan clearly identifying all participants' contributions, assignments, and deadlines will help cosponsored activities run more smoothly and equitably.

SPECIAL EVENTS

Special events and rewards can generate excitement for your program and good media coverage. Staging such events at times that permit live, on-site TV coverage often increases publicity tremendously. The noon or later-afternoon news programs are often interested in covering local events with their live mobile camera units. Consider something visual like children eating the new healthier school lunch, an anniversary celebration, a milestone occurrence, a bike race or other athletic event, a nutrition day or health fair, a food tasting, a free cholesterol screening, a testimonial dinner, or an event that ties in with a civic celebration, a holiday, or a seasonal theme. Award presentations offer an opportunity to thank those who have made special contributions of time, money, or resources to your project. A tip: high-quality engraved or beautifully designed invitations make a strong impression on those invited to your event and help put them in a festive frame of mind.

CELEBRITIES

Celebrities attract attention; the media want to interview them and the public wants to see and mingle with them. Hiring a media or sports celebrity, or persuading such a person to become involved as an act of charity, may help assure success for your venture. It certainly helps your advance publicity. Just be sure that the celebrity's public image matches the one you want to create for your program or event.

ADVERTISING

Advertising is purchased promotion in print, on broadcast media, or the Internet. It is used to draw potential buyers' attention, teach your customers something new about your product, change customers' attitudes, or remind them of past satisfaction with your product or company. Advertising exposes a large number of people to your message. You can better control the timing and quality of the exposure because you are a paying customer.

When you advertise, just remember the basics:

■ First determine the response you want from your audience;

■ Choose a message that will stimulate that response;

■ Find the medium that enhances your message; and

■ Keep the message consistent.

The choice of media depends on your target market, budget, and goals. Potential buyers must be exposed to an ad several times before they remember it, so advertising campaigns must optimize frequency and reach (how often the estimated number of people see or hear the ad). Some practitioners have been very successful in using advertising for their private practices; others have not. The approaches that have worked best are Yellow Pages, advertising and ongoing ads in local newspapers, and on local radio. The Internet is a growing source of contacts and revenue as well. Websites help to continually evaluate the effectiveness of different forms of advertising by asking every new client how he or she heard of your services.

To better evaluate the cost of advertising for a service, divide the average fee for an initial consultation into the total cost for the advertising. For example, if a radio campaign costs $1,000 per month and you charge $150 for an initial consultation, you will pay for the ad or break even with seven new patients per month, which is reasonable. In contrast, if the advertising costs $3,000 per month and you charge $150, it will take 20 new patients per month to break even and cover your advertising costs. That is a lot of added hours and expense!

FOUR KEYS TO SUCCESSFUL ADVERTISING

First, decide what you want your ad to do. There are then four keys to successful advertising (2,3,4):

1. *Stimulus/Response.* What response do you want from your audience? Select the appropriate stimulus to evoke that response. For example, if you want people to come to a diabetes education program, after you excite them about the program, you may offer half off registration for the first five callers.

2. *Surprise.* Never underestimate the element of surprise in an ad. Surprise grabs attention and makes a lasting impression. For example, your ad may say, "Did you know that 21 million Americans have diabetes?"

3. *Emotion.* Love, fear, sadness, and humor involve the audience and make your point with impact. Remember the little elderly lady in Wendy's "Where's the beef?" People are still talking about that ad many years later.

4. *Relevance.* Make sure your ad leaves your audience thinking, "They are talking about me!" If it does not, you have lost an opportunity, and perhaps a sale.

SELECTING THE APPROPRIATE MEDIA

Television delivers visual movement and impact, but the cost is high, and 15- or 30-second spots offer only limited time to convey your information. Radio airtime can be a cost-effective way to get your message heard frequently and you can choose the demographics by the type of programming, but radio often plays in the background and airing on the best stations is expensive. A lot of people read newspapers each day, but the competition for the readers' attention is fierce. Yellow Pages advertising can be very effective because surveys show that a high percent of adults consult their directory every month—at the time they are looking for something to buy. The most common errors people make when buying Yellow Pages advertising is placing ads that are so small they contain too little information or are not competitive in their category, or their ads are under the wrong category so response is light. Websites offer the opportunity to have vibrant color and adequate space and time to tell your story, describe what you sell, or entertain visitors. On the down side, website development, hosting, and management costs must be controlled, and the site must be adequately promoted in order to attract enough visitors to make it worth having.

WEBSITES

A website home page is where a business or individual provides current and potential customers with information about the firm, its brands (products or services), and other content of interest (2). Setting up a website can be accomplished fairly simply and inexpensively. But to have one that attracts attention and is commercially successful costs more and takes more effort. Some sites give brand exposure and sell products and conduct the transaction online. Others are only informational—they give extensive product or service information or nutritional facts. "Lifestyle" sites are specific to the needs of a particular target market and offer educational, entertaining, and sometimes interactive options (2). For example, a site for older adults could have nutrition information for healthy aging, 10 keys to healthy memory with a self-test online, and a discussion of Medicare coverage for prescriptions. Entertainment sites offer games, YouTube videos, e-books, and so on. Some sites have a mix of options.

There are two concerns with websites: the first is optimizing the site to improve search engine ranking (see Chapter 24), and the second is getting customers or Internet surfers to stay longer or come back to your site over and over again—a feature called "sticky" (2). Sites that are sticky often have engaging, interactive features, or recurring information like weather, sports scores, news, or stock quotes (2). Others offer games, horoscopes, raffles, or "thoughts for the day." Multiple navigational tools on a site (like icons to move around the site, an internal search engine, and a site index) are highly prized by visitors.

A domain name is a distinct URL Internet location. When deciding on a domain name, Internet expert Dennis Scheyer suggests using a descriptive but unique URL and an intuitive but distinctive one (2).

TELEVISION

Network TV is expensive for the small business owner. As mentioned in an earlier chapter, the marketing experts Rapp and Collins, authors of *The Great Marketing Turnaround* (10), believe that mass marketing on network TV is not particularly effective at stimulating customers to buy products, especially considering the relative cost. If you use network TV, check into buying one of these less-expensive options (2):

- *Pre-emptible time.* You pay for a certain time slot and your commercial will air then, unless someone else pays a higher price for the same spot, thus pre-empting you.
- *Run-of-station time.* You pay a certain price for the week, and the station places your spots in unsold time.
- *Distress time.* You wait until the last possible minute and buy unsold air-time at a lower price.

Buyer beware! If you purchase bargain airtime, monitor it carefully to make sure it delivers an audience worth your investment. For example, if you buy distress time on the late movie, be sure your ad runs in the first hour, not during the last 10 minutes (2).

CABLE

Sometimes referred to as narrowcasting (as opposed to network TV, which is broadcasting), cable is a good alternative for many small businesses that rely on local or neighborhood customers. Cable is less expensive, and many cable operators help you produce simple, low-cost commercials. However, your purchasing options will vary, depending on the age and sophistication of the cable operator's equipment, and you may find yourself relegated to one specific time slot for an entire week (2).

RADIO

When you advertise on the radio, if you choose the appropriate type of music or talk format, you can reach a specific demographic group and achieve frequency fairly easily. Ads must be particularly attention-grabbing to be remembered. With radio, as with TV time, the more popular stations and time slots are the most expensive because more people are listening or viewing at that time.

PRINT

The number of specialty magazines and journals has been steadily on the rise, meaning there is a newspaper, magazine, or journal for just about any group you would like to target, whether it is business-to-business or consumer-oriented. And people who buy those publications are actively looking for information (2). Consult the *Gale Directory of Publications and Broadcast Media* or other trade resources in your local library for rates, circulations, and ad specifications for consumer magazines, trade journals, and radio and television stations. See Table 13.1 for a listing of resources.

One possible disadvantage of print advertising is long lead times, which means that ads do not come out for two or three months and cannot be changed quickly. It also takes longer to build an audience when a publication comes out only once a month or once a quarter. Also, some publications may be cluttered with competitive advertising, making it more difficult for your message to stand out.

When choosing between newspapers and magazines, remember that magazines allow for more efficient targeting, but have longer lead times. Newspapers reach a broad audience quickly, but may not reach the people you are looking for when they are making buying decisions.

TABLE 13.1.   RESOURCES

Resource	Frequency or Publication Date
PR and Writing	
Bly RW. *The Copywriter's Handbook: A Step-by-Step Guide to Writing Copy That Sells*, 3rd Ed. New York: Owl Books	2005
Business Publication Advertising Source. Wilmette, IL: Standard Rate & Data Service	Monthly
Caples J. *Tested Advertising Methods*. Englewood Cliffs, NJ: Prentice-Hall Business Classics	1998
Consumer Publication Advertising Source. Wilmette, IL: Standard Rate & Data Service	Monthly
Curtin PA, Gaither TK. *International Public Relations: Negotiating Culture, Identity, and Power*. Thousand Oaks, CA: Sage Publications	2007
Gale Directory of Publications and Broadcast Media. Detroit, MI: Gale Research	Annual; also on software
O'Guinn T, Allen C, Semenik R. *Advertising and Integrated Brand Promotion*, 4th Ed. Mason, OH: Thomson Higher Education	2006
Pride W, Ferrell OC. *Marketing: Concepts and Strategies*, 12th Ed. New York: Houghton Mifflin	2003
Rapp S, Collins T. *The Great Marketing Turnaround*. Englewood Cliffs, NJ: Prentice-Hall	1990
Direct Mail	
Entrepreneur Press, Barnes R. *Direct Response Advertising Made Easy*. Madison, WI: Entrepreneur Press	2007
Nash E. *Direct Marketing Strategy, Planning & Execution*. New York: McGraw-Hill	1984
Simon J. *How to Start and Operate a Mail-Order Business*, 5th Ed. New York: McGraw-Hill	1993
Trade Shows	
International Exhibitors Association, 5103-B Backlick Road, Annandale, VA 22003	Ongoing; call 703-941-3725
Miller S. *How to Get the Most out of Trade Shows*. Lincolnwood, IL: NTC Business Books.	1992
Stevens R. *Trade Show and Event Marketing: Plan, Promote and Profit*. Mason, OH: Thomson Corp	2005
Trade Shows and Professional Exhibits Directory. Detroit, MI: Gale Research.	Annual

SIX KEY MEDIA CONCEPTS

Price is always an issue, but spending more money will not necessarily make your ads more successful. You can make your ad campaign work for you if you keep these six key media concepts in mind (2–4):

Concentration

It is usually more productive to concentrate limited funds instead of spreading them over a variety of media. Customers are more likely to remember you or your product when they see your message multiple times. Twenty-five radio spots are usually more effective than one TV spot or one large newspaper ad.

Reach

Reach is the number of people exposed at least once to the vehicle carrying your ad. For example, you may be able to reach 25,000 people through your local weekly newspaper. Reach accumulates as you add media, concentration, or frequency.

Frequency and Continuity

One of the jobs of your ad is to teach people, and people learn through repetition. That means frequent exposure to your message. So if you have to choose between one glossy 4-color image and 10 black-and-white ads, go for the black-and-white ones. The fact that your ad will run 10 times increases the chance that a prospect will see it more than once.

Visibility and Impact

If your ad is not memorable, it will not matter how many times you run it. It must grab your audience and get their attention! Do not throw your money away. Just remember the four essential considerations: stimulus/response, emotion, surprise, and relevance.

Awareness of Your Competition

Do not copy your competitors, but know what they are doing. If they have more money for advertising, look for a new message or target a different market niche. For example, if they are going after large catered affairs, go after small parties for people with incomes over $70,000. Know your competitors' strengths and weaknesses; know what they are doing that works.

Test What You are Doing

The owner of a large department-store chain once said, "I am wasting my money on 50% of my advertising budget—I just do not know which 50%."

Test your advertising strategy. It can be as simple as asking callers how they heard of your service, running the same ad in two different media, or using coded order forms.

DIRECT MAIL

Use direct mail when you know specifically whom you want to contact (usually either potential clients or referral agents). The average response rate to direct mail is 1% to 2%, which is higher than for most other forms of advertising. The greater your name recognition, the better the response. When dietitians are known in their communities, some report their response rate from direct mail to physicians and clinics as high as 30%.

Direct mail can be used to send a brochure, conduct surveys, announce new services, acquaint potential clients with your services, or sell your product or service. Mailings should be personally addressed, whenever possible, instead of "To whom it may concern" or "Occupant." Membership lists of your local medical society or national dietetic practice groups, the Yellow Pages, and shared business cards are good sources of names and addresses. Many organizations charge a fee and require an explanation of how their membership lists will be used. The Internet has a wealth of list companies that sell databases with names of hospitals, physicians by specialty, or business contacts for mailing labels.

Because an estimated 30% of all mail is thrown away unopened, what you put on the outside is very important. Pat Stein, RD, founder of NCES catalog, found that her response rate doubled when she changed from 1- or 2-color brochures to 4-color layouts. It also saves money if you are sending thousands of pieces to use a mailing service that sends the items by sorted bulk mail.

TRADE SHOWS

Trade shows are a one-on-one sales medium that can produce very attractive sales figures. According to the Small Business Administration, 54% of the qualified prospects who hear your pitch at a national trade show will turn into sales. The keys to success at trade shows are:

- careful selection of the shows and sales staff,
- attractive booth and location,
- a good sales pitch and system to qualify leads, and
- excellent follow-up. (See Chapter 35 for specific hints on how to market at trade shows.)

PROMOTIONAL AIDS

BUSINESS CARDS

Business cards are the most common communication tool used by business and professional people to promote services, facilitate networking, and provide a handy reminder of a phone number or appointment date. The typical card includes your name, credentials, title, place of business, mailing address with zip code, phone number(s) with area code, website, and email address. Colors, fonts, logos, layouts, and other design elements vary greatly as seen in Figure 13.2. Figure 13.3 shows letterheads, which are generally coordinated with the envelopes, cards, website, and other promotional materials to give a consistent branding.

LETTERS OR NOTES

Letters or notes are excellent ways to improve communication and promote referrals and client loyalty. Practitioners who send frequent letters show their concern and involvement. Telephone calls and emails also serve this function.

More frequent communication can also strengthen your ties with community or professional

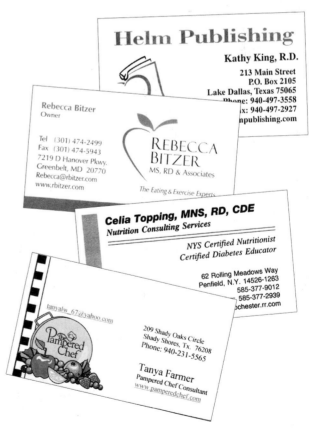

FIGURE 13.2. ■ Various design and color elements.

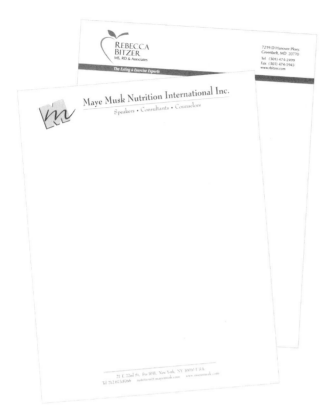

FIGURE 13.3. ■ Sample letterheads.

organizations. Letters to editors of newspapers, magazines, and journals give you a chance to air your views and educate others. Personal letters to community leaders, authors, and other individuals may help you identify allies and expand your network.

Ask one or more people to proofread and evaluate all of your important and potentially controversial written communication. All typed or handwritten correspondence should look as clean and professional as possible because they represent you and should convey the image you want to project. See Chapters 34 and 36 on writing.

RESUMES

Resumes can be powerful tools of self-promotion. A well-thought-out resume may give you a competitive edge in job negotiations. It may be used, along with a letter of introduction, to acquaint potential clients with you and your services. It may be sent to sponsors of speaking engagements or media interviewers to assist in introducing you, or included with a publishing or business proposal. You may want to write several different resumes representing your varied areas of expertise. A resume may be either chronological—listing your experience in reverse chronological order—or functional—highlighting your skills and responsibilities. Variations include the curriculum vitae or vita—an expanded version of a resume that includes published books

and papers—and the biographical sketch, which is written in paragraph form. All of these should be updated on a regular basis to fit new markets and reflect new skills and accomplishments. (For more on resumes, see Chapter 29.)

LETTERS OF REFERENCE OR INTRODUCTION

Letters of reference or introduction can lend credibility to you and your services. They are most effective when written by someone who knows your recent work but is also objective—perhaps a satisfied client or the head of clinical services. Such letters may be included with resumes to introduce you to potential clients or to offer new programs to established markets. They document your success with past ventures.

TRADE NAME

Using a trade name to identify a specific program, event, activity, or business helps you and others differentiate between programs and increases recognition in the minds of your target market. If you are in business for yourself, choose a name that is descriptive and easy to remember. You can use your personal name; a straightforward name, such as Baltimore Nutrition Services; or a catchy name, like Nutrition Thyme for a culinary class.

PUBLIC SPEAKING

Public speaking is a promotional opportunity of great value to dietitians. The public is willing and eager to hear information and guidance about nutrition. Speaking is an effective way to teach, influence, motivate others, and introduce a product or service. Public speaking, like media work, requires special skills and training. (For more information, see Chapter 25.)

GRAPHIC AND PRINT MATERIAL

Logos are pictorial symbols or names in stylized letters that stand for a product, service, event, or business. A logo can add visual interest and create a distinctive professional identity. It is used to improve audience recall or recognition by providing a cohesive, consistent look to all printed materials.

Use of your logo provides you with trademark rights in the United States. Federal registration, although not mandatory, is evidence of your exclusive right to use the logo. You can formally document your claim to your logo by registering it with the U.S. Patent and Trademark Office,

Washington, DC 20231. A logo that is used on a product, such as food or a software program, can be registered as a trademark; if a logo is used for a service, such as nutrition counseling, it can be registered as a service mark. A logo will not be registered if another logo design in the same basic category (such as health associations) is too similar. It is not difficult to register a logo. An application must be filed along with a fee and samples of the logo. A lawyer can conduct a trademark search and consult on the filing of the application. You can also request an application form and information booklet from the Patent and Trademark Office. It is the responsibility of the owner to defend the right to the logo and to pay for any legal action. Some sample logos are shown in Figures 13.2 and 13.3.

BROCHURES

Brochures are used to describe and promote your products, services, and programs. Brochures may be handed out at speaking engagements, included in materials given to clients, mailed to target markets or the press, or left in waiting rooms. Brochures are surrogates of you and your services. They should be attractive, well written, and easy to read. A public relations expert might help you improve the wording, and a graphic artist the presentation. It is usually worth the extra money to enhance the brochure's appearance with color, a photo or drawing, and good-quality paper since the quality of your work is often judged by the quality of your promotion. The importance of a professional look in all communications cannot be over-stressed. See Chapter 28 for specific tips on how to write a brochure.

PORTFOLIOS

Portfolios are visual presentations of the services you offer. They may be simple, such as a three-ring binder with color photos of your catering selections or samples of creative projects completed for clients. They may be sophisticated, such as a professionally created flip chart with graphs and sales projections. Using a portfolio in interviews helps potential clients better understand and visualize your services.

PROPOSALS

Proposals are comprehensive promotional and sales tools used to interest a client, administrator, or financial backer in your service or new program. Proposals can range from a simple one-page typewritten information sheet to a slide show or tasting session accompanied by a typeset, bound, multi-page document. The higher the stakes, the more elaborate the presentation. Proposals should be only long enough to interest the potential client and make the sale. Care should be exercised to ensure that good ideas and explanations are not so detailed that clients can carry out the projects without you. See Chapter 30 for more information on proposals.

POSTERS AND SIGNS

Posters and signs are potentially effective promotion tools, especially when used in hallways, storefronts, or cafeterias where the target market must pass them several times each day. They generally are not as effective in drawing business when placed randomly in public places, although libraries, supermarkets, and local businesses are often willing to accommodate you with space in their windows or on their bulletin boards. Posters should be designed to be eye-catching, to provide pertinent information (date, place, time), and, most important, to entice the reader to respond or to attend the program. A phone number or tear-off mail-in card may be included for those who want more information.

Banners draw attention and create name recognition. They create a festive mood and are a great promotional tool for large areas where crowds gather. They can be used at the finish line of a fun run, in a lobby during a wellness festival, or over the cafeteria door to promote a new line of light and natural foods, for example. Banners can be made with paper and paint; however, they can be reused many times if they are made from vinyl. Lettering, layout, and graphics all demand careful attention, perhaps from a graphic art professional. Remember that a program is often prejudged by the quality of the items that promote it.

OTHER AIDS

Other aids that can be used for promotional as well as educational purposes include photos and multi-image slide shows on laptops, videotapes, blogs, YouTube, and multimedia presentations. For instance, if you take a booth at a local health fair to promote your coordinated exercise and nutrition program, a two-minute videotape that automatically repeats would be a good way to stop traffic. If you are attempting to sell your kitchen design skills to a new client, a slideshow on your laptop might be the most impressive way to present what you have done in the past.

Computer graphics can enhance many forms of visual promotion. They need not be elaborate. You

CORPORATE CAREER COACHING WORDS OF WISDOM

Jean R. Caton, MS, MBA, RD, McKinley Coaching & Consulting LLC ; http://www.JeanCaton.com

What Is Success?

Success is a product of loving what you do, combined with hard work, self-confidence, and competence. My self-proclaimed successful career has been characterized by jobs for which I have great passion, derive personal fulfillment, and receive significant financial rewards.

How did I manage to have such a satisfying, successful, and diverse career? I sometimes still wonder. For someone who grew up in the 1950s and 1960s—when women's career choices included teacher, secretary, nurse, or wife—a career earning a six-figure salary in corporate America was certainly not one I envisioned. As Henry Ford said, "Whether you think that you can, or that you cannot, you are usually right."

My Career Path

After a short time as a teacher, I returned to college for a Master's Degree in Nutrition and worked for a while as a clinical dietitian. My next job presented me with many exciting new opportunities. I assumed the newly created position as Educational Coordinator in the Nutrition Department at a teaching hospital, designing and managing a dietetic internship from scratch with the department manager. It was this position that ignited my business career aspirations.

The best time to move ahead is when you are happy in your job. Do not wait until your career plateaus, you feel stuck, or until you outgrow your job. I returned to school for my second Master's Degree, a Master's in Business Administration (MBA), at the time a rather unusual step for females, especially registered dietitians. After completing the degree, I sold my condominium in Boston and moved to Chicago, packing all my possessions and my RD and MBA. These two credentials got me in the door for an interview, and subsequently, my first corporate job as product manager. I was naïve and fearless, still leveraging my success of previous jobs.

No one ever said it was going to be easy, and it was not. The work was extremely demanding, competitive, highly paid, and well matched to my intrinsic strengths. I went on to work the majority of my career in four Fortune 100 companies in increasingly responsible positions. I found the work of directing the design, development, and marketing of products ranging from medical devices (including enteral feeding pumps and electronic thermometers) to food ingredients to be exhilarating.

I have since graduated from corporate America, choosing at last to work on my own—a long-time desire that was detoured by my worry about paying the mortgage. Operating my own small venture is a whole new world. After 3 years on my own, the romantic myths have disappeared. Yes, I do things my way and I am my own boss and janitor. Working in a large corporation, with every resource at my fingertips and a large budget, is not the perfect preparation to having your own business.

My Coaching Tips

- Believe in yourself!
- Be competent: There is no substitute for having the depth and breadth of knowledge required to do your job well. Observe and learn from others, especially those at higher levels in the organization. Reading the professional literature and attending conferences is essential in a rapidly evolving field.
- Keep adding new skills to your professional toolbox: I admired those I saw at professional conferences who were good public speakers. I decided to develop this skill, so I volunteered as a spokesperson for the American Heart Association speaking to seniors about good nutrition. To this day, I am convinced they were more interested in the cookies and punch than learning what to eat to lower their cholesterol. Nonetheless, I learned how to speak to groups.
- Get involved—Volunteer: Participate in local and state dietetic associations. I continue to do so today. I have met a lot of people, some of whom have been instrumental in my career advancement.
- Do not go it alone—Find a mentor, coach, and advocate: Most successful people report that they have had one or more mentors supporting their career advancement. Coaching provides another way to assist you in your career progress. Advocates can do more than a mentor or coach. Advocates typically are in higher-level positions and can offer a hand up and positive word of mouth to people in positions who can make a difference. Seek out mentors, advocates, and hire a coach. Build relationships across department boundaries.
- Follow a career path aligned with your strengths. Assess your strengths and design a career roadmap aligned with them, not one where you have weaknesses to overcome.
- Take Risks: The move to a new city a thousand miles from home was a big risk. Little did I know that people in Chicago did not understand English—or at least English with a heavy Boston accent. But I have never looked back. I was fearless and

continued

continued

perhaps too naïve to be daunted by the impending demands of my new job. It was an opportunity of a lifetime to me.

■ Life Long Learning: Read technical professional literature and equally important, business magazines, newspapers (*Wall Street Journal* is a favorite), and business books to keep well informed and current. Speak the language of leaders, managers, and business.

■ Polish your executive presence and market yourself. Believing is seeing. Having a presence is an essential way to be recognized as capable. I always knew I was being judged by the way I looked, and how I acted, responded, and interacted with others. *Just doing a good job is not going to get you ahead*. You need a personal brand to describe what you stand for and need to market and promote your strength in a way similar to marketing a product.

■ Communicate with confidence. Did you ever make a comment in a meeting and have it be ignored only to have someone else say essentially the same thing and have the response be "good point!" I was never one to hesitate to speak up and yet I sometimes had a problem being *heard*. Like many women, I often spoke with too many details, qualifiers, and hedges. After receiving feedback from a meeting facilitator who pointed this out to me and suggested a great book on workplace communication I embarked on the challenge of becoming a more effective communicator.

■ Continually reinvent yourself: Reinvention involves ongoing formal and informal education and a willingness to embrace change.

■ Build relationships—Network: Networking is all about helping others, building bridges, giving before getting, and can even be fun. When you are in your own business, effective networking is an essential marketing tool. It is also the way over 70% of new jobs are found.

■ Break through your FUD (Fear, Uncertainty, and Doubt): It is not about being fearless. Everyone has fears of some sort. It is about recognizing when fear is holding you back—causing procrastination—when you are waiting to be told what to do or procrastinating until you know you can do it perfectly. When you experience self-doubt, as we all do at times, silence the negative thought. Focus on strengths. Figure it out as you go. Just do it!

might use a graphics imaging program on your personal computer to give a simple flyer a more professional appearance. Another program could produce colorful bar and pie charts for your sales presentation. You might hire a computer graphics house to create impressive three-dimensional effects for your DVD. Computer-generated slides are an inexpensive way to add a graphic element and color to a slide presentation. Computers can save you time and money in creating visuals, and computer graphics used appropriately can help convey a high-tech, up-to-the-minute image.

Giveaways, such as T-shirts, clipboards, notebooks, mugs, bumper stickers, gym bags, sweatbands, posters, and refrigerator magnets with company names or logos are popular promotion items. The more useful and practical an item is, the more it will be used and the more the name or logo will be displayed. Such items are sometimes sold as fund raisers rather than given away.

SUMMARY

Promotion is essential for every dietitian in carrying out marketing plans. But beyond that, it is an exciting challenge to your creativity. It takes effort to promote yourself, but what project of any worth does not take effort?

REFERENCES

1. Beckwith H. *The Invisible Touch*. New York: Warner Books; 2000.
2. O'Guinn T, Allen C, Semenik R. *Advertising and Integrated Brand Promotion*, 4th Ed. Mason, OH: Thomson Higher Education; 2006.
3. *Market Brand*. Wikipedia. Accessed February 6, 2008.
4. Bennett P. *Dictionary of Marketing Terms*, 2nd Ed. Chicago, IL: American Marketing Assocation; 1995: 4.
5. Beckwith H. *Selling the Invisible*. New York: Warner Books; 1997.
6. Arruda W. *Branding: All You Need Is Love*. Marketing-Prof.com. Available at http://www.marketingprofs.com/print.asp?source=%2F5%2Farruda20%2Easp. Accessed July 26, 2005.
7. Sanders T. *The Likeability Factor: How to Boost Your L-Factor and Achieve Your Life's Dreams*. New York: Three Rivers; 2006.
8. *Promotion: Solving the Puzzle*. Arlington, VA: Small Business Video Library; 1990.
9. Caples J. *Tested Advertising Methods*. Englewood Cliffs, NJ: Prentice-Hall; 1974.
10. Rapp S, Collins T. *The Great Marketing Turnaround*. Englewood Cliffs, NJ: Prentice-Hall; 1990.

PURSUING THE POTENTIAL OF THE MEDIA

14

Mary Lee Chin, MS, RD, and Joan Horbiak, MPH, RD

What do you want? A way to advance your career or private practice? Community support for your hospital event? New legislation? Visibility for your research or book? Better understanding of the new dietary guidelines? The media can bring all that about. In fact, no other institution or group has the power and reach of the media today.

MEDIA REACHES THE PUBLIC

As more consumers turn to the media for answers to diet and health-related questions, opportunities for dietetics professionals to reach consumers through local broadcast and print communications are unlimited. According to the 2006 Future of News Survey, conducted for the Radio and Television News Directors Foundation, 65.5% of Americans choose local television news as their top source for news over any other form of traditional or new media. The survey also found that 28.4% of Americans got their news from their local newspapers. And the Internet was third choice for news, weighing in at 11.2% of those surveyed (1).

The good news is that the prospects that you or a member of your organization will be called on for an interview—print or electronic—are skyrocketing. Over the past decade, rarely a day went by without food making big news. Health and how food impacts Americans' health have emerged as the single-most important focus of media reports about nutrition and food safety. That is the conclusion of a decade-long tracking survey by the International Food Information Council (IFIC) Foundation and the Center for Media and Public Affairs (CMPA) (2). Whether it is childhood obesity or reports on spinach recalls, Americans get most of their nutrition information from televisions and magazines, according to the American Dietetic Association's Trends 2002 survey. Other sources include newspapers, the Internet, radio, dietitians, doctors, family, and friends (3).

As the public's interest in nutrition grows, the media's search for dietitians with stories and reports also grows. According to Gina Selby, news producer for WB2 in Denver, "Right behind weather and traffic, medical and health news rank as top reasons why viewers tune in to watch television news. As a television producer, I am regularly looking for a dietitian who can comment, expand, and localize the latest health news. Sometimes we only have a minute and a half to convey the story. A dietitian who can give concise explanations is what producers and reporters look for. As a producer, my job is to also present the news in a simple, creative, and visually appealing way for viewers to understand. Having a dietitian who can present the news visually (i.e., using food examples or cooking demos) adds to the viewer benefit."

The media want to talk to you! But do not wait for the media to come knocking at your door. The success stories will come from dietitians who create rather than wait for media opportunities. The keys are to learn how the media work, what they want and when they want it, and to build media relationships. Learning the rules of the game can help you meet the Media Age head on and win.

THE RULES OF THE GAME

The rules of the game are based on years of doing, not theory. The rules are simple and may sound like common sense. But according to media producers, reporters, editors, and correspondents, there is a big difference between common sense and common practice when working with health professionals!

KNOW THE TYPES OF MEDIA

Your communication strategies must take into account the kinds of media available and the diverse ways in which different media organizations formulate news stories. Be prepared to capitalize on the opportunities offered by these differences:

Local television stations offer news shows with special health reports and community affairs programs.

Community cable stations can offer local news programming, community access channels, and public affairs programming.

Public affairs television stations can provide local news programming as well as a diverse mix of locally produced public affairs programming.

Newspapers have various beat reporters covering specialized issues for the hard news section, plus business, food, lifestyle, consumer, environment, and style sections offering soft news.

Magazines cater to targeted audiences with focused health, food, and diet interests.

Online magazines and websites offer a variety of specialized news information and, frequently, interactive programs.

Most issues can be marketed from a variety of angles or points of view. For example, a story could be covered as a business topic, a lifestyle matter, a consumer concern, a legal question, an editorial opinion, or a local or national issue, depending on how it is framed. You may want to shop around for a reporter who has a good understanding of your issue. In the end, an editor or news director will make the final decision on who covers your story for the media outlet. However, if you are actively promoting a story, as opposed to just reacting to a reporter's request for information, you are in a better position to approach a specific reporter with a good story idea.

Be sure your information is in a format suited to the medium you have selected. Types of news formats include hard news, soft news, face-to-face interviews, panel discussions, and news conferences. Understanding the media will enable you to provide information in the format that best meets each medium's needs. Determine whether your story is hard or soft news. *Hard news* follows the format of who, what, where, when, and how. Such news is timely and affects a great number of people. *Soft news* is treated as a feature story as long as it has value. Such information is less urgent, but must still have a "news hook" related to a timely topic. You may suggest a soft news feature story by writing or phoning an editor and presenting a summary that will grab attention and demonstrate the significance of the story. Or, you may provide the editor with a backgrounder as a feature sample. You must maintain exclusivity when pitching a soft news feature; only approach one media at a time, but move on quickly if that one turns it down.

KNOW WHAT IS NEWSWORTHY

The key to getting positive coverage from the media is to have a story that is really newsworthy and to tell the media about it. Every hour of every day, the media need to fill "news holes" with stories. Nanci Hellmich, the health reporter for *USA Today*, points out that dietitians need to look at what they do with a new perspective. "I am always looking for the new and interesting, but 'new' can simply mean a different twist on an old idea," she explains. "Dietitians work with creative approaches to what may seem like old, worn-out topics such as weight reduction, and they do not even recognize it. They routinely deal with the angst that we want to capture and write about." Fresh tips and tactics you have developed for your patients will also be new and beneficial for the public.

The media are interested in what you are doing, and they are even more interested in what you are seeing. Dietitians are in a unique position to spot and evaluate emerging trends, such as changes in the foods people eat and buy. Also, breaking nutrition news can have immediate impact: the spinach and E. coli scare, a hurricane's effect on water safety, or a new study on anti-oxidants and functional foods, for example. The media cannot always wait until top health authorities issue recommendations. Because you are a nutrition expert, your rapid response to breaking news is newsworthy. The media are hungry for stories filled with energy, grace, and humor. To appeal to the media, a good story should be both newsworthy and entertaining. Also keep in mind that simplicity counts more than wisdom. If you pitch a story in the style of a professional journal article, it will be rejected. Finally, a story must be timely and of current interest. Stories that follow a trend or buck a current way of thinking are attention getting.

You can find a wide variety of nutrition-related story ideas and resources in the Media section of the ADA's website, http://www.eatright.org. Check out the links to news releases and consumer education programs, among other areas. For more ideas, also see the "Tip of the Day" and "Monthly Feature," which are posted on ADA's home page.

BECOME A MEDIA TRACKER

Keep your eyes and ears open and your antennae out. New ideas and policies are often reported in small, in-house publications or presented in speeches and academic papers to limited audiences. Professional journals, newsletters, magazines, and articles are also launching pads for new developments or ideas. Stay in touch by subscribing to nutrition journals and newsletters. Reporters, especially health reporters, subscribe to the *New England Journal of Medicine* and *Science* magazine, and monitor breaking health news as it comes over the wire services and the Internet.

Monitor the popular press to assess what is important to the public. "Piggy-back" and focus your story on what is happening locally. Read your local newspaper and at least one national newspaper daily, such as *USA Today*, the *Wall Street Journal*, the *New York Times*, or the *Los Angeles Times*. Become a television media monitor. Television news follows and reports on consumer trends. If an issue is in the national news, think about its local impact. Local news outlets are always looking for sidebars to national stories. The trick is to stay ahead of your local station on story ideas.

Some of your best press coverage will come from watching, listening, and reading the media, and applying your stories to their issues.

DEVELOP A NEWS HOOK

A newsworthy story should have an interesting "news hook," or "peg." Hooks can be humorous, seasonal, of human interest, or scientific, but they must also be creative and practical. According to Jeanne Ambrose, editor of *Heart Healthy Living*, a Special Interest Publications of *Better Homes and Gardens*, "RDs who can write for a consumer magazine are in demand. Come up with unique ideas (we do not want 'been there, done that' stories) with good solid quotes and resources, and you get the gig."

Talk about lifestyle changes, not diets. In the past, magazines could present a different diet every month. Today readership polls show that diets are out and practical tips, recipes, and how-to's are in.

Articles in most daily newspapers describe national and local problems in human terms. To humanize a story, the lead paragraph often presents a victim or a beneficiary. Personal stories are also essential elements in television and radio news stories.

Any approach to the media that does not have a good story to tell is not likely to be of much interest to the reporters.

KNOW YOUR AUDIENCE

Once you have developed your story, it is time to shape your examples to meet the needs of your audience. Who are you going to reach with your information? What do you know about them? Nothing angers the media more than a "one-size-fits-all" approach. Each publication, newspaper, and television or radio station has a different focus and needs. Target audiences have different interests . . . and you better pay attention to them. Jeanne Ambrose of *Heart-Healthy Living Magazine* states, "For instance, we will not run a story about Buttery-Rich Indulgent Desserts because our target is the 40-plus female, and we will not be featuring stories about newborn babies (unless there is a heart angle), nor will we be focusing on stories that suggest ways to avoid exercise. The key is to be able to match the writing style of the magazine. Read and study the magazine. Request writer's guidelines. Send a professional query/proposal. More often than not I get writers asking me for assignments. I do assign stories on occasion to writers I love, but my biggest need is NEW ideas. Send me a bulleted list of ideas with proposed sources and a sidebar suggestion, and then, maybe, we will talk."

Do your homework. Analyze and tailor the details of your story to meet the needs and interests of your medium's audience. And never pitch a story or give an interview without first reading the publication or watching or listening to the show. Remember, *amateurs think of the story while professionals think of the audience.*

KEEP IT SIMPLE!

An important fact to remember when giving interviews is that people do not remember much. One classic research study showed that audiences will forget 75% or more of what you say in 24 hours or less. To be most effective, develop a clear, simple speaking style. Plan to express one quality message. Have no more than two or three key points to convey. Write them down. Take out the jargon. Use conversational language and put some zip into your delivery. Work to make your material simple, direct, fresh, quotable, and easy to understand. If you really want to make your point, you had better make it short, and you had better make it simple. In fact, complex messages are trashed by the media.

Dr. David Hnida, the medical correspondent for CBS Television News, frankly points out, "Viewers today want extremely practical information—it needs to be of service in their lives. Stories or reports that are presented as too complicated or research-oriented, I just blow off!"

Producers and reporters agree that it is especially beneficial to the viewers when interviews feature a dietitian who can break down the medical jargon and explain the story in everyday lingo. So just say "no" to nutritionese. The use of technical words causes confusion. The truth is that most people are not as comfortable with science as we are. We speak of the RDAs and RDIs. What does this mean to the average consumer struggling to make healthier food decisions? In this day of the television remote control, mention a stanol-enriched diet, and you will be zapped. Say "genetically engineered," and they think artificial, manufactured, or not natural. People shop for food, not nutrients, and they crave easy-to-digest information. The fastest way to put your audience to sleep is to speak in a language they do not understand. Be concise. Crystallize your thoughts into a few hard-hitting, quotable sentences. Do not be an information dump. With the media, less is more.

MAKE YOUR MESSAGES SNAP, CRACKLE, AND POP

If you want your words to have impact, give your audience something they can see. People remember 50% more of what they see and hear than what they hear only. You can also paint a picture with words. For example, describe a serving of meat as the size of a deck of cards, rather than saying it weighs three ounces. Draw attention to the taste and texture delights of a vegetable medley rather than its relative fiber content. Do not bore your audience with the statistic that "37% of the average American's calories come from fat." Shock them with the fact that a client consumes the equivalent of a can of Crisco per week! Do not overlook the power of sound. Sizzle burgers, stir-fry seafood, chop vegetables, blend drinks, pop corn, crack eggs, and whip egg whites. And remember, you are your own best visual aid in interviews. Look good and use winning moves to accent your message. Pound your fists, point your fingers, lean forward, raise your eyebrows, and smile like the actors in toothpaste commercials! But please do not rock back and forth—such movement is distracting and a sign of nervousness.

Use a visual to make the story come alive. Sound, visual images, and action are the spices that add pizzazz to your messages.

PRACTICE THE PLEASURE PRINCIPLE

People have received more than the recommended allowance of bad news about food. According to the ADA Nutrition Trends Survey of 2002, health professionals think of food and nutrition as interchangeable. Consumers however, see food and nutrition as two separate things: food is exciting and enjoyable, while nutrition is what gets in the way of good food. Too often, consumers receive nutrition messages with worry, anger, guilt, helplessness or confusion (3).

When developing a story or being interviewed, your job is to bring back the joy of eating. When giving advice, do not insist on perfection. Tell people not *what* to do, but *how* to do it. Address what concerns the consumer, keeping in mind the reasons shoppers give for not eating more healthfully: time constraints (30%), the high cost of healthy foods (27%), lack of concern (23%), and conflicting information about what is healthy (21%) (4). And then give positive, practical advice to help them surmount these barriers and achieve positive changes. Take words like *never, must, always, should,* and *should not* out of your vocabulary. Positive messages are more persuasive in helping consumers make healthy food choices. And keep in mind the 2006 IFIC Foundation Food & Health Survey that when it comes to Purchase Priorities, "taste and price win out over healthfulness as top factors influencing food and beverage purchase decisions"(5).

MAKE THE MOST OF TELEPHONE INTERVIEWS

Many print and radio reporters conduct their interviews by telephone. Telephone interviews can be the most difficult because there is no personal interaction and no body language to read. Review these tips before your next "phoner":

- Slow down. Talking too fast is the #1 reason for being misquoted in phone interviews. Many reporters still take notes by hand. Others type rapidly trying to get everything you say. Do not make them struggle. Occasionally, ask if you have made yourself clear or if you are speaking too fast. They will appreciate the courtesy. If you hear a reporter typing when you are saying one of your sound bites, slow down to let the reporter catch up. Then say it again.
- Use cheat sheets. Keep a card or handout next to the phone with the key message points and phrases you want to work in during the interview.
- Shut out background noise. Find a private room away from pets, children playing, and the television. Do not drink, eat, or chew gum during a telephone interview. Give the interviewer your undivided attention.
- Avoid speaker and cell phones. Speaker phones make you come across remote and distant. Cell phones fade in and out and drop calls. Worse yet, you will wind up yelling questions and an-

swers at each other. Use a land line and disable your call waiting. Speak directly into the telephone and keep the mouthpiece about one inch from your mouth. Stand up and you will find it easier to project your voice and stay more focused.

■ Do not let your guard down. Since we talk on the phone daily, it is easy to be more casual than we might be if the interview were face-to-face. After a while on the phone, you may forget you are talking to a reporter who can quote everything you can say. That is when mistakes can happen.

BUILD GOOD MEDIA RELATIONS

Review past media coverage of the issues you target. Spend some time in the public library or the reference room of your local newspaper. Review how the national and local media have covered the story. "Be familiar with the publication," insists Marti Meitus, food editor of the *Denver Rocky Mountain News*. "It is irritating," she continues, "to get a pitch from someone who obviously has not read the paper, has no clue about the objective of the section, and offers me a story idea that I wrote about last week. In this day and age, when you can read everything online, there are no excuses."

Find out if the local media have covered your topic. If so, track bylines to see who wrote the articles. If not, suggest stories when you approach reporters with ideas. And find a local angle that will make local readers more interested. Select the media that will best reach your audience. If your story is aimed at a broad audience, select television, a daily or weekly newspaper, or popular radio. For targeted audiences, contact specialty journals, trade publications, or special sections of the newspaper. If your sphere of influence is local, select local media. If it is statewide, select regional media. Community-based, African-American, Asian-American, and Hispanic newspapers, radio, and television can be used to reach ethnic markets. If your influence is national in scope, select a national publication, wire service or broadcast medium.

KNOW LEAD TIMES

Be sure your information is timely and meets the deadline of the selected medium. For newspapers and television, check with the receptionist who answers the phone to find out deadline times. Do not call during the few hours before deadline.

Think ahead when working with magazines. "Quarterly magazines have nearly a one-year lead time, as do many monthlies. Magazines are always struggling with seasonal stories because they often have to shoot photos a year in advance if they want to include pumpkins in October (ever try finding a pumpkin in May?), fresh cranberries or snowy sports in winter, or fields of tulips for a springtime issue," says editor Jeanne Ambrose of *Heart Healthy Magazine*.

PITCH THE MEDIA: PROACTIVE STORY PLACEMENT

The media are constantly on the look-out for good stories and credible people to quote. If you want to get their attention, send a notched Rolodex card with your name and area of expertise in bold letters across the top. Members of the media live by their Rolodexes. Success in pitching stories with local media depends on building strong relationships with reporters and editors. Assignment editors and city editors usually have the final word on doing a story. If you have cultivated a relationship with a reporter, who can make a strong pitch to the editor in favor of your story, success is more likely.

Briefly outline your story, starting with a strong attention-getting lead and supporting bullet points. Send or email (do not email attachments) to the appropriate print reporter or assignment editor. Follow up with a telephone call a few days later. Identify yourself and ask if it is a good time to talk or if you can make arrangements to contact them at a more convenient time. Make sure you have all your information at hand, know what you are going to say, and get to the point quickly. Busy reporters will appreciate your succinctness.

If you do not know which reporter to contact, send your story idea to the newspaper's city desk or the television station's assignment editor. For radio, direct your letter to the producer of the show you are targeting. Reporters are inundated with faxes and press releases. Skip these avenues of approach unless you have already spoken with a reporter who has asked you to send the information.

Generally, do not use the phone to make your first contact with a reporter unless you have a breaking news story. When a reporter expresses interest, send your information, making sure to spell names and addresses correctly. Allow time for the information to arrive. Then follow up with a phone call to arrange the interview and the story.

When reporters express no interest in your story, thank them for their time and ask if they would be interested in being contacted in the future about significant nutrition stories. If a reporter is vague about doing your story and asks you to call back later, make arrangements to call back once. If the reporter is still vague, express polite thanks and say

TABLE 14.1. CONTACTING BROADCAST MEDIA			
Medium	Format	Contact	Lead Time
Television	News: Studio interview	associate producer, assignment editor	6 weeks to 2 months
	News: on location in a city	assignment editor	48–72 hours a.m. reminder
	News: on location in a small town	special representative	5 days to 48 hours reminder call
	Women's programs	associate producer	6 weeks to 2 months
	Talk shows	associate producer	6 weeks to 2 months
	Consumer interest spots	associate producer	6 weeks to 2 months
	Public service announcements (PSAs)	director of public service or community affairs	1 month
Radio	News: studio interview	program director	6 weeks
	News: event announcement	program director	2–3 weeks mail
			1–2 weeks call
			2–3 days reminder
	Talk shows	show host or producer	1 month to 6 weeks
	Call-in shows	show host or producer	1 month to 6 weeks
	Public affairs programs	show host or producer	1 month to 6 weeks
	Public service announcements (PSAs)	director of public service or community affairs	2–3 weeks

that you plan to take the story to another media outlet. If it is a good story, this may be just enough to heighten the reporter's interest in taking action.

Do not be discouraged by initial rejection of story ideas. Persistence and, above all, good stories pay off. Work to establish personal contacts with the journalists who are most likely to place your stories. Some information that will be useful in selecting and contacting broadcast and print media is presented in Tables 14.1 and 14.2.

RESPONDING TO UNEXPECTED MEDIA CALLS: REACTIVE STORY PLACEMENT

What do you do if a reporter calls unexpectedly and you do not know the reporter or it is a controversial issue?

First, ask the reporter questions. Questions elicit information, lead to greater control, and can help you decide if they are the right person or if you should agree to do the interview. In fact, you have

the right to ask as many questions as reporters ask you. These questions are not hard and fast guidelines, however they are a beginning list:

- What is the direction or thrust of the story?
- What issues do you want me to address?
- How did you happen to contact me about this story?
- What is your story about?
- Who else are you interviewing?
- Have you interviewed anyone else? What did they say?
- What is your deadline?

Once you have obtained the answers to these questions, decide whether you are fully prepared to speak to the reporter. If it is a simple situation, handle it promptly. If the interview will cover a sensitive topic and you need time to prepare, ask to call back. If you are not prepared to speak, tell the reporter that you need to gather your thoughts and some information, and agree on a time for you to call back. You can also buy time by saying, "I wish I could talk to you right now but I am on my way to a (meeting, or a patient consultation, etc.). I would be able to call you back tomorrow."

If the reporter leaves a message, return the reporter's calls promptly. Not returning a reporter's phone call is considered the same as saying "no comment" in most newsrooms. The words "registered dietitian refused to comment" looks evasive in print. Although there may be limits on what you can say, the goal is to demonstrate that you are willing to help the media get the answers they need. If you cannot do the interview, have a referral list of registered dietitians, or university or health experts who you can recommend for interviews.

TABLE 14.2. CONTACTING PRINT MEDIA		
Format	General or Holiday Release	Lead Time
Newspapers: Daily	General	1 month
	Holiday	2 months
Newspapers: Weekly	General	6 weeks
	Holiday	8–10 weeks
Consumer magazines	General	6 months
	Holiday	7–8 months
Trade publications: small	General	3 months
Trade publications: large	General	4–6 months

The contact for all print formats is the editor, feature editor, or a specific editor (e.g., food, fitness, lifestyle, health, science, medical, etc.).

LEVERAGING YOUR MEDIA SKILLS

Dietetic professionals with media skills are in demand and are utilizing those skills in a variety of career opportunities. Stephanie Smith, Communications Director for Western Dairy Council describes her job: "My communication position demands skill and experience with the media. I create nutrition-related story ideas and key messages, pitch story ideas to reporters, write press releases, provide background information, answer questions and serve as spokesperson. These activities have helped solidify me as a go-to source for the media, enhancing my employer's image and my profession's image, along with my own professional standing."

Opportunities exist for dietetic professionals to work through the Internet. Kathleen Zelman, nutrition editor for WebMD states, "More and more consumers turn to the internet for answers to diet and health-related questions. Dietitians can write educational content; analyze nutrient composition; write columns, blogs, feature stories; monitor community boards; or be the professional behind a diet program. People with busy schedules and other issues find support and success at the growing number of diet programs on the internet. Studies have shown these programs can be as effective in weight loss as long as clients feel connected and supported."

MAINTAINING GOOD PRESS RELATIONS

Understand how the media work. Paper overload, telephone tag, and breaking news events are all the daily realities of a reporter's life. Never ask to have a story read or sent to you for approval before publication. After a story is completed, leave a short message or send a note letting the reporter know the positive response you have received to the story. This is not a thank you note, but a "job-well-done" note. Also, keep in touch with the media, and not just when you want something.

Keep your credibility with the media by maintaining the highest professional ethical standards and avoiding conflict of interest issues. You can learn more by referring to the Code of Ethics in the Practice section, and the Conflict of Interest Policy on the ADA's website: http://www.eatright.org. Professional Work Ethic:

- Demonstrate integrity in all professional and personal actions supporting ADA's code of ethics.
- Project a positive professional image and attitude.
- Provide—and, when necessary, seek out—accurate information when acting as a source for the media, the public, or any other audience.
- Avoid conflicts of interest and promotion of self and business.
- Provide full disclosure when a real or potential conflict of interest (personal or financial interest) arises.
- Maintain scientific integrity when promoting products and services through the media.

Maintain the media's reliance on you as a polished nutrition resource by honing your communication skills. Sharpen your media skills by constant practice and by consulting "Working with the Media: A Handbook for Members of the American Dietetic Association," produced by ADA's Public Relations Team, which can be downloaded from http://www.eatright.org.

The most successful press coverage does not just happen. Know what you want the coverage to be, and work with reporters so they will understand your position. In the end, the article or newscast will be the responsibility of the reporter. Unless you are a journalist, you will not be able to write the article, headline, or script, but, the more you know about what you want, the better your chances of achieving it.

CASE STUDY 14.1

ONE DIETITIAN'S MEDIA SUCCESS STORY

Liz Weiss, MS, RD, co-author, The Moms' Guide to Meal Makeovers *and co-founder, http://www.MealMakeover Moms.com*

Back in the early 1980s, I attended the annual meeting of the American Dietetic Association in Washington, DC. While there, I heard an inspiring dietitian by the name of Carolyn O'Neil speak about her work as a nutrition reporter for CNN. Intrigued by her unique and exhilarating career, I decided that I, too, wanted to work in television. The prospect of reaching thousands, or perhaps millions of TV viewers with sound diet and nutrition advice set me on a new career course. I enrolled in the Nutrition Communications program at Boston University, and by 1986, had my Master of Science degree in hand. Soon after, thanks to an internship with the health reporter at the CBS affiliate in Boston, I landed a job with none other than Carolyn O'Neil. I packed my bags, headed south to Atlanta

continued

continued

(a minor shock for a Yankee such as myself), and joined the CNN Nutrition News unit as an associate producer.

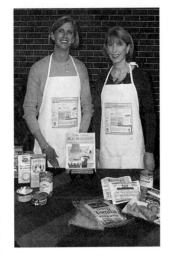

Looking back on my 5 years with CNN, I can honestly say it was one of the coolest jobs a dietitian could ever dream of having. Sure, I was working 10- and 12-hour days and making just $16,000.00 (thankfully by the time I left, my salary had more than doubled, but bear in mind that TV salaries are still fairly low), but the non-stop action and personal career growth made it all worth it. As dietitians, Carolyn and I shared the vision of promoting fellow registered dietitians. With a mandate to produce five nutrition stories a week and a 30-minute weekend program called *On The Menu*, we had the opportunity to showcase more dietitians than I can surely even remember. A quick sampling: Evelyn Tribole, author of many books, including *Eating on the Run*; sports dietitian Nancy Clark; Linda Van Horn, a leader in diet and cholesterol research; Robin Kline of the National Pork Council; Mary Creel, editor at *Cooking Light* magazine; Kathy King, former consultant at the Greenhouse spa; and Janet Helm, PR dietitian extraordinaire.

We traveled the country bringing the world of nutrition to life for our viewers with entertaining stories and news they could use. Our coverage changed with the times. When the issue of salmonella in eggs and poultry was first reported, our focus shifted to food safety. As new research on the link between dietary fats and blood cholesterol made front-page news, we covered the low-fat and fat-free diet craze. When consumers began to demand better tasting, more gourmet fare, innovative chefs made their way on to CNN. I too changed with the times and was promoted to senior producer. I even dabbled in reporting and learned how truly difficult it can be to be to stand there and face the camera!

I left CNN in 1992 and went out on my own as a freelance producer and reporter. At that time, my resume was quite different from most other TV producers given my background in health and nutrition, so doors opened and interesting "gigs" came my way. While I continued to work for CNN, producing stories from my new hometown of Boston, I was also hired by a former CNN colleague to cover nutrition stories for the weekly PBS show, HealthWeek. During those years, I attended the Cambridge School of Culinary Arts (I am a big

"foodie") and also started a side business producing nutrition education videos with such titles as *New Nutrition for Pregnancy*, *Baby's First Spoonful: Tips for Starting Solids*, and *I'm Not a Baby Anymore: Tips for Feeding Toddlers*, all available at http://www.NutritionVideos.com.

Having worked in TV and video for 15 years, and feeling kind of antsy, by 2002 I was ready for a new venture. As the mother of two young boys, I became increasingly aware of the growing crisis of childhood obesity and the challenges busy families face getting healthy meals on the dinner table night after night. Watching my sons' friends clamoring for soft drinks and junk food and refusing all things green, I knew it was time to educate fellow parents about easy, nutritious ways to feed their families better. My personal success feeding my boys a healthy, kid-friendly diet, coupled with my writing skills and my love for cooking, got me thinking it was high time I wrote a book. Having worked alone as a freelancer for many years, I knew I would be more successful (and have a lot more laughs) with a cowriter at my side, so I teamed up with fellow mom and dietitian Janice Newell Bissex (she is on the left in the photo above). Together, we wrote *The Moms' Guide to Meal Makeovers: Improving the Way Your Family Eats, One Meal at a Time* (Broadway Books, 2004), which was a finalist in the 2005 IACP Cookbook Award in the Health & Special Diet category, and we founded www.MealMakeoverMoms.com. On our website, we created lots of features, including a Moms' Club, a bi-monthly newsletter, a customized supermarket shopping list, and a discussion board.

Writing the book was the hard part; promoting the book was where the fun began. We understood which kinds of stories print and broadcast journalists would find interesting and newsworthy, and subsequently had great success getting attention for our book. Aside from the timeliness of the book, we created a series of cooking classes for fellow parents called *Meal Makeover Mom Cooking Parties*. Reporters were wowed by this concept, leading to coverage by CNN, *The Boston Herald*, and WHDH-TV (the NBC affiliate in Boston). The *Today* Show also featured our book, as did *Parenting*, *Child*, *The Boston Globe*, *Newsweek*, and many more. During all of this craziness, we were approached by the editors of *Nick Jr. Family Magazine*, and now write the monthly recipe/nutrition column, *Meal Makeover*.

Through years of media experience and mentoring from dietitians like Carolyn O'Neil, I turned my love of dietetics into a career in communications. I enjoy it all: writing for magazines, creating new content for my website, producing nutrition education videos, working as a spokesperson, and now, writing a second book! And since Carolyn is doing similar things, we are still sharing ideas and providing each other with support

continued

continued
and encouragement in the often-challenging world of nutrition communications.

You too can work for the media and with the media. Want to appear regularly as a live guest on one of the local network affiliates in your area? Sure, why not? It is unlikely you will get paid for your work, but if you are in private practice, the payoff could be more clients. Looking for more media attention for your website, dietetics practice, or book? Create new "hooks" to get the media looking your way. And do not forget, as you find success along this exciting way, to share your experience and knowledge with other dietetic professionals. Over the years, dozens of dietitians have contacted me for advice on careers in communications or just to brainstorm on ways to promote their product or service. I am always happy to help and look forward to even more phone calls and emails in the future!

SUMMARY: RELAX, HAVE FUN, AND ENJOY!

We have saved the most important advice for the last. That is, relax and enjoy yourself. And please do not take things personally. You will see a return on the energy and resources you expend in your media effort. A media appearance confers a level of professional credibility that advertising cannot buy.

If you pitch a story and it does not get picked up, you will learn something that you can use the next time. Kathleen Zelman of WebMD counsels, "Do not give up. Sometimes it takes several pitches before you are successful. Creativity wins the race. Polish your creative skills by paying attention to the world around you, and try your hand at clever takes on ordinary subjects."

If you see working with the media as an exciting, stimulating challenge, you can get the opportunity to touch and change the lives of hundreds—if not thousands—of people with sound, credible, useful, and interesting nutrition news.

REFERENCES

1. The Radio Television News Directors Foundation. *RTNDF's 2006 Future of News Survey*. Bob Papper; 2006.
2. International Food Information Council, *Food For Thought VI*. Reporting of Diet, Nutrition, and Food Safety; 1995–2005.
3. American Dietetic Association. *Nutrition and You: Trends 2002*. Chicago, IL: American Dietetic Association; 2003.
4. Food Marketing Institute (FMI) and *Prevention* Magazine. *Shopping for Health 2005: Whole Health for the Whole Family*.
5. International Food Information Council, IFIC Foundation Food & Health Survey. *Consumer Attitudes toward Food, Nutrition, and Health: A Benchmark Survey 2006*.

15

WRITING A MARKETING PLAN

Kaye Jessup, MS, RD, and Kathy King, RD, LD

THE BIGGER PICTURE

The marketing plan defines your product, the group of individuals most likely to use the product, and how you plan to let them know the product's features and benefits. A detailed formal plan is most helpful in a large organization to coordinate the marketing efforts of the business and for a smaller business when it is first starting. However, every business and project needs a marketing plan in order to assess the market and its changes, evaluate new product ideas, and steer the path of the business. Each year, the plan should look back and identify client profiles of major accounts as well as evaluate promotional strategies and tactics, particularly the ones that did not work as expected or the ones that performed unbelievably well (1). Consultants suggest that the yearly plan should be kept in a 3-ring binder and then archived with the previous years' plans. Looking back, you may find trends, successes, and problems that you had overlooked when assessing only one year.

MARKETING PLAN VERSUS BUSINESS PLAN

A business plan spells out what your business is about: what you do and do not do, and your ultimate goals (2). It encompasses more than marketing, like location, staffing, financing, strategic alliances, and the mission—the purpose of the venture; it provides the framework in which your marketing plan functions (2).

People may use a separate marketing plan for the introduction of each new product or as a tool to coordinate the function of the whole business. The purposes of the marketing plan are (1–3):

- To offer a brief explanation of why this plan was produced—whether to start a business,

introduce a new product, change the direction of the department, and so on.
- To offer a rallying point—you want employees and customers to feel that there is a leader at the helm who has assessed the past sales and thought about the future and planned for new opportunities and threats.
- To offer a chart for success—the plan helps you decide what you want to do so you are not pulled off course so easily, and you can record what has not worked and why, so the failures do not have to be repeated.
- To capture the numbers and research that lead you to the plan's conclusions and decisions— this means people can come and go, but the plan has the points of agreement that lead the way.
- To provide the opportunity for high-level thinking—a time for analysis and reflection that is so necessary for planning for the future.

Dietetic professionals must learn about both plans to survive the growing competition and changes in the health care and food industries. The following pages will guide you through the writing process.

WRITE THE PLAN FOR ITS READERS

Unless the plan is for your personal use, it is crucial to know who will be reading and approving your marketing plan. You want to write your plan to show the dimensions of the business venture, but you also want to write it in the language of the ultimate decision makers. Find out what their "hot buttons" are and how they like information written and presented. For example, if they are CPAs, include detailed financial information.

The key components of a marketing plan and some tips on assembling it are outlined below. Your organization of the elements may vary, but the information should be straightforward, easily understood and provide the business with direction for at least the coming year.

BEFORE YOU SIT DOWN TO WRITE

It will save you a lot of time if you are writing a plan for an ongoing business to collect the information you will need ahead of time. This will minimize delays and interruptions to the writing process. Information you will need (1):

- Latest financial reports (profit and loss statement, budget, balance sheet, and so on) and sales figures by product for current sales and last 2 to 3 years.
- List each product and its target market.
- List employees and their titles in an organizational chart—unless it is a really small business with only a couple employees and a chart will not be necessary.
- The marketplace from your point of view: assess your competitors, location, demographics, distribution channels, and latest trends in the area.
- Ask your staff or consultants to write down any points to consider, anticipated problems, or opportunities that should be pursued.

ELEMENTS OF A MARKETING PLAN

Plans can have many different formats and sections, but there are usually six or so sections that are covered (3,4):

   I. Executive Summary
  II. Identify the Target Market and Product Line
 III. Environmental Analysis
 IV. Marketing Strategies and Objectives
  V. Tactical Marketing Programs
 VI. Budgeting, Performance Analysis, and Implementation

I. EXECUTIVE SUMMARY

Write a concise, clear statement that gives an overview and defines the primary purpose of your business or department. This is the most frequently read component of the marketing plan, and it is usually written last. Answer the following questions:

- What business do you want to be in (or are you in)?

- What needs do you wish to serve?
- What clients do you wish to serve (client profile demographics)?
- How will you go about offering your product or service?

II. IDENTIFY THE TARGET MARKET AND YOUR PRODUCT LINE

- Identify your chosen target market(s) using specific demographic characteristics; it may vary for different products.
- Identify needs of each target market. What do they want or need out of life? What motivates them?
- What are you going to sell? Describe it and make it "real" to the reader. You may compare or contrast it to more familiar products.
- What makes your product unique in the marketplace? Explain its competitive advantages and positioning. List any companion products that could be added as sales increase.

III. ENVIRONMENTAL ANALYSIS

This section should describe the organization's relationship to the present market, current target markets, competitors, and the marketplace where your business is located. These statements can be written in paragraphs or bulleted (1):

1. Strategic assumptions—identify four trends that are or will affect you or your target markets in the next year; and then next 2 to 3 years.
2. Competitive forces—Are competitors doing well and growing? What are they selling as compared to what you offer? List competitors and their product characteristics.
3. Economic forces—What trends or economic issues are affecting your business or product line?
4. Legal, regulatory, or political forces—Are there any new regulations that provide positive or negative influences (for example, Medicare coverage of new diagnoses or cuts in reimbursement)?
5. Technological forces—Are there any major emerging technologies that will make your services obsolete? Or increase your reach and success?
6. Sociocultural forces—Are there any trends that you could exploit to your advantage like home-delivered meals for busy executives?

MARKET RESEARCH

Market research of the environment must be done initially to determine the feasibility of the business idea and whether the time and conditions are right for your business idea to be a success. Market research has been defined as the systematic, objective and exhaustive search for and study of the facts relevant to any idea or problem in marketing.

When conducting a formal investigation of the market, two types of data can be gathered to help analyze the business idea:

Primary data are original data gathered specifically for your project. For example, standing in a store and observing people's buying habits is a way of collecting primary data. A focus group is another way of gathering primary data. If you are a beginner, primary data collection is not recommended, unless you are going to investigate something relatively simple, like calling medical offices and clinics to see if they already refer patients to a Registered Dietitian for counseling or you ask cafeteria customers about their food likes and dislikes. Primary data-gathering tools must be carefully designed to obtain answers that have meaning to your study.

Secondary data are data that already exist. You must decide what types of information you want and then locate it. Reference librarians can help you locate certain information. Examples of secondary data are the number of physicians practicing integrative medicine at the local hospitals, the number of drug rehabilitation homes within a ten mile radius that could be consultant accounts, the names of local broadcast media, or names of managers at public relations firms with food accounts. Such data can help you establish the position of your product in the marketplace (who will buy it) and determine if there are other similar audiences that should be included in your marketing strategies.

The profile of your customer can often be drawn from secondary data. Such information will lay the foundation for your marketing strategies. Customer profile data include such demographic information as gender, age range, education level, and diagnoses. Depending on your business idea, you may need other information, such as data on food product manufacturers or ethnic restaurants in the state or the local area. Incredible amounts and types of market research information are available. You just need to define what information you want and then ask knowledgeable people where to find it.

Secondary information is readily available in libraries, local Chambers of Commerce and at state, federal, and local governmental agencies. A growing source of information is computer search engines and database services (often available in libraries). A fee may be associated with some of the information searches. A detailed profile of your target patient or client account is an important component of your business and marketing plan.

If you need primary data beyond the very simplest level, consider hiring a market research company. It will most likely save you money in the long run. Market research can be done on many levels, and if it is incorrectly conducted on the wrong target or too small a sample or with the wrong questions, it can lead to misleading conclusions.

CONDUCT A SITUATIONAL SWOT ANALYSIS

This involves learning about the internal and external environments of the company or organization through library research, professional journal articles, and government sources, plus having interviews with Chamber of Commerce members, professional peers, referral agents, colleagues, physicians, customers, competitors, company officials, job-search firms, and, possibly, advertising agencies. The goal is to learn about the company's potential, its proposed products and target markets, competition, and the industry in general, plus specific ideas about the feasibility of the business idea.

Put your data into a manageable format to be analyzed and interpreted. One approach is to use the format of the SWOT analysis. SWOT stands for (4):

- Strengths—What do you do very well? These are competitive advantages or core competencies that give the organization an advantage.
- Weaknesses—These are limitations a firm has in developing or implementing a marketing strategy.
- Opportunities—These are favorable conditions in the environment that could work in your favor if acted on in the right way.
- Threats—These are conditions or barriers that may prevent an organization from reaching its objectives even with planning and effort. (See Chapter 2 for more discussion.)

You may use a SWOT analysis for each business idea, such as location, competition, and demographics. Or, one SWOT analysis can be prepared for the whole concept, as shown in Table 15.1. It may take more time to SWOT each component of your business idea, but when you prepare your final analysis, your SWOT charts will be very useful in assisting you to make decisions based on an organized set of information.

TABLE 15.1. SWOT ANALYSIS FOR LOCATING NUTRITION CONSULTATION PRIVATE PRACTICE	
Strengths	**Weaknesses**
1. In professional office building next to hospital 2. Adequate space in office, well laid out 3. Access to building is user-friendly	1. Office next to food court smells of pizza 2. Rent is $1.50/sq. ft. more than planned
Opportunities	**Threats**
1. Medical director of nutrition-support team has office on same floor 2. Hospital installed a new service referral program and will include nutrition consultation service	1. Hospital Nutrition Services Department is starting outpatient consultation service

IV. MARKETING STRATEGIES AND OBJECTIVES

A. What niche will your product or service fulfill?

B. Business Image: What five attributes do you want your image to convey to your target market (1 being the highest).

____ High quality   ____ Customized service
____ Convenient   ____ Staff expertise
____ People-oriented ____ High Status
____ Affordable price ____ Staff courtesy
____ Other

Image objective: How will it be measured (survey of past customers, exit interview, etc.)?

C. Target market objective: What market share (percentage) are you striving for?

D. Overall marketing strategies: Which one do you plan to pursue for your various target markets?

- Sell more to the same market (get current customers to buy more at one time or more frequently)
- Find new markets (find new people who have not bought before)
- Develop new products for existing customers
- Develop new products for new customers
- Use techniques to maintain status quo (used in times of economic decline)
- Cost control (contain or cut costs to maintain profit)
- Market exit (when leaving a market that is no longer profitable or to redirect the company)

E. How many total customers are you seeking for this coming year? What percentage of new customers are you seeking? What percentage of retained customers?

F. Financial—What is the financial arrangement?

____ Cost center
____ Cost recoverable
____ Profit center

What is the financial objective (customer sales, profitability, ratios, etc.)?

THE MARKETING MIX

The marketing mix is important as you investigate business marketing strategies, and set your goals and objectives. There should be considerable details regarding each element of the marketing mix. Product, place, price, and promotion are dynamic elements whose synergy yields sales, referrals, and increased business. Carefully evaluate their roles in the development of your business idea. In marketing a service where relationships are crucial and the purchase is intangible, there are three more P's: people (bedside manner, relationship building, and provider's reputation are important), physical environment (since there is no product to observe or hold, the ambiance, décor, and comfort where the service is rendered becomes more important) and process (the professionalism, delivery, and communication clarity affect the success of the service) (2).

Product

Whether you are talking to a banker or a client, always describe your product in terms of the benefits it delivers (i.e., saves time, helps make you more healthy, kids love it, etc.) rather than just listing its features (i.e., it is blue, lightweight, low fat, etc.). If the benefits are things that people want, that can translate into sales. In defining your product's features and benefits, you must also be able to define its USP, or *unique selling proposition*. Define in writing what differentiates your product or business idea from the competition.

Another important phase of product evaluation is to plot the phase of the product on the product life cycle (PLC) (see Chapter 2). There are four phases of the product life cycle: introduction, growth, maturity, and decline. A company's marketing success often depends on its ability to understand and manage the life cycle of its product. The PLC is important to understand because the phase your product is in can indicate what marketing strategies to use.

Products Objective:

What products will you add, retire, reposition, redesign, or create this year? Which stage of the PLC is each product in?

Place

In evaluating place or distribution, consider the following:

- Is the place/location where the product is available affordable and convenient to your customers? Do you have to pay grocery store slotting fees to get your food product on the shelf or give up 55% to have a distributor carry your book? Must you create a mail-order business to sell your product or can you subcontract with other companies that sell directly to your markets?
- If you sell a service, is its delivery accessible to clients? Do you take the service to them, or do they come to you? Does the location offer wheelchair access, bus transportation, and parking?
- Is the space attractive, but not overdone? Clients need a clean, comfortable space that looks successful?
- Are you considering changes in the location or decoration? If so, carefully examine all of the above points and your budget. Will the expenditure enhance the environment in proportion to the expense?

Place Objective:

Where are your products available now? Are there any new locations that will open new doors for the products like an online shopping cart or a new fitness center?

Price

Establishing price is an ongoing challenge because it is crucial to the success or failure of any business. In establishing prices within an organization, consult the administration about your role. Does the administration expect you to be a cost center (a non-revenue producer), to break even or make a profit? Sometimes, programs or services are purposely priced lower and used as a strategy to attract patients to feed into other profit-making services.

Prices and the image they convey should not be too low, or according to numerous marketing experts, the consumer does not respect or value the product or service. See Chapter 11 for more details on pricing.

Price Objective:

What is your pricing strategy? Will you change any prices or offer any incentives this year?

Promotion

This is essential to the continued success of a business. For this example, there are two major types of promotion: paid advertising and public relations. Paid advertising means placing prepared messages or ads where they will be seen by the target market that you have determined to be the most likely to utilize your product. The objective of paid advertising is to inform consumers and referral persons about your product and to motivate them to come in or refer someone to your product. Public relations includes participating in health fairs, placing stories with reporters, doing radio and TV interviews, and holding open houses, seminars, and continuing education programs. See Chapter 13 for more details on promotion.

Choosing the most appropriate mix of promotional activities is important because such activities cost money. Remember that to make money, one must spend money *wisely*. In selecting promotional activities, consider the following:

- What are your target markets and who are your customers? Use the client profiles you have established from primary and secondary research. Examples of target markets for a medically supervised weight-management program are physicians, nurses, the target consumer, professional organizations, HMOs, PPOs, insurance carriers, and corporations.
- The next step is to identify where your target markets seek information. Ask questions like: Which magazines do they read? Which radio station do they listen to and at what times? At what times do they watch TV? Which newspaper do they read, and which sections do they read first? There are so many questions you can ask to identify the best places and times to attract the attention of your target customers. In dealing with the media, ask similar questions as you investigate pricing, placement of ads, and the like. They have much information regarding their readers and viewers.
- The mix and level of promotional activities change based on the product's phase in the product life cycle. An example is shown in Table 15.2.

TABLE 15.2.	PROMOTIONAL ACTIVITIES APPROPRIATE FOR THE INTRODUCTION PHASE OF THE PRODUCT LIFE CYCLE

Direct Response Marketing

- Print advertising—heavy
- Radio/TV—heavy (if affordable)
- Direct mail—introductory information to target markets
- Public relations—press releases, contact media for news story coverage

Physican Referrals: *these build slowly; it may take 8 to 18 months to see results from these strategies.*

- Telephone—one call per week to physicians' offices to educate physicians and staff about the program
- Print—articles in hospital newsletters and advertisements in local medical association publications
- Grand Rounds—presentation by medical director to medical staff
- Medical section meetings—meet with each section about the program

Word of Mouth: *spread the word in the hospital community first.*

- Print—articles in employee newsletters
- Informational programs—department presentations

Promotion Objectives:

What is the level of brand awareness?

How much traffic has increased to the website or clinic?

How many product demonstrations were conducted this year? What percentage ended in a sale?

V. TACTICAL MARKETING PROGRAMS

This is where the nuts and bolts of the marketing plan are laid out. The action plan should outline the specific activities required to implement the marketing plan, who is responsible for performing these activities, and when the activities should be accomplished based upon a specified schedule (4). This action plan will have timelines and ac-

tivity grid to assign activities, key persons, and due dates.

KEY OPERATING INDICATORS (KOIs)

Ongoing evaluation strategies must be determined for your product and monitored at regular intervals, whether daily, weekly, or monthly. This management function is necessary to identify and correct problem areas and operational weaknesses. Be proactive! Key operating indicators are important to discuss during the interview phase of marketing research. Suggested areas in which to establish key operating indicators are marketing, product quality operations, and finance. Key operating statistics are often expressed as ratios. Table 15.3 shows some KOIs for a medically supervised weight-management program. Once the

TABLE 15.3.	SAMPLE KOIs FOR MEDICALLY SUPERVISED WEIGHT-MANAGEMENT PROGRAM

Marketing

- *Inquiry—Conversion Rate*: Of the number of people who call for information, how many actually come in for an orientation? This figure would indicate the program's effectiveness in translating a telephone inquiry into a face-to-face orientation visit.
- *Sign-Up Rate*: Of the number of people who attended an orientation, how many actually signed up for the program? This figure would suggest how effectively the program closes the sale.

Quality

- *Attendance Rate*: Of the total number of people enrolled, how many actually attended the class? This is one indicator of the quality of the program and the effectiveness of the instructor.
- *Drop-Out Rate*: This is the number of patients who leave the program before completion divided by the number of patients who start the program and is a measure of how effectively the program keeps patients active in the program.
- *Labor Cost per Group*: This is the labor cost for both full- and part-time employees divided by the total number of class meetings during the period, expressed as a dollar amount. As the program grows, labor cost per group is expected to decrease.
- *Finance —Return on net revenue*: This is the profit divided by net revenue for the period and is a relative measure that allows management to determine if the program is operating above or below the expected range of profitability.

key operating indicators are determined for your product, develop or adapt forms to facilitate systematic documentation.

VI. BUDGETING, PERFORMANCE ANALYSIS, AND IMPLEMENTATION

FINANCIAL INFORMATION

This part of the marketing plan is the area that will ultimately "sell" the plan to those who have the final power to approve it. Businesses must make money, or at least break even, to continue operating. Decision makers may require that your business and marketing plan contain the following types of financial information (they are presented in the order in which they are usually developed):

■ A "break-even" analysis indicates the amount of revenue (sales) required to pay all expenses incurred by your product. Break-even is discussed in Box 15.1.

■ A pro forma income statement presents projected revenue, expenses, and income for several scenarios. Normally, it will present the most likely scenario, a scenario at 10% less revenue, and a scenario at 10% more revenue.

■ A budget (financial plan) presents the target revenue and costs in a monthly and whole-year format. This document may also have supporting sub-schedules for revenue, personnel, marketing, and operations that show specific items in detail. Budgets are guidelines for monitoring the current year's revenues and expenses. They also serve as the foundation for future budget planning. Budgets are prepared for the fiscal year (FY). A fiscal year always consists of 12 months, but it may start with any month. A fiscal year may run from January 1 to December 31, or from July 1 to June 30, or from October 1 to September 30. It does not matter which 12 months you select, but you must be consistent. If you are part of a larger organization, the fiscal year will already be established.

BOX 15.1 | *Break-Even Analysis*

The purpose of a break-even analysis is to determine the amount of revenue (sales) necessary to pay all expenses incurred by the business. In preparing this analysis, you must determine the cost of goods sold and all other expenses that are associated with the business. This is normally done as follows:

1. Variable expenses tend to change directly with the amount of revenue, and include such items as the cost of goods sold, hourly labor, copier/office supplies, credit card fees, and cash over/short. These are normally expressed as a percentage of revenue (a video that sells for $60 and costs you $30 will have a cost sales of 50%: $30.00 ÷ $60.00 = .50 = 50%). These cost relationships remain essentially constant regardless of the revenue volume. If you have multiple products and/or services, it is important to determine a cost for each, as in Table 15.4.

2. Fixed expenses tend to not change directly with the amount of revenue, and include such items as the management salary, utilities, rent, and insurance.

These expenses tend to change due to nonrevenue relationships (i.e., electricity is a greater expense in the summer months in Texas.).

3. Segregate expenses into variable (expressed as a percentage of revenue) and fixed (expressed in annual dollars).

4. Select a revenue volume for each type of goods or service that you will provide. In the early planning stage, it is often easier to think of what percentage of total revenue each product will represent. If you use a total revenue number of $100, then the percentage of the product and its dollar amount are the same, as shown in Table 15.5. Do not worry if your actual revenue volume is higher. The percentages will remain valid regardless of the revenue.

5. Calculate total expenses with the following emphasis:

Variable: Percentage of expense and profit
Fixed: Total dollars
Prepared by Eric P. Jessup

TABLE 15.4. COST PERCENTAGES

Product/Service	Cost %
Nutrition consultation	0.0%*
Cookbooks	25.0%
Videos	50.0%
Educational materials	15.0%

*The cost of this product is the registered dietitian's time and expertise, which is fixed and not included in the variable cost of the sales.

TABLE 15.5. REVENUE PERCENTAGES AND DOLLARS

Product/Service	Revenue %	Revenue $
Nutrition consultation	41.0%	$41.00
Cookbooks	20.0%	$20.00
Videos	19.0%	$19.00
Educational materials	20.0%	$20.00
Total	100.0%	$100.00

PERFORMANCE STANDARDS AND FINANCIAL CONTROLS

A comparison of the financial expenditures with the plan goals should be included in the project report (4):

- What percentage of the promotion budget will the major product roll-outs be this coming year?
- Use a standardized reporting form to report the expenditures for each project and compare it to the approved budget.
- Weekly reports should be made by the marketing director or overseer when costs are over the budgeted amount and for any redirection of budgeted funds to cover the costs.
- At some interval (probably quarterly), any new product should be evaluated for profitability. Product development costs should be distributed over several years (depending upon the product and its costs) and the quarterly income and expenses should be compared.

MONITORING PROCEDURES

To analyze the effectiveness of your marketing plan, compare your actual performance against the plan objectives that you set out to accomplish. Monitoring procedures could include (4):

- A perpetual comparison of the action plan against the actual activities conducted. In the beginning it should be monthly for the first year, followed by quarterly for long-term projects.

- Each project team is responsible for determining what changes must be made in procedures, product focus, or operations as a result of the comparisons.

SUMMARY

Effective marketing is one of the most important factors that contribute to the success of a business. A marketing plan is a part of the business plan, or it can be created for each new or redesigned product or service. A good plan sets the course, it hones your effort and resources to only those expected to be most effective, it plans what to do and who will do it by when, and then it requires ongoing and final evaluation on its effectiveness.

REFERENCES

1. Moran G. 23 Hours to a Great Marketing Plan. Entrepreneur.com. 2005. Available at: http://www.Entrepreneur.com/article/0,4621,270382,00.html. Accessed July 13, 2005.
2. How to Create a Marketing Plan. Entrepreneur.com. 2007. Available at: http://www.entrepreneur.com/article/printhis/43018.html. Accessed March 23, 2007.
3. Know This Tutorial: How to Write a Marketing Plan. Know This LLC. 1998–2005. Available at: http://www.knowthis.com/tutorials/marketing/marketingplan1/0.htm. Accessed July 13, 2005.
4. Pride WO, Ferrell OC. *Marketing Concepts and Strategies*, 12th ed. New York: Houghton Mifflin; 2003.

APPLICATION TO PRACTICE

MARKETING HEALTHY FOOD AND THE FOOD INDUSTRY

16

Catharine Powers, MS, RD, LD, Mary Abbott Hess, LHD, MS, RD, LD, FADA, and Mary Kimbrough, RD, LD

In the not-too-distant past, the terms *healthy food* and *healthful food* were associated with bland, boring, and unappetizing food. Dietitians were considered the "food police." You ate either a good meal, or a healthful meal, but it was seldom the same meal.

HEALTHY EATING HAS WHOLE NEW MEANING

Today, eating well has taken on a new meaning. Healthful food can and should taste good and look as appealing as traditional fare. There are many opportunities for chefs and dietitians to collaborate toward the common goal of preparing great-tasting, nicely presented, well-balanced meals. In other words, people can have their cake and eat it too, albeit a small portion of the cake! Additionally, surveys show that not only do consumers want good healthy fare, but they are also willing to pay for it. The opportunities for dietetic professionals with culinary proficiency have exploded in all areas of foodservice—from fast food to fine dining, as well as schools and medical facilities.

The popular press and the newly reformed consumer like to give the impression that marrying culinary skills with healthful cooking is innovative and new, and often the expertise of the dietitian is a forgotten element. Yes, there is some innovation, but it is hardly a new concept. Dietitians did know about food and were experts of food at one time; we understood where it came from, what to do with it, how to advise our clients about it, and even how to enjoy it. We understood that people eat food, not just nutrients. Over time, however, the profession of dietetics focused more on clinical nutrition and less attention, resources, and continuing education has

been given to food and food service. However, you cannot effectively teach or even talk about nutrition and healthful eating practices without understanding how to prepare food. The two concepts are connected and interdependent.

PARTNERING WITH CULINARY PROFESSIONALS

If the dietetic professional represents one side of the healthful eating coin, the flip side and the ally or partner, is the culinary professional. In the past, chefs and cooks often dismissed efforts by well-intentioned but culinarily naïve dietitians as "too many cooks spoiling the broth." But this is no longer the case. Culinary professionals know that if they are to succeed, they must respond to demands from the popular press, trade journals, their own professional organizations, their peers, governmental regulations and, most importantly, their guests for healthful meals and options. For some managers, owners, and chefs, the quest for a greater emphasis on healthful cooking has taken a truly personal slant; many who have had personal health problems are especially keen to implement changes on their menus. Culinary philosophies can turn 180 degrees because the general manager has had a heart attack.

Many dietetic professionals now recognize the importance of dual training and certification in nutrition and the culinary arts. Numerous culinary schools have added culinary nutrition degrees to fill this need. Self-study programs, such as Helm Publishing's *Professional Cooking*, fill the growing need for upgrading culinary skills. The American Dietetic Association's Commission on Dietetic Registration now recognizes culinary education as eligible for continuing education and professional development. Continuing education portfolios can focus on upgrading culinary skills and knowledge using assigned codes for various aspects of culinary expertise.

FOODSERVICE OPPORTUNITIES

The opportunities to market your services within the commercial foodservice segment are bountiful. Many operators, managers, and chefs are anxious to implement some sort of healthful eating and dining program but lack the time, financial resources, staff, and expertise to do so.

Americans continue to spend a significant portion of their food dollars on meals eaten outside the home. Dining out has become a way of life for many and is no longer just for special occasions. Business travelers report health problems attributed to a lifestyle that includes high-fat, high-calorie restaurant meals. They have become more vocal about their needs, and restaurants have become more responsive to their rising demands for healthier options. Commercial foodservice operators such as restaurateurs need help, but there is mounting pressure for non-commercial foodservices, like school and senior feeding programs, correctional institutions, group homes, and others to provide healthful foods. Those same restaurants trying to respond to their guests have gotten lost in a sea of conflicting reports, misinformation, and consumer confusion. And the legislating of nutrition, including regulation of trans fats, disclosure of calories and changes related to labeling is being forced on them, whether or not they want to provide this information to guests.

A great many cooks and chefs are ready to form new partnerships with health and nutrition professionals, but are we ready to join with them? Our opportunity to impact school meals, health care, food manufacturers, and commercial foodservice markets is *now*, and we should not let it pass us by.

WHAT YOU HAVE TO OFFER THE FOODSERVICE INDUSTRY?

What you have to offer is your culinary as well as other dietetic expertise. Depending upon your interest, education, and experience, you may have considerable or minimal culinary expertise. Few of us are truly experts in all aspects of dietetic practice, so be realistic in assessing what you have to offer. Your services could run the gamut from nutritional calculation of menu items or a simple menu evaluation to a complete recipe-development project. When consulting in this area, remember your role and tailor your services to the expertise of the people with whom you are working. When working with highly trained culinary professionals, respect their expertise and offer guidance on ingredient substitution, menu balance, portion size, and nutrient related issues. Enhance their creativity, do not stifle it. When dealing with someone with less training, step forward with more input on better

---

CASE STUDY 16.1

DAYS OF TASTE, CULINARY PROGRAM FOR KIDS

Robin Plotkin, RD, LD, Culinary and Nutrition Communications Consultant, www.robinplotkin.com

One of my very first clients as a culinary and nutrition communications consultant was the American Institute of Wine and Food's Days of Taste (AIWF) Program. (http://www.aiwf.org/dallasftworth). Days of Taste (DOT) is a national discovery-based program of The American Institute of Wine & Food, modeled after a French program called "Journée de Gout," which also means "Days of Taste." The first Days of Taste took place in New York City in the fall of 1995, after evolving from many early AIWF initiatives examining issues of health, nutrition, and feeding children, and collaborations with other organizations.

Designed for fourth and fifth grade students to learn about food and how it weaves its way through daily life

from farm to table, it has become a signature program of The AIWF. Through the program, students have the opportunity to explore the nuances of taste through the five senses with a tasting component guided by a chef, a visit with a local farmer to discover the wealth and variety of products grown and sold locally, and prepare

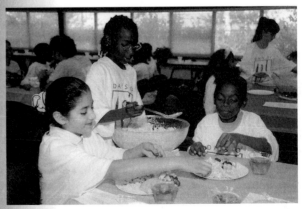

continued

continued

a Harvest salad using fresh produce they purchased themselves at the Dallas Farmer's Market. Volunteer culinarians and other volunteers share their enthusiasm for fresh ingredients, cooking, and love of food. The program teaches kids the concept of "from farm to table"— one that is difficult for kids to grasp these days.

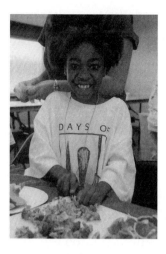

In the Dallas/Ft. Worth area, DOT had previously been run by volunteers, however, the committee was ready to hand it over to a paid professional to handle the work load and grow the program. My mentor, Mary Kimbrough, RD, LD, recommended me to the AIWF board. I am proud to say that I am starting my fifth year as the Director for this wonderful program.

In this role, I report to the Chairman of the AIWF-Dallas/Ft. Worth affiliate as well as two cochairs of the Days of Taste program. In addition, I am in communication with the National office of AIWF and other chapters around the country. I am fortunate enough to work with a supportive and dedicated team of AIWF volunteers. They truly believe in the Days of Taste program.

Because I was the first paid person in this position, I was able to create the position to be what it is today. The main responsibilities of this position include coordinating 225 volunteers annually as well as eight schools for a total of 400 to 500 kids, plus teachers and chaperones. The registered dietitian volunteer base has grown over 200% in the last 4 years. In addition, I facilitate the chef and grower trainings, coordinate the volunteer thank you party, solicit cash and in-kind donations, work with the media, promote the program year round and solicit new volunteers. Logistically, it is a challenge, but with one very well executed Excel spreadsheet, it can be done!

In addition, I field all questions and emails related to the program and correspond with the National office with regard to program data and documentation. I sit on the National education committee with others who are proponents of Days of Taste. I have been asked to present at the National meeting about the success of the Dallas/Ft. Worth program.

As part of my role, I am responsible for the execution of the strategic development in terms of growth of the program. In an effort to continuously expand the reach of this program, we recently partnered with a local grocery store (Central Market) to pilot 20 classes in 2008. These 20 additional classes will allow us to reach 1,000 kids.

Recently, I learned about the $10,000 Champions for Healthy Kids Grant, offered by the General Mills Foundation, in partnership with the American Dietetic Association Foundation and the President's Council on Physical Fitness. In an effort to expand the program objectives to include physical fitness, I applied for the grant and, at this writing, am waiting to hear if we are one of the grant recipients.

For more information:

American Institute of Wine and Food: http://www.aiwf.org

American Institute of Wine and Food Dallas Ft. Worth Chapter: http://www.aiwf.org/dallasftworth

cooking methods, recipe development, and ingredient selection.

RECIPE ANALYSIS (NUTRIENT CALCULATIONS)

Whether you are assisting in the development of an operation's recipes or are evaluating the menu, providing nutritional calculations of recipes is a valuable and often lucrative service. It is often easier for a chef to relate to a recipe analysis and use it to make modifications than to conceptualize a healthy recipe.

The process of recipe development and evaluation will take several steps: develop the recipe, calculate the recipe, make modifications, recalculate the recipe, and so forth. Recipe calculation calls for a specialized database, so you may need to buy a more sophisticated program or spend some time customizing the database you use. Complete data for stocks, dried cherries, sundried tomatoes, specialty meats, and imported sauces and fishes may not be found in traditional databases.

Recipe calculation also calls for an understanding of how ingredients will react during preparation. For example, when marinating items, how much of the marinade will be absorbed, or how much alcohol is burned off from heating or flaming a product? How much fat will be released when meat is roasted or grilled?

Recipe calculation services are used by many segments of the industry and can be a primary part of your practice or a source that supplements your income. Fees can range from $25.00 to over $250.00 per recipe. More is usually charged if the recipe will be published on the package or is complicated with several sub recipes combined in the final presentation. Some dietitians charge by the hour for calculating time; most charge per recipe. Remember that when providing this service you will be held responsible for the accuracy of the data you provide. Nutritional calculations require more than simply inputting numbers from a database based on an ingredient list (most high school students could do that). Take the time to develop expertise at nutritional calculation before you offer this as a professional service.

STANDARDS OF OPERATION

Before starting the actual recipe evaluation and development, it is important to set standardized nutritional criteria. There are no set rules or absolute values. The nutritional criteria will vary depending on the style of operation. For example, a spa might have a lower caloric limit, and a sports training facility might have a higher caloric limit. It is important for both the patrons and the food-service operators to have specific values or guidelines based on sound rationale.

One potentially difficult area in implementing a healthy cuisine or menu into an operation is setting standards of practice, or agreement and evaluation procedures. We all know that what is done on paper (such as a printed recipe) and how food is actually prepared may not be the same. Are all recipes standardized? Are employees literate and trained to prepare standardized recipes? It is important to protect your credibility by setting evaluation standards.

RECIPE EVALUATION, REVISION, AND DEVELOPMENT

Evaluating Existing Recipes

Some items that are prepared and served in restaurants can be identified as healthful and will meet the defined nutritional criteria without any major changes. Examples of such items may be clear or vegetable soups, grilled fish, pasta with marinara sauce, and some salads and fruit desserts.

When evaluating recipes, look for the following:

- Recipes that use lower-fat main ingredients, such as lean meats, fish, poultry, grains, and legumes.
- Recipes that have light sauces, such as fruit and vegetable coulis, natural reductions, and alternatives to roux, such as arrowroot or cornstarch as thickening agents.
- Recipes that use lower-fat cooking methods: poaching, simmering, broiling, grilling, roasting, hot smoking, stir-frying, or dry sautéing.

- Portion sizes that are appropriate and adequate based on documented yield of prepared food.
- Recipes that have a higher percentage of whole grain products or vegetables as compared to meat or cheese.

Modifying Existing Recipes

Many traditional or classical recipes can be adjusted or modified to meet the defined nutritional guidelines. One word of caution: when modifying recipes, be careful not to compromise flavor, texture, or appearance. Customers have expectations based on menu descriptions. The kiss of death is "this is not too bad—for healthy food."

When adjusting recipes to meet nutritional guidelines, look to the following:

- Modifying portion sizes, particularly with the main item.
- Substituting ingredients that are lower in fat, sodium, or sugar, and/or higher in flavor or nutrient density.
- Using alternative techniques, such as smoke roasting, dry sautéing, and poaching.
- Including fruits and vegetables, including small salads, on the main plate to increase the volume and perception of a generous plate presentation while reducing calories and fats from other sources.

Creating New Recipes

Using the chef's skills and your knowledge of the nutrients in ingredients, together you can create and develop new and exciting recipes that meet the nutritional criteria you have set. New recipes can be marketed from the start as healthful alternatives and will not invite comparisons to traditional items.

When creating a new recipe, keep the following points in mind:

- Use the freshest ingredients available.
- Use lean meats, fish, and poultry.
- Include ingredients rich in fiber, antioxidants, and phytochemicals.
- Keep sauces light and flavorful, and use moderate amounts.
- Use low-fat cooking techniques.
- Use low-fat and moderate sodium and sugar products when possible.

INGREDIENT SELECTION

Nutrition consulting services can include advice and guidance on product selection and development of purchasing specifications. Providing a wide range of healthful alternatives to standard products will help professional cooks and chefs understand how a dietitian with in-depth knowledge of foods can assist in the development of a healthful menu.

An interesting approach to this service might be to develop comparison or selection grids that compare different items within a product line. Comparison criteria might include taste, color, texture, usability, fat content, calories, sodium, and overall palatability. Items that lend themselves to comparisons are regular and reduced-fat cheese, alcoholic and nonalcoholic beverages, commercially prepared soups and bases, and various grades of meats or cuts (prime versus choice beef, or free-range/pasture-raised versus factory-raised poultry).

Also arrange tastings to broaden the kitchen staff's flavor repertoire and update menu selections. Interesting and useful items to taste include flavored or infused vinegars and oils, sun-dried fruits and vegetables (cherries, blueberries, strawberries, cranberries, tomatoes), chilis, chutneys, or prepared sauces, cheeses, flavored waters, herbal teas, and different type of grapes, apples, pears, tropical fruits, or less familiar grains (quinoa, spelt, amaranth) and legumes.

Tastings may be expanded to include others in the organization. Consider including the chef, the sous-chefs, the maitre 'd or dining room manager, lead servers or waiters, cafeteria supervisors, or others as appropriate.

STAFF TRAINING

Many healthful dining programs fail because of inadequate staff training and support. The kitchen and service staff must buy into a program's philosophy wholeheartedly to keep momentum high.

Training for the back-of-the-house staff might include the following points:

- Basic nutrition information that will explain why changes are being made. (Staff members need to understand the whys of the change to relate to the hows.)
- Portion control and ingredient-measuring techniques for standardized recipes.
- Proper cooking techniques and the need for conscientious application every time a dish is prepared.
- Translating customers' special requests into specific menu items (such as broiling fish instead of sautéing, frying, or cooking a la meuniere).
- Importance of careful ingredient and technique control, especially while preparing foods for patrons with food allergies, intolerances, or special diets.

Training for the front-of-the-house staff needs to emphasize basic nutrition information to communicate more accurately with guests, as well as information about cooking techniques and ingredients. Only then can the waitstaff help guests meet their individual needs and more accurately communicate customers' special needs and requests to the kitchen staff. Some guests and clients have true allergies, intolerances, or medical conditions that are influenced by food choices, so the person asking if there is cream in the soup, or if a menu item has nuts, needs a correct response. Sometimes busy servers do not bother to check, especially if it is a new food item on the menu and may give an incorrect response, not realizing the potential of creating a medical emergency.

Simply having a dietitian as part of an operation provides credibility and reliability for any promotion related to healthful dining. The dietitian becomes a source of information for marketing and generating local support.

"SELLING" HEALTHY FOOD ON THE MENU

A natural extension of recipe development and menu revision is working with the manager or operator to determine how the new information will be communicated to guests and potential customers.

There are several schools of thought concerning how best to identify healthful items on menus and even controversy about identifying healthful options. One classic approach relies on symbols or icons to designate items on a menu as healthier alternatives. Symbols assist guests in making selections without a lot of server assistance and eliminate guesswork. They are also clear and concise. Nonetheless, the jury is out regarding the overall benefit of symbols. Many operators report that customers say they want healthful options but do not select identified healthful options because they think they will not taste as good as other menu items. Interestingly, when some restaurateurs removed the "healthy" symbols and claims from their menus, the same healthful items actually increased in sales, presumably because they were stigma-free.

Another approach is to design a separate menu or section of the menu for healthier items. All courses from soups to desserts, and even beverages, are segregated. The obvious benefit for the guest is that healthier alternatives are easier to find. The great disadvantage of having a separate menu is that the guest must specifically request it to see the healthier alternatives. It is possible that more people might order these items if they were within the main menu.

Some operations, particularly fast food and quick service chains, have the nutritional information for menu items that they can provide to a customer upon request. It is helpful to many consumers to be able to plan their food choices based on the nutritional information that is available on a website or in the operation.

Another approach is to offer, but not highlight, the healthful alternatives. This approach is based on the reasoning that special labeling sends a negative message about the rest of the menu and may lead guests to wonder, "If these items are 'healthy,' does that mean the rest of the menu is 'unhealthy?'" This reinforces the old "good food/bad food" approach to eating. A more positive approach is to let the items speak for themselves and rely on a combination of the guests' knowledge and personal interest in healthful selections and the servers' ability to promote the items appropriately, for example by explaining that a soup is prepared without added cream. Many customers will request dressing or sauce on the side or lightly dressed salads.

Yet another approach is to offer "small plates" or reduced portions of entrees. The problem here is often pricing because a guest may expect a 4 oz. portion to be priced at half the price of an 8 oz. portion. Typically, the half portion is priced at about 75% of the larger portion, reflecting overhead, dishwashing, service, utensils, and labor cost factors independent of the difference in portion size. For many patrons, a better choice may be sharing an entrée, ordering two appetizers or a salad and an appetizer as an entrée, or splitting desserts.

TAKING THE SERVICE TO THE CUSTOMER

INDEPENDENT RESTAURANTS

Let us look at the specific needs of the commercial foodservice industry that cry out for the assistance of a dietetic professional who knows food. There is great business potential in independent restaurants. Such restaurants are usually small and often have limited resources. They cannot afford to hire a full-time dietitian, but may be willing to hire a consultant.

The easiest way to begin consulting with such restaurants is to assist them with menu modifications and recipe evaluation. The best place to begin is at a restaurant where you are a frequent customer. Arrange a meeting with the owner, manager and/or chef to discuss your (or your client's) desire

for lower calorie meals or healthier alternatives and turn it into an opportunity to assist. If you know the operation, their customer base, and their basic operating philosophy, you will have a distinct advantage.

Other networking opportunities can evolve by joining a local chapter of the American Culinary Federation (AFC) and/or the American Institute of Wine & Food (AIWF). By becoming active in these groups you will meet chefs, restaurateurs, and those most active in your local food community who are potential users of your services. You can become known through those organizations as a culinary nutrition resource. Author Mary Kimbrough is currently the Chairman of the Dallas Chapter of Les Dames d Escoffier. Mary Abbott Hess has been national president of AIWF and chairman of the Chicago Chapter.

Nutritional concerns are viable marketing and profit-generating tools. Building relationships with the food community is key. Demonstrating your interest in good food and the pleasures of the table help the food and culinary community to embrace the dietitian as a food professional. Attending local food events and participating in culinary programs also adds to your credibility and creates opportunities to market your expertise.

Once you have identified potential foodservice clients, put together individual proposals to meet each operation's needs. Present all the consulting services you can offer, such as reviewing menus, staff training, and assistance with marketing to specific groups including senior-citizen centers, weight-loss programs, and other likely candidates. You are offering a service that the commercial foodservice market wants. Some restaurants also want assistance putting together catering menus or menus for meetings tailored to specific groups. What is appropriate for a senior citizen breakfast or a dinner for the local chapter of the American Heart Association?

Consider, for example, aligning the restaurant with a hospital outpatient wellness center, weight-loss center, or health organization. Arrange for the chef to provide cooking demonstrations or classes for the community. Bring groups into the restaurant to experience healthful dining at a new level. Market the restaurant through cooking competitions, food tastings, and media interviews that promote healthy dining.

RESTAURANT CHAINS, HOTELS, AND RESORTS

Another segment of the commercial foodservice industry that may want your services is restaurant groups or chains. Beyond single dishes, special brochures, and cooking demonstrations for customers, the dietetic professional and restaurant chain can develop a unique relationship and varied list of services.

Hotels and resorts can use your services in more than their restaurants. Getaway weekends with themes are becoming more popular. Combine your expertise with the chef's skills and innovation to put together a series of getaway weekends that include cooking demonstrations, nutrition seminars, exercise workshops, and other lifestyle enhancers. If a venture of this sort is developed for a hotel chain, it can be marketed across the country.

Several hotels are now marketing healthier bedtime treats. Rather than sending their guests to bed with a high-calorie, high-fat snack, they send a healthy alternative: fresh fruit, fresh-squeezed juice, or a specially created house item. Others are expanding room service options to include healthier light meals such as smoothies, yogurt, fruit, or other options. If you have ideas for food options you would like to be available to you, why not turn those ideas into a business opportunity?

Do not forget to tie into the hotel fitness center, a natural potential for seminars, private consulting, and product promotion. Make recommendations for additional profit opportunities for the hotel or resort. Natural extensions in the fitness center include creating a juice and smoothie bar, healthy snack items, offering body-fat testing, and developing a menu for the restaurant that is "sponsored" by the fitness center.

Many hotels host conferences that can use special food and/or nutrition seminars for programs such as spouse activities or lifestyle-enhancement seminars. A series of seminars that could interest a range of guests might include "Healthful Entertaining," "How to Survive Business Lunches," "Staying Fit on the Road," and "Eating to Increase Your Productivity."

Resorts, including cruise ships, spas, island resorts, ski resorts, and dude ranches, also present some unique marketing opportunities. Menu consulting and recipe development opportunities can be found in any of these entertainment arenas, but to realize the fullest potential, you need to look beyond the standard fare. Complete service packages are often more enticing to such organizations, which may not know they need or could benefit from your services.

These services can range from menu consultation to seminars, cooking demonstrations, fitness-center evaluations, nutrition consultations for guests, wine tastings, and employee wellness programs. Keep in mind that people will often pay more for services when they are on vacation or on business than they would at home.

Carefully Present Your Ideas!

There are many ways dietetic professionals can incorporate aspects of the culinary field into traditional avenues of practice to enhance their marketing potential. But heed a word of caution—when presenting a proposal, tell what you will do *but do not present your plan or idea with details*. Be aware that given this information, the client can implement your ideas without you and avoid paying for your services. Do not sabotage your sale by giving it away!

HEALTH CARE FOODSERVICE

The food served in health care has long had a reputation for being unappealing and bland, but today many facilities are changing that image. Even with budgetary constraints, hospital administrators understand that the quality of food service in a hospital adds immeasurably to the image of the facility and to patients' and families' satisfaction. Certainly, health care foodservice is challenging—adding unique and special dietary restrictions to the budgetary, staffing, training, and other limitations of other non-commercial operations. Patients are often acutely ill and on many medications that make enjoying food difficult. Creating appealing food for a multiplicity of dietary restrictions is a major challenge.

However, foodservice was once an area of great pride, and innovation is again making great strides under the direction of many dietetic Food Service Directors in collaboration with culinary professionals. Today, many innovations that are focused on quality foods are happening in the health care arena. Culinary teams lead by certified or culinary trained chefs are partnering with the registered dietitian Food Service Director to create nourishing quality meals. The traditional tray-line is being replaced by the room service model where patients are able to have some control over what they eat and when. Patients can order what they feel like eating when they are ready to eat and not when it is convenient for the hospital staff. As hospitals and other health care operations are trying to differentiate themselves from the competition, patients often look to auxiliary services. The food served is certainly an area for differentiation, and good food is always appreciated. The days of strict diets have been replaced with a more liberalized approach to the menu.

Since as many visitors, staff, and family members eat at hospitals, there is an expectation that good-quality, delicious food should be available throughout the hospital's food service sites. Patients and staff know which hospitals have good food and this can be a factor in selecting where to be treated or where to work. With the increased knowledge, experience, and demands of the patients, families, visitors, and the hospital staff regarding food choices, many health care food service directors hire experienced culinarians to manage their production units. In fact, when the situation is analyzed, they cannot afford not to hire a professional chef. The increase in patient and employee satisfaction, the increased revenue from the cafeteria and catering, and the savings from limiting mistakes can often pay for a professional's salary. This is a case of doing the right thing correctly.

There are many marketing opportunities within health care that can bring the culinary and nutrition worlds together. Once you have made a hospital's food healthy and delicious, invite the board, medical staff, and auxiliary for lunch. Show off the new fare at catered functions, and invite the local media to taste the food and interview satisfied patients. Invite guest chefs from local restaurants or hotels to appear at fund raisers, promotional activities for the hospital foodservice, or educational activities for the outpatient center. Give cooking demonstrations to send a sound nutrition message and draw new clients. Become a part of the local food community by offering your facility for meetings and food events to showcase what you serve. This helps attract staff and creates a positive image of the facility for the public.

OUTPATIENT COUNSELING

It is almost impossible to discuss diet modifications or nutritional concerns without discussing food and its preparation. When dealing with patients or clients, it is helpful to translate theory into practice. The public wants to know what ingredients they can substitute, how they can change traditional recipes, what cooking methods are recommended, which yogurt is best to use, how many grams of fat are in specific products, and the like. It is clear that people are dealing with food—not theory—and that talking about food is more useful than "teaching nutrition."

SCHOOL FOODSERVICE AND OTHER LARGE-QUANTITY FEEDING OPERATIONS

Students and institutional residents of all ages appreciate the strides foodservice directors are making to serve food that is more nutritious and appealing. Many food establishments are adding salad bars, baked potato bars, soup and salad lines, vegetarian and stir-fry entrees, homemade whole-grain breads, low-fat entrees and dairy products, lite salad dressings, and grilled and petite meat portions. Display cooking, moving the final stages of preparation to the front of the house, has become popular in colleges, hospitals, and most onsite foodservice operations.

New food options can be promoted in newsletters to parents or residents, on websites, on bulletin boards and posters, on table tents in the cafeteria, and in presentations to classes or group meetings. Again, it helps first to instruct the cooking and serving staff, residents, and teachers on the nutrition benefits and reasons for change before introducing the change.

Dietetics professionals can teach good food habits directly to students or through class curricula from preschool through graduate school. Nutrition presentations, cooking demonstrations, food and wine tastings, catered parties, and holiday or theme meals are all popular with retirement residents.

TEACHING IN CULINARY SCHOOLS

The American Culinary Federation (ACF) requires 30 hours of nutrition studies for their chef certification program. Dietitians in various localities have developed nutrition-education programs for chefs and have worked with local ACF organizations for sponsorship and promotion. From such programs many other opportunities have followed.

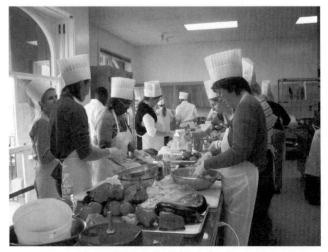

FIGURE 16.1. ■ Cookshop at Washburne Culinary Institute in Chicago.

CASE STUDY 16.2

FOOD ROOTS LLC

Mary Kimbrough RD, LD, and Mark Haley, Owners, Food Roots LLC, Dallas TX
www.foodroots.com

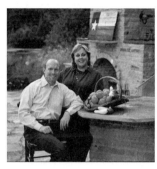

Culinary tourism makes unique and memorable food and drink experiences a part of the overall travel experience. It can be the major focus of a trip, or just a portion of a planned trip. Travel with a food and wine emphasis has become a growing niche market in the travel industry, some featuring recognized chefs, others focusing on foods and cooking of the destination, and some sponsored by food or wine organizations. Some culinary tourism is planned for day trips, while others involve several days or weeks.

Many tourists seek activities that connect them with their tour destination especially from an insider's perspective. Culinary tourism connects people with the local food scene by their participation in cooking classes, trips to local markets and food sources, and fine dining. Culinary tourists are interested in being educated about food and wine and many are concerned with making healthful choices in their daily lives.

Food Roots LLC is a boutique culinary tour company located in Dallas, Texas, focused on providing custom culinary tours for professional organizations and corporate groups. Food Roots grew out of an experience of founder Mary Kimbrough, RD, LD. Mary was setting up a wine tour in California and could not find a single resource to give her connections to the tour venues she was seeking. Understanding the need for culinary tour organizers with knowledge of the local area and connections to unique venues, Mary founded Food Roots with business partner Mark Haley to provide custom, behind-the-scenes culinary tours. Excellent local resources and contacts using industry insiders allow customization of tours for particular groups. The tours are an exciting and fun way to see, touch, feel, taste, and understand the source of local food and wine in Texas, and meet growers and producers of artisanal foods and wines.

As a dietitian, Mary wanted to integrate her knowledge of food and passion for food education in the culinary tour experience. She started with the philosophy that making excellent food part of our daily lives is a continuous journey. Food Roots helps people on that journey by involving them in the source of their food, the roots of their nutrition. A Food Roots experience is interesting, interactive, and educational. It connects people with the farmer, the rancher, the grower, and the producer. They all have a story to tell and hearing their stories can help people change the way they interact with food.

While tours are customized for particular groups, a typical Food Roots tour might look like the one pictured in Figure 16.2.

SUMMARY

Dietetics is a profession that proclaims its practitioners as food and nutrition experts. Culinary knowledge and skills are an essential component of most areas of dietetic practice. The public needs information and guidance about food choices to attain optimal health. Translating nutrition knowledge into food choices and creating and serving healthful, delicious food is the realm of the culinary nutritionist. Developing and using food expertise is an ongoing challenge and a perfect opportunity for lifelong learning and a satisfying career, all while enjoying the pleasures of the table and calling that "work."

BIBLIOGRAPHY

Culinary Institute of America. *The New Professional Chef,* 8th ed. New York: John Wiley & Sons; 2006.

Culinary Institute of America. *The Professional Chef's Techniques of Healthy Cooking,* 3rd ed. New York: John Wiley & Sons; 2008.

Davidson A. *The Oxford Companion to Food.* New York: Oxford University Press; 1999.

Gielisse V, Kimbrough M, Gielisse K. *Good Taste: A Contemporary Approach to Cooking.* Upper Saddle River, NJ: Prentice Prentice Hall; 1999.

Glassner B. *The Gospel of Food.* New York: HarperCollins Publishing; 2007.

Hess MA, ed. *Portion Photos of Popular Foods.* Chicago: The American Dietetic Association and Center for Nutrition Education: University of Wisconsin—Stout; 1997.

Jacobi D, Simmons M, Hess MA. *Williams-Sonoma Essentials of Healthful Cooking.* Des Moines, IA: Oxmoor House; 2003.

Ostmann BG, Baker J, eds. *The Recipe Writer's Handbook.* New York: John Wiley & Sons; 2001.

Smith AF, ed. *The Oxford Companion to American Food and Drink in America.* New York: Oxford University Press; 2007.

MARKETING HEALTH CARE: ACUTE AND OUTPATIENT SETTINGS

17

Chris Biesemeier, MS, RD, LDN, FADA

In health care, cost containment and expense reduction have been at the forefront for many years, and this will continue in the future. Achieving positive outcomes and demonstrating results are as important as ever. Now there are two additional areas of focus: providing quality care and ensuring patient safety. Providers are using an approach to care known as evidence-based practice (EBP) that promotes the achievement of positive outcomes and clinically significant results. With EBP, providers implement recommendations from national practice guidelines that have been developed through systematic reviews of the literature, or when research is lacking, that are based on consensus statements from national experts. The expansion of health care technology has brought with it new and exciting opportunities to meet all of these targets. Technology and marketing facilitate dissemination of guidelines to providers and also to patients and payers.

MARKETING SUCCESSES

COMPETITION STIMULATES MARKETING AND NEW PROGRAMS

There is vigorous competition for health care business. Hospital marketing departments are focused on promoting the high-quality, individualized care their hospitals provide and on differentiation of their services from those of other institutions. Hospitals continue to forge networks and partnerships of many kinds, in order to have the market share that is needed for survival. Aligning with physicians, both primary care providers and specialists, continues to be important. New services have arisen to fill identified needs:

- bariatric surgery programs,
- women's pavilions,
- geriatric clinics, and
- cancer centers.

Hospitals are reaching out to the communities they serve with an array of health and wellness programs, and they are working with schools to reduce the prevalence of overweight children.

WHY MARKET NUTRITION SERVICES?

Simply said, providers and payers are busy and have many issues vying for their attention. If dietitians do not market their nutrition services, they may be overlooked and may not be recognized for their expertise and contribution to the organization. In addition, market research allows dietitians to identify their customers' needs and develop programs and services to meet those needs. Clinical outcomes and cost-benefit data can be used to demonstrate the impact of medical nutrition therapy (MNT) and nutrition care, supporting new programs and expansion of existing services.

GETTING STARTED

Marketing yourself and your department within an institution should be a part of your personality, professional presence, and job description. Primary targets are likely to be administrators, physicians (both primary care providers and specialists), and other providers such as nurse practitioners, physician assistants, payers, groups of employees, the community, and, of course, other dietitians. Less traditional targets also should be considered, such as exercise physiologists, personal trainers, physical therapists, dentists, and dental hygienists.

Marketing activities can be fun and rewarding, but take time and financial resources. While dietitians may have some time to devote to marketing, it is likely to be limited. This makes it important to define core nutrition services and the targets

135

for these services in order to maximize return on time and energy invested. Although valuable, marketing activities do not always generate revenue, so a balance between marketing and managing the existing workload must be established in order to ensure that budget goals can still be met. In the hospital setting, dietitians often do not have their own marketing budgets. However, hospitals usually have marketing departments with budgets allocated to promote the hospital and its services to both existing and potential customers. The opportunity for collaboration exists. Nutrition continues to be an area of media focus, and marketing departments like to capitalize on the public's interest in food, and the prevention and treatment of disease by diet. Ideas for promoting nutrition services include:

- writing a column for the local newspaper,
- supplying nutrition experts to the media (TIP: Ask if your marketing department provides media training. This can be a way to build your own skill set and market your programs, too),
- participating in health fairs,
- sponsoring nutrition seminars for colleagues or the community,
- conducting cooking classes and grocery store tours, and
- developing a website and posting patient-education materials and links to other health-related sites.

Dietitians need both organizational awareness and a network of influence in order to identify needed programs or services and to obtain approval for implementing them. Organizational awareness can be accomplished by:

- attending management and other meetings,
- reading hospital newsletters,
- attending bedside patient-care rounds and case conferences,
- participating on quality-assurance teams, and
- volunteering for committees.

During these activities, ideas for services are likely to be mentioned. In addition, they offer an opportunity for the dietitian's expertise and skills to be on display.

Marketing requires discipline. The outcomes and cost-benefit data that are important to share with target groups have to be available when the need arises. The only way this can happen is for dietitians to set up systems for data collection and analysis ahead of time. Opportunities to market programs and services can arise quickly, and if data are not available, opportunities can be lost.

OVERVIEW OF THE HEALTH CARE ENVIRONMENT

MEDICAL NUTRITION THERAPY

Coverage for Medical Nutrition Therapy (MNT) has expanded considerably and now includes a Part B benefit for Medicare recipients with diabetes mellitus and non-dialysis kidney disease with many private third-party payers offering coverage of these as well as other diseases and conditions. Expansion of coverage to additional diagnoses continues to be a goal, as is expansion in the number of MNT sessions covered. The tightening national economy and changes in state budgets continue to have an impact on health care. Workers at many companies no longer have health care benefits, and in some states, large groups of people have been removed from Medicaid eligibility, leading to increased numbers of uninsured. These uninsured individuals turn to emergency rooms for acute illnesses and often neglect care for chronic conditions, increasing the likelihood of long-term health care problems.

ACUTE SETTING

In the acute setting, most insurance companies have followed the lead of the Centers for Medicare and Medicaid Services (CMS) in implementing fixed-rate reimbursement systems based on primary diagnosis (Diagnosis-Related Groups, or DRGs) with adjustments for bed type (for example, intensive care unit [ICU], non-ICU medical/surgical, or maternity), and negotiated discounts. Lengths of stay seem to have stabilized over the past few years, perhaps due to reaching the lower limits of what is feasible and still provide quality care. Patient acuity is higher than ever, resulting in patients who are sicker during hospital stay and sicker at discharge. Discharge nutrition teaching is limited to providing "survival skills," and post-discharge care is often provided by family members. When skilled care needs exist and there is insurance coverage, patients may be discharged to skilled or rehabilitation facilities or receive intermittent visits from home care providers. Low risk and diagnostic procedures are routinely performed in special care centers, for example, surgery centers, magnetic resonance imaging clinics, and radiology clinics.

During the past few years, health care has experienced the front end of the nursing shortage, fueled by the aging of the baby boom generation. Not only are there fewer nurses as more retire, but there are fewer educators of nurses, creating the paradox of long waits for admission to nursing schools in some areas. The situation is worsened by the more limited physical abilities of the existing nurse work force, attributed to its own aging. Adding to the physical demands of nursing is the need to care for a patient population that includes much heavier patients.

DIETITIANS IN ACUTE CARE

The number of dietitians working in acute care is relatively stable; however, dietitians with experience and specialized training, such as those in pediatrics, intensive care, and nutrition support, are especially in demand. Seeking more autonomy and pay, some dietitians have chosen to obtain specialist certifications or more education outside of dietetics, for example, as nurse practitioners and physician assistants. Workloads are heavy, though generally manageable with prioritization, and dietitians are working smarter by using the tools of technology, including the Electronic Medical Record (EMR).

PATIENT SAFETY

As noted, patient safety is a priority, and initiatives to increase patient safety are underway. As an example, the Joint Commission on the Accreditation of Health care Organizations (JCAHO) has defined national patient safety goals and a list of unapproved abbreviations that are not permitted in medical records. Automated medication order entry and tracking systems are being used to reduce medication errors. The demands of regulators and payers for quality have led to public access to health care quality measures, permitting cross-facility comparisons. Criteria for centers of excellence have been created, and facilities eagerly seek the designations in order to obtain higher reimbursement and more referrals for services.

MARKETING BASICS IN THE CLINICAL SETTING

The specifics of a marketing plan for each target group like in-house clinics or physicians will differ. One approach might work for a prenatal diabetes program with whom a relationship already exists, while another strategy will be needed for a new bariatric program. However, the central tenet of effective marketing is to learn about the selected target's existing practice and services; discover the gaps they are experiencing, that is, their areas of need; and present possible solutions to meet these needs. Those are the programs and services that you provide. Background information, such as types of patients served and patient volumes, is often available from a variety of sources. However, a great way to identify needs and to present possible solutions is in a face-to-face meeting. Meetings provide opportunities to gather information and plant the seeds for ongoing collaboration and partnerships.

Proposals for programs and services should be simple and easy to understand (see Chapter 30). Although dietitians may be familiar with terms and activities commonly discussed in our profession, others may not grasp them as easily. A helpful idea used in business is to limit a proposal to the amount of information that will fit in a one-page typed memo. Using bullets rather than paragraph format helps guide the reader's eye to key concepts. In the proposal, clearly state the benefits of your program for both the target program and participants. When possible, suggest a trial or test period for a new service or program. Not only will this appeal to the customer, but it allows you the opportunity to observe and refine your program or service before committing all your resources.

In health care organizations, approval to implement a program or service may require working through several layers of organizational structure. This complexity in decision making increases the likelihood that multiple changes will be made in the original proposal. However, by including people in the planning phase who are impacted by a program, buy-in is increased, and potential obstacles to a program's success can be addressed during planning, rather than during the approval process. All in all, perseverance is often needed. Some proposals may have to be presented multiple times before they are accepted.

The next section highlights specific examples of programs and services that dietitians might consider in the acute care and outpatient settings. Collection of positive data on the effectiveness of nutrition intervention or patient satisfaction is one of the most valuable marketing tools.

ACUTE CARE SETTING

The American Dietetic Association (ADA) Nutrition Care Process and Model (NCPM) provides the framework for nutrition care in the hospital, as in other care settings. Each part of the NCPM also provides insight into program development and enhancement, along with opportunities to market nutrition care and services. The NCPM focuses on the relationship between the patient and the dietitian at its center. The outer rings of the NCPM describe the attributes of the dietitian providing care and the external environment in which nutrition care is provided. Nutrition screening and referral are the triggers for care, while outcomes management promotes implementation of services, performance improvement, and demonstration of positive patient outcomes. The four steps of the actual Nutrition Care Process (NCP) define a systematic method for care provision, ensuring consistency in the process while promoting the critical thinking that leads to individualized care and achievement of patients' goals. (See the American Dietetic Association Nutrition Care Process and Model on its website: http://www.eatright.org/ada/files/NCPM_G_11.pdf.)

Nutrition Screening

Dietitians are responsible for implementing systems that improve patient care thus better insuring positive outcomes. Nutrition screening is performed within 24 hours of admission to identify risk factors that indicate impaired or possibly impaired nutrition status. Nutrition screening is often completed by emergency room, pre-surgery, or unit-based staff, using a paper or online checklist that is a part of the admission process. Online systems have the advantage of being able to generate automatic referrals for patients who need nutrition intervention. Paper systems may require a consult, a step that can be overlooked when things get busy. Monitoring compliance with nutrition screening policies is often part of ongoing performance improvement activities. Incomplete compliance with policies leads to delays in patients getting needed nutrition care as well as issues during accreditation surveys.

The author's facility completed a transition from a paper system to online nutrition screening. The transition period provided an opportunity to review nutrition screening policies in all areas, ensuring understanding of screening criteria and processes, and reinforcing compliance with procedures. Dietitians met with their unit managers to review audit data and, when needed, to develop action plans to increase compliance. The dietitians and unit managers met with unit staff to provide feedback on performance throughout the implementation period, resulting in a successful transition and much-improved audit results. During implementation, the author determined that the emergency room was not included in the initial plan for use of this portion of the EMR. By demonstrating the impact this would have on compliance with nutrition screening standards, she was able to support expansion of use of the online admission process to this area.

In some institutions, nutrition screening has been shifted to the preadmission setting. In these facilities, patients who are scheduled for elective surgery are assessed anywhere from a few days to a few weeks before they are admitted to the hospital. Nutrition screening is completed by center staff or by a diet technician assigned for this purpose. Updates at the time of admission ensure that any recent changes in nutrition status are identified.

Nutrition status may worsen during hospitalization in patients who are reasonably well-nourished on admission. Dietitians can train nurses, social workers, occupational therapists, speech pathologists, enterostomal therapists, geriatric nurse specialists, and discharge planners to be alert to indicators of nutrition problems and to request nutrition consults when they identify indicators. Many facilities have implemented nutrition rescreening procedures to allow routine monitoring of this group of patients, leading to rapid nutrition assessments and intervention when needed.

It is common for enteral feeding tubes and central lines for nutrition support to be inserted in the outpatient setting. A nutrition screening protocol can be implemented that allows all patients having nutrition support tubes and lines placed to receive automatic nutrition referrals to the dietitian. Facilities with EMRs may create protocol sets of physician orders that are diagnosis or procedure-specific with consults to the dietitian for nutrition assessment and intervention for patients having tubes or lines placed.

Nutrition Care

Patients with impaired nutrition status receive a nutrition assessment. The result of nutrition assessment, according to the NCP, is one or more nutrition diagnoses, written in "PES" (problem, etiology, and signs/symptoms) format, and a nutrition intervention plan to address the nutrition diagnoses that are based on evidence-based practice guidelines or protocols. The nutrition intervention plan includes:

- a nutrition prescription that states the patient's individualized recommended dietary intake of energy and/or selected foods or nutrients, based on reference standards, the patient's condition, and nutrition diagnoses;
- specific, measurable, and timed goals or expected outcomes for each nutrition diagnosis;
- a set of interventions aimed at eliminating the cause or etiology of the nutrition diagnosis and/or improving the signs and symptoms that led to the nutrition diagnosis; and
- plan for monitoring, evaluation, and reassessment. (See the case example in Box 17.1.)

The American Dietetic Association (ADA) has published Standardized Nutrition Language (SNL) that includes specific terms for nutrition diagnoses

| BOX 17.1 | *Cardiology Patient with Heart Failure* |

DESCRIPTION OF CASE

- 67-year-old white male, lives alone in an apartment, is on disability
- Anthropometric measurements: Height—5'6", Weight—135 lbs.
- Heart failure diagnosed 2 months ago, has experienced a weight loss of 20 lbs. from dyspnea, shortness of breath, and inability to consume large meals
- Unable to shop or cook, uses many processed foods with high sodium intake

SAMPLE PES STATEMENTS

Inadequate oral food/beverage intake (P) related to poor appetite and early satiety (E) as evidenced by recent unintentional 20-lb weight loss (S)

or

Inadequate oral food/beverage intake (P) related to inability to shop for food and prepare meals (E) as evidenced by recent unintentional 20-lb weight loss (S)

SAMPLE NUTRITION INTERVENTIONS

1. Food and/or Nutrient Delivery:
   - Meals and Snacks
   - Modify distribution of food:
     - Three small meals and small afternoon and evening snacks
     - Liquids after meals
   - Supplements
     - Medical Food Supplement—4 ounces twice daily with snacks
     - Commercial product: (name of product)
2. Coordination of Nutrition Care:
   - Collaboration with Social Worker
   - Referral to Meals on Wheels

and interventions. Consistent use of the NCP and the SNL leads to improved quality of care, as dietitians focus on patients' intake problems and interventions to alleviate these problems. Documentation following the NCP supports the flow of nutrition care and demonstrates dietitians' critical thinking skills. Use of SNL terms promotes clear communication among dietitians within a facility, from one setting to another, and from one facility or region of the country to another. Nutrition outcomes can be more easily monitored, laying the groundwork for large-scale nutrition outcomes projects.

Clinical Practice Guidelines and Protocols

Using Evidence Based Practice (EBP) as the gold standard for nutrition care, dietitians need to be key members of the teams that develop protocols and protocol orders—made possible through marketing to professional peers. Clinical practice guidelines and protocols are used to ensure consistent provision of care to patients with a specific medical diagnosis or who are having a selected procedure. They are often used for complex patients who require multiple interventions by many members of the health care team. In facilities using an EMR, they may be supported by protocol order sets. Protocols specify the care to be provided for each diagnosis or procedure on each day of hospital stay, and they define daily goals and discharge preparation outcomes to be achieved. Variances in expected care processes and in the achievement of expected outcomes are documented and lead to rapid responses to address changes in the patient's condition. Patterns of and reasons for variances are usually evaluated at selected intervals, leading to refinements in the protocols over time.

Ideally, facilities use national, evidence-based practice guidelines and systematic reviews of the literature to develop their own protocols. This is true at the author's facility where new protocols and order sets, as well as revisions in both, require this high level of supporting evidence before they are approved for use in the EMR.

The ADA Critical Illness Evidence Based Practice Guideline (CIPG) is a tool that defines evidence-based dietetics practice for critical care patients in the acute care setting. The CIPG Algorithm outlines the flow of nutrition care according to the NCP and lists specific recommendations for assessing energy needs, selecting the type and route of feeding, and monitoring and evaluating the implementation of nutrition interventions and the outcomes achieved. Each CIPG "Major Recommendation" has a notation of strength of the recommendation for practice (for example, strong, fair, weak, consensus, or insufficient evidence). Each recommendation also includes a summary of its supporting evidence and is linked to ADA's Evidence Analysis Library (EAL). The EAL is an extensive resource for dietitians who want to review the evidence behind their practice, or who need data for a member of the team or a facility protocol revision. It is updated on a regular basis.

At the author's facility, the implementation of the CIPG was preceded by a review of the evidence on the EAL and a self-assessment of adherence to the CIPG by each dietitian, using a checklist that was developed by the author. The dietitians were able to understand the rationale behind recommendations and ask questions to clarify their understanding. Protocol orders were adjusted to conform to the CIPG.

All critical care dietitians began attending daily team bedside rounds, to ensure that they were present to share monitoring data and make recommendations for nutrition care when the team was making its decisions and writing orders. The increased visibility was immediately evident in improved patient care, enhanced recognition by the team for the role of the critical care dietitian, and satisfaction of the dietitians with their new roles. Adjustments in daily routines and workloads were needed, but these adjustments were accomplished, allowing priorities for nutrition care to be realigned.

Nutrition Support Teams

The use of nutrition support teams can be a cost-effective way to monitor the selection of patients for nutrition support, adherence to established guidelines for product selection and recommendations for infusion, and patients' response to nutrition intervention. The visibility and recognition of a nutrition support team highlight the importance of nutrition therapy in achieving positive clinical outcomes and cost savings. In many institutions, nutrition support teams are well established, while in others, they are not. At these institutions, the marketing challenge is to convince administrators to allocate staff and resources to the development and ongoing operation of the team.

At the author's institution, a large academic medical center, the nutrition support team manages patients on parenteral nutrition support across the care continuum. Unit or team-based hospital dietitians manage enteral feeding during the hospital stay. Dietitians who are experienced in monitoring enteral nutrition in both the inpatient and outpatient settings provide discharge teaching on home enteral nutrition support care protocols. They also monitor, evaluate, and reassess enterally fed patients after discharge.

Creation of a home enteral nutrition teaching and monitoring program is an example of a marketing success. Program development occurred over several years and required ongoing attention to accomplish. The hospital's marketing department created a set of attractive brochures that are used to market the program to physicians and patients and family. A physician champion was identified and adjustments in dietitian assignments were made to allow adequate time for their enteral nutrition support activities.

Discharge Planning

Discharge planning procedures vary from one institution to another. They may include the activities of a team or only one or two individuals. Discharge planning may be completed on all patients or only for selected groups, such as oncology or geriatric patients. Dietitians should review their facility procedures and identify ways to increase their involvement. Active involvement ensures quality patient care and is a way to promote postdischarge follow-up, including scheduled appointments with the outpatient dietitian. Ideally, these appointments can be scheduled prior to discharge to coincide with return physician appointments. Some facilities use tools in the EMR, known as discharge wizards, that facilitate provision of routine discharge nutrition guidelines to patients and allow entry of individualized recommendations for patients with complex discharge nutrition regimens.

Reimbursement for Nutrition Services

Any effort to market nutrition services in the acute-care setting should focus on the quality impact of the program or service, its effect on patient safety, and the opportunity to reduce costs of care. The examples described above provide ways to demonstrate this focus. Current systems of reimbursement for hospital care limit dietitians' ability to generate revenue by billing patients for their services. While some facilities do still "charge" for services, these charges do not generally produce revenue, but rather are a method to track productivity. However, dietitians who work in facilities that participate in pay-for-performance programs may be active in quality initiatives that result in additional reimbursement to their facilities. Many hospital-based dietitians generate revenue through their work in outpatient clinics affiliated with their acute care facilities.

Outpatient Nutrition Care

Hospital patients often need nutrition education to modify their food selections, change eating and nutrition-related behaviors, and manage their health. Nutrition education provided in the hospital generally focuses on survival skills and answering patients' questions. Comprehensive nutrition education and nutrition counseling are more appropriate to the outpatient setting, where clients usually feel well enough to participate during appointments and classes and have the capacity needed to manage their self care.

As noted above, reimbursement for outpatient MNT has improved in recent years. Many insurance companies provide partial or complete coverage for MNT sessions. In addition, Medicare Part B coverage for diabetes mellitus and non-dialysis kidney disease is available for patients with this type of outpatient insurance. It has taken time for some hospital dietitians to become Medicare providers and begin providing Medicare Part B MNT. There are numerous reasons for this, including lack of understanding of the system for reimbursement by both dietitians and outpatient billing staff. At some facilities, dietitians still provide MNT for covered Medicare services at no charge or as an out-of-pocket charge. Both situations are problematic, and neither should continue. It is important to provide patients who have Medicare Part B insurance with the MNT benefits to which they are entitled. In addition, use of the MNT benefit demonstrates to CMS that dietitians support it, indirectly endorsing the ADA's work to expand the Medicare Part B benefit to other diagnoses. Pay-for-performance programs present additional opportunities for dietitians to receive higher payment for MNT, as does billing for team conferences and non–face-to-face care, for example phone calls and email messages to resolve nutrition problems.

Evidence based MNT practice guidelines have been developed for several conditions, including type 1 and 2 diabetes mellitus, disorders of lipid metabolism, nondialysis kidney disease, oncology, adult weight management, and pediatric weight management. Each guideline provides an algorithm for nutrition care that follows the Nutrition Care Process, defines recommendations for MNT, and provides evidence to support these recommendations. Guidelines specify the number, length, and duration of MNT sessions, although patients with complex conditions and multiple diagnoses may need additional MNT sessions to reach their therapeutic goals and outcomes. Use of MNT guidelines is mandated for dietitians providing MNT to patients with diabetes mellitus and non-dialysis kidney disease under the Medicare Part B benefit.

OUTCOME DATA

Tracking and managing nutrition outcomes have been advocated for many years. However, surprisingly few dietitians actually do this important work. While time in busy clinics is always limited, outcomes data can be used to improve the quality of nutrition care provided, market services to physicians and other providers, and demonstrate the value of MNT to payers. Each ADA practice guideline has an accompanying Excel spreadsheet that can be used for collecting and compiling individual patient data into useful summaries for performance improvement and marketing activities. And the ADA has formed a Dietetics Practice Based Research Network (DPBRN) that facilitates member involvement in practice-based research (TIP: ADA members can join the DPBRN on the ADA Research website at http://www.eatright.org/cps/rde/xchg/ada/hs.xsl/ho me_115_ENU_HTML.htm. The spaces in the address are actually underlines. There is no cost to join).

In a multi-site practice-based research project that assessed dietitians' ability to implement an MNT protocol, the Lipid Management Nutrition Outcomes Project (LMNOP), data collected by dietitians providing MNT to patients with dyslipidemia revealed that approximately one-third of the patients in the study received only one MNT session and had no follow-up lipid data. In patients who did have follow-up appointments and lab data, improved eating behaviors and lipid values were achieved, results that were not attributed to changes in medications. In addition, weight loss occurred. LMNOP showed that in order for MNT to be effective, it must be provided over multiple sessions. In addition, lipid data must be evaluated over time, to identify the impact of MNT and the refinements in the nutrition care plan that are needed to achieve goals. These data are marketing gold mines for our profession and your practice.

SEIZING OPPORTUNITIES

Identifying the need for outpatient nutrition programs and services can result from networking with physicians, managers, and administrators. Mention of new programs and services can stimulate an idea for a nutrition component that might not have been planned. At the author's facility, a chance conversation with an administrator led to the submission of a proposal to provide MNT services for a new bariatric surgery program that was being developed. A co-proposal for a presurgery weight loss program was also submitted. In another case, an email message asking about use of the Dietary Approaches to Stop Hypertension or DASH diet and possible dietitian availability led to scheduling the dietitian in a weekly hypertension clinic, and cross-referral of hypertension patients with diabetes to the nutrition clinic for more in-depth MNT.

Annual benefits fairs provide a great opportunity to market nutrition programs and services to employees. At the author's facility, the nutrition clinic cosponsors the "America on the Move" program, working to enhance employees' overall health while increasing visibility of the clinic. Employees can also participate in what is known as the "Go for the Gold" program. Participation includes an annual health risk appraisal (HRA). On employee request, health coaches review the results of the HRA and recommend ways to decrease health risk. Ensuring that the health coaches understand the criteria for MNT and know how employees who meet established criteria can access these services via physician referral is another way to market MNT.

Nutrition services and MNT can be promoted to physicians and their patients via direct marketing campaigns. A campaign can provide physicians with materials for their patients, including talking points, basic educational materials, posters, and brochures for the office waiting room. Criteria for MNT and referral forms to the registered dietitian can be included for patients with complex conditions. Partnering to provide nutrition care in this way is a win-win for everyone (TIP: Materials for a direct marketing campaign are available on the ADA website at http://www.eatright.org/cps/rde/xchg/ada/hs.xsl/advocacy_8115_ENU_HTML.htm).

SUMMARY

Dietitians have much to offer through the nutrition care and services they provide. However, it is important that physicians, administrators, payers, and patients understand the value that we take for granted. Successful marketing strategies in the acute care and outpatient settings ensure this happens. Each situation is unique. Therefore, it is up to each of us to assess our own environment, evaluate the options, make plans, and take action—with the understanding that we will not always have a map to follow. Developing and marketing new and existing programs and services are fun and challenging at the same time. The take-home message is that nutrition care and services provided by registered dietitians and dietetic technicians improve the quality of care provided, reduce the costs associated with health care, and improve patients' quality of life.

BIBLIOGRAPHY

American Dietetic Association Nutrition Care Process and Model, 2003. Available at: http://www.eatright.org/ada/files/NCPM_G_11.pdf. Accessed March 28, 2007.

American Dietetic Association Evidence Analysis Library. Available at: http://www.adaevidencelibrary.com. Accessed March 28, 2007.

Litt A, Mitchell. *ADA Guide to Private Practice: An Introduction to Starting Your Own Business*. Chicago, IL: ADA Publications; 2005.

American Dietetic Association. *The Medicare MNT Provider* (monthly newsletter).

American Dietetic Association. *MNT Works Kit*. Available at: http://www.eatright.org/cps/rde/xchg/ada/hs.xsl/advocacy_8115_ENU_HTML.htm. Accessed March 28, 2007.

American Dietetic Association. *Nutrition Diagnosis and Intervention: Standardized Language for the Nutrition Care Process*. Chicago, IL: ADA Publications; 2006.

18

MARKETING WELLNESS AND HEALTH PROMOTION

Kathy King, RD, LD, and Jean Storlie, MS, RD

After 39 years working in wellness and disease prevention, it boggles my mind that it has taken so long for these concepts to be accepted and implemented by American medicine, business, and government. In fact, it was the public and a few aware, forward-thinking business owners and health professionals that first embraced the idea that eating well and making good lifestyle choices could actually affect one's health and help avoid some diseases. I remember hearing physicians say in the 1970s that wellness was not cost effective for a medical practice—how could a doctor make a living keeping people well? In the beginning, some businesses too often treated wellness programs as just a perk for their top executives, or the message was wrong—it appeared that businesses wanted employees to get healthy in order to save the employer money on health insurance. —Kathy

Today, wellness is being promoted as the answer to the growing health care crisis, and according to the Wellness Councils of America (welcoa.org), more than 81% of businesses with 50 or more employees have some form of health promotion program, the most popular being exercise, smoking cessation, back care, and stress management (1). According to David Anderson, PhD, "of the $5,000 per employee the average employer spent on health care in 2001, more than 95% was spent on diagnosis and treatment, with maybe 2% to 3% being invested in early detection (screenings) and no more than 1% to 2% in prevention. This reactive approach persists despite evidence that up to 50% of health care expenditures are lifestyle related and therefore potentially preventable" (2). U.S. health care costs doubled from 1990 to 2001 and they are projected to double by 2012 (3). The U.S. spends more on health care than any other nation in the world but ranks just 37th in the health of its population (4).

Wellness is a proactive concept that focuses on healthy habits and disease-prevention practices (5). Throughout the last two decades, the role of wellness in the practice of dietetics has expanded into private practice, corporate, university, hospital, clinic, school systems, government, culinary, churches, and community settings. Wellness programs are targeted to a wide range of audiences: employee groups, hospital and clinic patients, restaurant and grocery store patrons, community groups, students, and many others. In some instances, dietitians are the only provider of services and programs, and in others they provide the nutrition expertise for an interdisciplinary team. Many dietetic professionals have broadened their skills and expertise into such complementary areas as:

- wellness program design and management,
- personal fitness trainer,
- health coach,
- spa nutritionist,

- counselor for smoking cessation and stress management,
- sports nutritionist,
- massage therapist, and
- exercise assessment and instruction.

Nutrition intervention is one of many strategies they use to promote health and well-being.

THE STARTLING STATISTICS

- 40% of U.S. adults get no physical activity; only 14% meet the standard of brisk walking for 30 minutes per day, five times per week (6).
- Cardiovascular disease is still the biggest killer and it is one of the most preventable diseases (1).
- Two out of every three U.S. adults are overweight or obese (7).
- Individuals who are obese have 30% to 50% more chronic medical problems than those who smoke or drink heavily; they have higher health care utilization rates (8,9).
  - 36% higher inpatient and outpatient spending
  - 77% higher medication spending
  - 11% higher annual health care costs
- Between 1990 and 2004, the number of obese adults in Massachusetts rose 80%, and Blue Cross Blue Shield of Massachusetts found that with every 1% increase in body mass index, an individual's annual health care costs goes up $120.00 (10).
- Stress-related absence accounts for half of all sickness from work (11).
- Each smoker costs an employer an additional $3,856 a year in health care costs and lost productivity (12).
- According to an insurance executive, diabetes care is the most expensive chronic disease for an insurance company to cover (13).
- According to an Employee Benefit News report, a person with a diagnosis of high blood pressure costs $1,240 more in medical services, expenses, premiums, etc., than a person without that diagnosis (14).

WHAT CAN A GOOD WELLNESS PROGRAM DO?

For many companies, medical costs can consume half or more of corporate profits. "Some employers look to cost sharing, cost shifting, managed care plans, risk rating, and cash-based rebates or incentives; but these methods merely shift costs. Only worksite health promotion stands out as the long term answer for keeping employees well in the first place" (15). By now we have the proof that good wellness programs do cut health care costs as well as produce a variety of other results.

- Employers who invest in worksite health promotion programs can see a return of $3 to $6 for every dollar spent over a 2-year to 5-year period; savings are seen in lower medical costs, absenteeism, worker's comp claims, short-term disability, and presenteeism (lower on-the-job efficiency due to health problems) (16).
- In a review of 42 articles on the cost savings of wellness programs, they found the following (17):
  - 28% reduction in sick leave absenteeism
  - 26% reduction in use of the health care benefit
  - 30% reduced worker's comp claims and disability management
- On average, health care claim costs for IBM employees who exercise one to two times a week are $350 a year less than those who do not exercise at all (18).
- An analysis of GE Aircraft employees showed that medical claims submitted by the company's fitness center members decreased by 27%, while claims made by nonmembers actually rose by 17% (19).
- Canada Life Assurance Company of Toronto reported that turnover rate for wellness program participants was 1.8% as compared to the company-wide average of 18% (20).
- Union Pacific Railroad found that 80% of its workers believed the company's exercise program helped increase their productivity, and 75% felt it helped them to concentrate better at work (21).

SUCCESSFUL MARKETING STRATEGIES IN WELLNESS SETTINGS

The marketing strategies dietetic professionals use in wellness depend on the practice setting, the target audience, and the background and focus of the dietitian who is promoting the services. Although worksite wellness and private practice are probably the most developed wellness opportunities for dietitians, they are not the only settings in which nutrition practitioners have established practices.

To develop a broader perspective on how dietitians market wellness services, Jean contacted 17 dietitians who had practiced wellness for more than 5 years. Most of these dietitians practiced in more than one setting, using a base (such as a university, physician's office/clinic, hospital-based program, or private practice) from which they branched into other settings (such as freelance writing, workshops, speaking, and consulting to business, food manufacturers, or sports teams). They served employee groups, students, community groups, healthy individuals, athletes, and consumer groups.

When the respondents were asked to identify their most successful marketing strategy, they ranked referrals highest, followed by public speaking and publishing. Networking through membership and active involvement in various organizations were cited as critical strategies for building a referral base. Some dietitians used constant media exposure in local markets as the cornerstone of their marketing programs. Conducting promotional events, exhibiting, listing in the *Yellow Pages* and other directories, cold calling, and direct mail techniques were cited as less-effective marketing techniques, but they did work for some products or services.

The common theme throughout the survey respondents' stories is a commitment to and a passion for both living and professing a wellness/fitness lifestyle. This makes them role models for their clients, who aspire to increased levels of wellness. They exude a caring and sharing attitude, and they demonstrate upbeat, enthusiastic personalities. When encountering low moments in their personal and professional quests for wellness, they said that perseverance, a tough skin, a sense of humor, and spiritual beliefs were essential.

MARKETING WORKSITE NUTRITION PROGRAMS

Employers are trying harder to tackle the root causes of health care cost increases through consumer-driven plans, employee education, and creating positive employee behavior changes through condition management and wellness programs (23). In the Hewitt Report (2005), 83% of the companies surveyed offered condition management programs

---

CASE STUDY 18.1

FOODPLAY PRODUCTIONS (HTTP://WWW.FOODPLAY.COM)

Emmy Award–winning FoodPlay Productions was founded over 26 years ago by dietitian and entrepreneur, Barbara Storper, MS, RD, and so far, it has reached over 3 million kids with its healthy food and fitness messages. It is a Massachusetts-based multimedia nutrition education company that presents touring theater shows and keynotes across the country, and now sells children's books. Barbara rolled her love of fun, theater, kids, and nutrition into a labor of love.

FoodPlay partners with state health departments, the U.S. Department of Agriculture, Centers for Disease Control and Prevention, Harvard Pilgrim Healthcare Foundation, and others. Together they bring the power of live theater and interactive resources to turn on kids

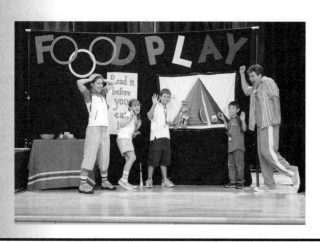

to healthy eating and fitness. From 2008 to 2010, the theater show, sponsored by Intermountain Healthcare and underwritten by SelectHealth, is touring 225 Utah schools (30,000 students). Each school will receive a comprehensive follow-up school resource kit, including fun, hands-on lesson plans, and reproducible activity sheets. They provide partners with turnkey nutrition education programs customized for maximum exposure and outreach. Research shows this approach works well with kids.

FoodPlay Productions won the 2006 National Excellence Award given by the Produce for Better Health Foundation for the ground-breaking partnership, The "Fresh Adventures at Hannaford – FOODPLAY Tour." Barbara won the 2006 "Distinguished Alumni Award" from Columbia University Teachers College, as well as "Outstanding Nutrition Entrepreneur" from the Nutrition Entrepreneur Dietetic Practice Group of the American Dietetic Association in 2005.

According to an article in *Today's Dietitian,* "It's not all fun and games for Storper. She's contributed to a range of scholarly and professional journals; held consultancies with prestigious educational and nonprofit organizations and government agencies; and given keynote conference presentations to dozens of leading dietetics and education conferences. In addition, Storper directs local interns in their community rotations. She's been an advocate for media responsibility as well, lobbying the Federal Trade Commission and the FDA to eliminate misleading advertising that negatively influences children. And through entrepreneurship seminars, she encourages other dietitians to discover their creativity and use their passions as a foundation for successful businesses" (22).

(like diabetes and heart disease management), 56% offered weight management programs, 30% offer incentives to encourage employee participation in wellness programs, and even 64% provide coverage for bariatric surgery (23).

Marketing worksite wellness services involves two levels of selling. First, the company's management must buy into the program enough to sponsor it. Management's support is critical for obtaining the necessary resources and establishing policies that permit employees to participate in the program (such as time away from the job to attend classes). Once management approval is secured, the employee population must be sold on the program. Marketing and promotional strategies need to be carefully crafted for each corporate setting to maximize participation rates, which are critical to both short- and long-term success. If a majority of employees do not participate, the impact of the program will be diluted, and programs that fail to make an impact on quantifiable objectives tend to have short lives. Regardless of whether an external consultant or an employee is selling a worksite nutrition program, these two tiers of selling are critical. Both new and existing programs need constant attention to marketing at both levels to remain successful.

WHEN SELLING TO MANAGEMENT

Careful preparation is crucial to marketing your wellness program to management. Taking the following steps will enhance your chances of success:

1. Learn as much as possible about how wellness is currently structured within your target company before making a sales call. If you know someone who works there, ask questions about the work culture and employer's support of healthy lifestyle choices or issues—there may already be a stress management or other ongoing program.
2. Target the highest management level you can reach. In small-size and medium-size companies, start with the CEO. This level of management may be harder to reach in larger companies, unless the CEO is a wellness advocate.
3. If upper-level managers are inaccessible, start with the human resources, training and development, or medical departments.
4. Go into the sales call armed with facts.

   ■ Managers want to know the costs, benefits, and expected outcomes of worksite nutrition programs and of all health-promotion programs in general.
   ■ Before a sales meeting, research the company to learn about the demographics of the employee population. Identify the number of sites and other factors that can affect the design and delivery of a worksite nutrition program.
   ■ Tailor a proposal that speaks to the needs and existing structure of the company. Include statistics that document the cost effectiveness of the program.
   ■ Demonstrate your track record as a program provider.

WHEN MEETING WITH MIDDLE MANAGERS

When you meet with middle managers, provide documents that clearly and concisely build an argument for why a worksite nutrition program can make a positive difference in their company. Since they will face the challenge of selling your program upward, you need to convince them to sponsor the program idea, then arm them with the tools they need to sell it to their superiors. Identify who will be involved in making the final decision to purchase nutrition services. Focusing a great deal of time and energy on someone who only influences a decision can be a futile effort. Try to become acquainted with both the influencers and the final decision maker. Work cooperatively with everyone involved, addressing the concerns that each party raises. Be careful not to become entangled in internal controversies and rivalries.

SALES CALLS WITH UPPER-LEVEL MANAGERS

Plan to spend no more than a half-hour with a busy executive. You may be given only 10 to 15 minutes, so be well prepared. A polished proposal that succinctly outlines the program concept, critical logistical considerations, costs, and expected outcomes is essential when presenting to upper management. Keep to the point and allow plenty of time for interaction. Top managers typically have take-charge personalities—they may want to lead the discussion.

Identify objectives for each sales call. For example, if the first sales call is an exploratory discussion with a middle manager, a realistic objective might be to gain enough information so you can draft a proposal. Close each meeting with a clear understanding of what the next steps are (for example, you will submit a proposal for preliminary review and the manager will schedule a follow-up meeting to introduce you to the decision-maker or other influencers). After each sales meeting, plan a follow-up strategy.

Karen Reznik Dolins, MS, RD, had an experience selling worksite nutrition services to Merrill Lynch that illustrates the importance of persistence and follow-up. She contacted the company soon after the National Cholesterol Education Program guidelines were issued, and they hired her to conduct a seminar on the subject for their medical staff. Although they expressed an interest in contracting her services to deliver a program to their 10,000 local employees, they did not act on it. For 3 years, she kept in touch with them periodically. Finally 3 years later, her timing was perfect. They had just budgeted funds for wellness, the medical director remembered her favorably, and she was able to sell them on her ideas. Karen says that this experience taught her that perseverance is everything. "Never forget a contact," urges Karen, "and never let them forget you."

CASE STUDY 18.2

BREAKING INTO WELLNESS

Katherine Tallmadge, MS, RD, Private Practitioner, Author, Corporate Wellness, Washington, DC

Working in the corporate wellness world has been a goal of mine for at least 10 years (Fig. 18.1). It finally happened, but only as a result of many different career moves coming together.

I had been in a traditional private practice since 1984 in Washington, DC. But I believed that expanding my counseling and wellness services into the corporate world would be a way to stretch myself professionally and creatively, to reach more people, have more impact, and earn more income. But it eluded me for so long; I was intimidated and unsure I could navigate the corporate arena and avoided trying seriously for many years. It is only now looking back on my experiences that I can see clearly how it finally happened for me.

First, to succeed in the corporate arena, you not only have to be extremely competent, knowledgeable, organized, and confident, you have to *look* the part, too. And that means having visible accomplishments that corporation executive's respect. That meant, for me, being published. Having been a regular columnist for a major newspaper (*The Washington Post*) and magazines (*SHAPE, Vegetarian Times, eDiets.com*), authoring a respected and highly quoted diet book (*Diet Simple: 192 Mental Tricks, Substitutions, Habits & Inspirations*), and regularly appearing in local and national media venues caused the corporations to look more favorably upon me. Though, I feel my book gave me the extra competitive edge and confidence boost I needed. But how did that happen in the first place?

INTERNAL PROMOTIONS TO EMPLOYEES

Securing management support will get your foot in the door; getting employees to participate will keep it there.

Even the best program can go unnoticed if managers and workers do not know what is offered and how to take advantage of it. When marketing a worksite nutrition program to employees, it is important to identify target segments within the employee population, such as women, minorities, blue-collar workers, or retirees. If a needs analysis was conducted, use the results to learn about the employees' needs and interests.

Company-wide marketing strategies alone may not be effective in achieving high participation rates. Focused communications that reach the targeted groups and speak to their needs will maximize participation (for example, presentations at

I returned to school to earn a second Master's in Journalism and Public Affairs, I began publishing freelance articles in *The Washington Post* almost immediately (though, honestly, no editors seemed to care about the Master's!). Eight years later, in 2002, I published my book, a culmination of my 18 years of private practice.

Having the column in a national newspaper and my book made getting into the corporate world so much easier. Promoters of my program like to say "author of . . ." Journalists interviewing me as an expert love to refer to me as an author. Even editors of magazines who may hire me to write articles or columns appreciate the fact that I have written a book. It's a huge bonus—up there with a Master's degree in terms of helping you get your foot in the door.

One of my first corporate clients was a large national broadcast media company. I'd worked with them for many years as an "expert" whenever they needed a balanced nutritional point of view on the air. Years earlier, I met one of their producers when she was working for a local TV station. They did a weight loss series during sweeps week featuring me and the ideas in *Diet Simple*. This producer then moved from the local station to a national network and kept using me as her expert (I later became an ADA spokesperson, which added to their desire to use me in their news pieces). So, I guess it was an easy choice when they decided they'd like an employee wellness program featuring nutrition counseling. In fact, the head of the bureau—not human resources—initiated the first contact.

Luckily I was prepared. The year earlier, I decided to be serious about corporate outreach. I had met with a

continued

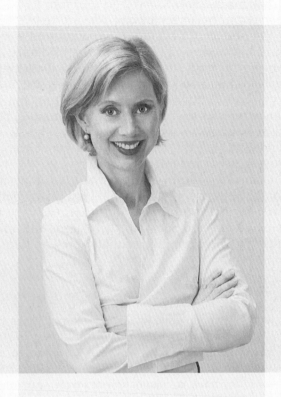

Improve Health, Wellness, Vitality & Performance NOW!

with Katherine Tallmadge

"One of the best presentations we've ever had!"
—White House Athletic Center

Katherine Tallmadge, M.A.², R.D.

Nationally recognized health, wellness, diet and nutrition expert, speaker, noted author, and columnist, Katherine Tallmadge, works with individuals and organizations to improve health and wellness

Katherine's interactive, motivational, inspirational, fun, information-packed sessions focus on your needs, your challenges and your concerns. Her real life experience, proven track record and practical how-to solutions will provide the boost your organization needs.

Tallmadge has designed and delivered presentations for clients such as: The White House Athletic Center, The Smithsonian, National Geographic, Pricewaterhouse Coopers, National Association of Manufacturers, and many more.

- **National Spokesperson** for the American Dietetic Association

- **Adjunct Professor,** George Washington University

- **Author of Diet Simple:** *192 Mental Tricks, Substitutions, Habits & Inspirations.* LifeLine Press, 2004 (ranked in the Amazon top 10)

- Bi-weekly "Diet Smart" columnist for ***The Washington Post***, regular columnist for *SHAPE* and *Vegetarian Times* magazines, and eDiets.com

- **Frequent guest in the media** (CNN, *USA Today*, *Newsweek*, The Television Food Network, among others)

- *Good Housekeeping Magazine* named *Diet Simple* as a top three diet program along with Weight Watchers

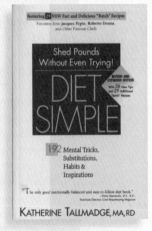

PersonalizedNutrition.com • DietSimple.info • Katherine@PersonalizedNutrition.com • (202) 833-0353

FIGURE 18.1. ■ Promotional flyer for Katherine Tallmadge.

continued

marketing consultant who advised me on brochures and other marketing materials I would need to reach and work successfully with corporations. With his help and the help of my graphic designer, we put together a beautiful brochure which could be sent by snail mail or as a PDF file (see example). I had also put together a questionnaire for my corporations to fill out to assess their needs, which I used for my corporate speaking engagements. I drew up a contract, asked for a 50% down payment and was ready to go.

Another bonus was the fact that in 2002 I had spent 6 months designing an online weight loss course for Barnes & Noble University. This course formed the basis of all of my corporate work. I turned it into a workbook (with the help of my graphic designer), and gave it to each corporate wellness participant as a companion to my book.

My "course" was very popular at the national network. I gave a talk, which was the "lesson of the week." Then, the participants would schedule themselves with me that day for their individual sessions. During many of my talks, I would bring in guest speakers. I brought in a dietitian from USDA to discuss the new food guide pyramid, a research scientist to discuss "superfoods," a stress management expert, a psychologist, personal trainers, and several cookbook authors and chefs for cooking demos. Having been in

Washington, DC, throughout my education and career means I know most everyone! I pulled upon their expertise and my clients really appreciated my eclectic offerings. My colleagues also appreciated the work and the exposure.

Most of my corporate work has come from my contacts in the media world or private practice clients. One client was the president of a medium-sized firm in the Washington, DC, area. He asked me to work with his employees. And when the president of the company endorses you, you are in!

As a result of this experience of offering nutrition programs in corporations, I have also been able to offer full-fledged wellness programs complete with personal trainers, stress management experts, and professionals in allied fields so that every health need of my clients is covered. I find this the most exciting aspect of the work. Instead of just recommending to my private clients to see this or that professional and hope they follow my advice, in a well-rounded corporate program, I provide the experts and am assured my clients are getting the kind of care they need to keep them healthy and happy the rest of their lives—which also improves the program outcomes.

I have to admit, I am not much of a marketer. I have achieved my success by loving what I do, doing a good job, nurturing relationships, and regular media exposure.

department meetings to reach employees in their work groups or offering an introductory session over lunch for people with diabetes to explain the upcoming condition management program).

One target audience that requires special attention in launching a worksite wellness program is management. Meet with managers and supervisors to identify any concerns they have about how the program might affect their work unit. They may resent and resist the program because they perceive it as a disruption. Alleviating these concerns at the onset and tailoring the program to the needs of each employee work group will prevent serious problems later. Sell the program from the top down.

An employee wellness committee fosters grassroots support, which is useful in marketing a program. Members provide valuable insights into the needs and interests of their coworkers, and they can help distinguish between effective and ineffective communication strategies. Members can play a role in the actual implementation of program promotions by volunteering to distribute materials, speaking on behalf of the program, and assisting in planning and conducting promotional events.

Joan Horbiak, MPH, RD, sets up a nutrition task force with every corporate client to guide her in tai-

loring her program to the company's needs. She believes that her most effective marketing technique is being an excellent speaker. Therefore, each year she attends a formal training program in New York to enhance her speaking skills, and she gets herself in front of a group as part of her sales process. Joan provides two free presentations: the first to sell management (a targeted sales tactic), the second to generate employee participation (a value-added service intended to improve her ultimate outcomes).

Table 18.1 presents strategies for internally promoting a worksite wellness program with its newest services on the Web and in disease management.

MARKETING HOSPITAL-BASED HEALTH PROMOTION PROGRAMS

While hospitals have tremendous resources for building health-promotion programs, traditional hospital systems also have a number of economic, legal, political, and philosophical barriers that inhibit the success of wellness programs (24). Due to ever-tightening fiscal conditions, complex organizational structures, and an orientation to crisis medical intervention, hospitals sometimes have difficulty

TABLE 18.1. MARKETING WORKSITE WELLNESS	
Reaching Employees	**Keeping Management in the Loop**
Initial kickoff	Introductory session/retreat on wellness, productivity, and health insurance cost
■ Letters from the CEO and managers	Strategies discussion and employee group on corporate culture
■ Small group meetings/promotion	Active involvement in the wellness program
■ Kickoff event	Status report on the program successes and challenges
■ Keynote speaker	Result reports
■ Health fair	
Website and group/individual	
■ Interactive assessments	
■ Education modules	
Disease management	
■ e-Counseling	
■ Diet follow-up online	
Promotion tools	
■ Posters	
■ Flyers/check stuffers	
■ Lunch nutrition table tent	
■ Weekly web "Healthy Points of Interest"	
■ Brown bag luncheon speakers	

positioning wellness effectively within their organizations. And if a program is not positioned effectively internally, it has little chance for success externally. For this reason, leaders in hospital health promotion have recognized the importance of strategic planning in marketing hospital health promotion programs. Strategic planning efforts hinge on the answers to three critical questions: Who are we? Where are we going? How will we get there?

Important questions to answer in strategic planning for hospital health promotion include: How does the hospital strategically position health promotion within the organization? What is going on in the market? What is the program all about as a business unit?

Many community hospitals position health promotion as a community-outreach service. It is viewed as an attractive way to build goodwill, enhance the community's loyalty to the hospital, and strengthen relations with large employers. In light of this mission for health promotion, direct profits may not be as important as the more intangible benefits, such as public relations. Other hospitals have profit motives for health promotion, which affects how the program is marketed.

Interpreting market conditions involves a thorough understanding of existing, as well as potential, competition. Knowing what factors will influence a given segment of the market to buy wellness services can be the most important determinant of long-term success. After identifying market segments, it is essential to gather information that will reveal their purchasing motives through focus groups, interviews, or surveys.

As Table 18.1 depicts, hospital health promotion programs may target a number of markets, and offer a wide range of services. Matching internal capabilities to the needs and interests of the buying groups is the cornerstone of creating an effective marketing plan. The ability to design specific promotion and sales strategies that communicate the benefits and features of a program in a manner that motivates purchasing behavior is what distinguishes successful from unsuccessful hospital wellness programs.

Years ago, selling nutrition counseling services to healthy populations represented a departure from the way nutrition was traditionally offered through the hospital (that is, only through a physician's referral or a hospital stay). Marketing nutrition counseling as a stand-alone product line, capable of producing revenue, enhanced the institution's image and actively cross-sold other hospital services. Many healthy populations desired nutrition information and personal guidance in the areas of weight control, heart health, sports nutrition, and food allergies.

The critical success factor in marketing these services was not the type of services, credentials of the provider, or sales strategy (although all three factors played influential roles), but rather the delivery of the service that is put into place. Realizing that to reach healthy audiences one has to cater to hectic schedules, personal appointments should be offered during evenings and weekends, as well as during the day. Clear directions for parking and locating the counseling center (which can be quite confusing in large hospital complexes) have to be provided. Because image and service are very important when serving healthy populations, and nutrition counseling is an optional service, care is given to the ambience and setting for counseling. A receptionist often greets clients. The facility should feature an attractive waiting room and pleasant, private counseling rooms. By making the dietitians accessible between appointments and accepting credit cards as a form of payment, they further cater to clients' needs.

The primary promotional strategies usually are:

- an article in the hospital newsletter (for employees to refer friends and family),
- local articles in newspapers, church bulletins, and corporate employee newsletters,
- word-of-mouth referrals from satisfied customers,
- physician referrals,
- free media appearances,
- minimal newspaper advertising, and
- participation in hospital-sponsored publicity events to enhance their visibility.

All these strategies promote preventive nutrition counseling services as a profitable and viable business venture for the hospital.

MARKETING IN PRIVATE PRACTICE

Over the years, thousands of dietitians in private practice have been successful in selling private counseling sessions to well populations. The most successful marketing strategies in private practice are:

- encouraging word-of-mouth referrals from satisfied clients to friends, family, and colleagues;
- networking and handing out business cards, brochures, or flyers;
- marketing to physicians, nurses, and clinic managers;
- marketing on your website;
- becoming a recognized expert in a field like obesity, diabetes, celiac, polycystic ovary syndrome, or heart disease, so that you are the person everyone thinks of when a diagnosis is made;
- writing a book, cookbook, or smaller pamphlet on a content area;
- joining American Dietetic Association's referral network;
- appearing in local media;
- writing newspaper and magazine articles, especially on your areas of expertise—make sure you get a by-line or one-line bio at the bottom with contact information;
- joining local professional or health and fitness groups—offer an exciting 20-minute brown bag lunch nutrition presentation to introduce what you do;
- speaking at community, sports, professional, church, and school meetings;
- attending and speaking at health fairs and fun runs; and
- sending out press releases when you do speak or publish.

For over 12 years, Evette Hackman, PhD, RD, consulted private clients, most of whom sought her services for support of their wellness goals, rather than for help in coping with an illness. She found that constant media exposure in her local market was the most effective marketing strategy for her. In fact, she said that if a month went by when she was not in the media, her patient load dropped. To keep herself in the media, Evette wrote a bimonthly column in the daily newspaper, developed relationships with local media contacts, and served as nutrition editor for *Shape* magazine. She sent out press releases regularly, and, as a result, she was frequently invited to appear as a guest expert on local television and radio shows.

CASE STUDY 18.3

MARKETING A PRIVATE PRACTICE

Rebecca Bitzer, MS, RD, & Associates, Greenbelt, MD,
http://www.rbitzer.com

I am the owner of a large nutrition counseling practice in Maryland. My main office is located near Washington, DC, with easy access to clients who either live or work in the Washington metropolitan area. My office is located on a suburban street that is filled with physician offices, which makes my office easy to find with free parking. It is in a lower-middle class section of Maryland, which is more unusual. Typically, Maryland nutrition counseling offices are in more affluent areas.

This makes price a big factor. Many of my clients are able to come to my office for Medical Nutrition Therapy and use their health insurance plan to cover a major portion of my fee.

Over time, I have increased the size of my practice to seven registered dietitians, specializing in various areas of nutrition, which makes us much more marketable (for example Certified Diabetes Educator, ACE personal trainer, Eating Disorder specialist, and Spanish-speaking nutritionist). This allows physicians to refer a wide variety of patients to us. With so many on staff, we are able to provide extended office hours with early morning and evening hours 7 days per week. Also, because we have a large staff, patients do not have to wait a long time for their first consultation.

continued

continued

MARKETING

In the beginning, my biggest marketing mistake was trying to reach individual customers. I have spent a lot of money over the years advertising via newspaper, phone book, and even radio ads. Also, if I was lucky, I would get a client or two by marketing directly to consumers at health fairs and speaking engagements (churches, schools, rotary clubs), but from my experience, these were not cost-effective ways to get clients. I finally decided that I had to reach many more motivated clients with a strong desire to see a registered dietitian. I decided to market my services directly to physicians who would refer their clients to me.

PHYSICIANS

I learned quickly that physicians were interested in delegating time-consuming nutrition counseling to a registered dietitian. My first marketing campaign to physicians focused on how they could save time and money by referring patients to me. I sent out a large mailing to physicians in the Maryland and Washington, DC, areas. I followed up by "pounding the pavement." I drove around to all the local physician offices and dropped off my promotional materials, which consisted of a brochure, flyer, healthy food product, water bottle with my business name on it, and business cards. I asked to make an appointment with the physician to discuss my services.

Occasionally, I did make an appointment, and this usually proved to be the best method because the physician connected my name and face with my professional service; hopefully, that ensured he/she would refer patients to me. Also, I think it showed that I was willing to go the extra mile by meeting with the physician. I would usually bring a small fruit basket or some healthy snacks to help make my visit more memorable and to leave a favorable impression with the office staff. I made the appointment short and sweet (now that I have grown my business and I understand how busy a medical office can be).

When I met with physicians, they kept asking, "Does medical insurance cover your services?" and "Do you accept medical insurance?" This convinced me that physicians in my area were concerned about making the cost of my services affordable to all of their clients and I have worked to improve insurance coverage for my services. I continue on-going contact with my referring physicians via the phone, FAX, and office visits to make sure they are happy with my services and will continue to refer to my practice.

NUTRITION ENTREPRENEURS DPG

Another very helpful way I established my private practice was to get involved with a local group of nutritionists who mailed out a list of "Registered Dietitians in Private Practice" in the Chesapeake Bay Area. Being associated with other registered dietitians also helped establish my credibility. Similarly, I became involved with the national Dietetic Practice Group (DPG) Nutrition Entrepreneurs, which works to make registered dietitians widely known as the nutrition expert. This was an excellent way to meet other registered dietitians from across the country and share ideas about bringing our businesses to the next level. It has given me many opportunities to share missteps and successes. We learn from each others' mistakes and inspire each other to move forward with our careers.

INSURANCE COVERAGE

My next marketing campaign focused on how to get insurance companies to pay for nutrition counseling services. I contacted many insurance companies and asked to become a Provider. I figured that if physicians wanted my services covered, then I should investigate how to make that happen. After spending many hours contacting insurance companies to get applications (this was all very new 20 years ago), I successfully became a provider for New York Life Care and Maryland Independent Physicians Association (MDIPA). I remember that in order for me to become a MDIPA provider, I had to submit three letters from physicians who were using my services and a letter of need to explain why my services were needed. This was another difficult step because I had not been in practice very long and I had not actually seen very many patients at this point, but I continued to jump through hoops to get things done. Once I was a provider for these two insurance plans, I sent out a flyer to physicians again, this time I focused on physicians who were providers for these insurance plans, and referrals started to come more quickly. Even today, one of the first questions people ask is, "What insurance plans cover your services?" (See the case study on selling to insurance agencies in Chapter 10.)

MARKETING TODAY

I think it is important to remember that today my business is based upon physician referrals. I do not market my services directly to the general public. Over the years, I have heard many registered dietitians complain about the poor reimbursement for Medical Nutrition Therapy and the enormous hassles of accepting insurance. However, I have found my niche with insurance coverage and have been able to grow my business based on the willingness of physicians to refer their patients.

continued

continued
Over the years, I have revised my marketing materials many times. I have changed the name of my business a couple of times. I had a clever business name for years but it never seemed to catch on, probably because I was established and physicians were in the habit of referring their patients to my last name and insurance referrals are routinely written to a professional, not as often to a business name. So, I have changed my name back to Rebecca Bitzer, MS, RD, & Associates, and even though it is a mouthful to say, it seems to be working. For this most recent marketing campaign, I hired a graphic artist and a professional writer to make a more professional package. I included my photo to help associate a person with a name and, lastly, I added a few testimonials from physicians.

I hope this inspires you to start or expand your private practice.

MARKETING SPORTS NUTRITION SERVICES

Dietitians have increasingly become involved in providing sports nutrition services to a wide range of athletic populations: high school, college, professional, Olympic, masters, and recreational athletes. Nutrition services are delivered through individual counseling sessions, group education, training programs for coaches and sports medicine professionals, and nutrition columns for newsletters and popular magazines. See Chapter 23 for more details on marketing sports nutrition.

When a dietitian works with an athletic team (from high school to professional), the athletic trainer or coach typically plays a key role. Therefore, when marketing nutrition services to athletic teams, it is important to build relationships with coaches and athletic trainers. Speaking at conferences for these professionals and writing in their trade publications will help build visibility. A mailing to local coaches and trainers followed by a personal sales call can be an effective way to explore the level of interest in your area and generate qualified leads. Once a contact is established, keep in touch. If a coach shows no interest the first time, call again a few months before the next year's season begins.

Dietitians provide individual counseling services for athletes through their private practices, sports team contracts, sports medicine clinics, and physicians' offices. When marketing to athletes in a private-practice setting, it is important to maintain a high level of visibility among consumers, particularly those active in sports and fitness. Exposure in media that are targeted to athletic populations and focus on athletic events will augment marketing during one-on-one counseling. When marketing nutrition as part of a sports medicine clinic or physicians' practice, establish a relationship with the professionals on staff, as well as the clients, to improve your referral network.

MARKETING CONSUMER-ORIENTED PROGRAMS

Consumer-oriented nutrition programs have considerable potential for success in today's marketplace. Supermarkets, restaurants, and employee cafeterias are ideal locations to influence eating behavior (see Chapter 21 on marketing in supermarkets).

Pending legislation may force restaurants to comply with stricter requirements when using descriptive terms, like "light" and "heart healthy," on their menus. Since restaurant owners do not know how to find a dietitian who can help them comply with the new regulations, it is up to dietitians to market their skills to restaurateurs. It is best to start with local, single-owner operations. Before making a sales call, become well acquainted with the restaurant—its patrons, menus, and (if possible) kitchen capabilities. When scheduling a sales call, try to reach the local manager or owner between lunch and dinner service. Sell your services in terms of tangible benefits (such as drawing in new customers, improving satisfaction among existing customers, increasing food sales, and avoiding regulatory risk). Present specific ideas about what you can offer. For example, you could propose to analyze the existing menu items and provide advice on the appropriate use of descriptive terms, or consult with the chef to develop a line of health-oriented menu items. If you have culinary training, that is a major plus.

TRENDS THAT AFFECT NUTRITION AND WELLNESS

To quote Naisbitt, "trends, like horses, are more easily ridden in the direction they are already moving" (27). Keeping abreast of trends that affect the future of the wellness movement is critical when marketing wellness services and programs. Wellness grew

CASE STUDY 18.4

MARKETING A FAITH-BASED WELLNESS PROGRAM

For 12 years there have been successful faith-based wellness programs being used in Black churches across the country to encourage more healthful eating, especially including more fruits and vegetables. Today, that program is called Body & Soul and it is available in states such as California, Delaware, Georgia, North Carolina, and Virginia, and is administered nationally through the American Cancer Society (25). In California, all state-funded churches are required to offer this program as part of their community programming, since studies show that African-Americans have the highest risk for chronic diseases such as hypertension, diabetes, stroke, and cancer (26).

These programs are successful according to people who work with them because:

■ Leaders in the church buy-in first and lead the way by example and words to head off any distrust of the program.
■ Advisory boards made of members adapt the educational messages to the ongoing Sunday school classes, prayer meetings, choir practice, age groups, potlucks, and other familiar get-togethers in the church.
■ Messages are given by the preacher or guest speakers with many hands-on activities used to expose members to enjoying more fruits and vegetables in food demonstrations, food tasting, grocery store tours, health screenings, health fairs, picnics, videos, articles in the church bulletins, or nutrition seminars.
■ A food policy is developed by each church to outline the types of foods that can be served at its church functions.
■ Influential church leaders are recruited as peer counselors and trained in motivational interviewing skills so they can call all church members at least monthly and encourage them to include more fruits and vegetables.

It is very smart—they recruit leaders who change their nutrition habits and beliefs, make them role models and peer counselors, and use immersion therapy to change the culture of the most significant social and spiritual affiliation the person has in her or his life. It works because of numerous people's unselfish commitment and because of the special place the church holds in the hearts of many African-Americans. Check out www.bodyandsoul.nih.gov/.

out of larger trends and continues to be influenced by forces that shape health care, the economy, corporate America, and even society like the aging Baby Boomers. Within a climate of change, there are both opportunities and threats to consider. As the costs of health insurance and acute care steadily rise, it appears that the need for corporate wellness and health promotion programs will continue.

KEY LINKAGES FOR PROMOTING THE NUTRITION ASPECTS OF WELLNESS

Since wellness is an interdisciplinary field, building and maintaining relationships with professionals outside the dietetics profession expands a dietitian's base of resources and expertise and enhances the potential for referrals. Connection to a larger network also stimulates new learning and makes it easier to stay at the cutting edge.

SUMMARY

A wide range of marketing strategies can be successfully employed to promote a wellness practice. The success of a given strategy will depend on the setting in which the practice is based, the services offered, and the target audience. The following hints will enhance your attempts to market your wellness practice:

■ Realize that referrals are critical. Credentials, establishing a solid reputation, and building relationships will foster both client and professional referrals.
■ Use strategic alliances (or partnerships) as springboards to other opportunities.
■ Know your numbers; be able to quote statistics on cost savings, loss of productivity due to poor health, return on investment, and so on.
■ Sell to the decision makers.
■ Get additional training if necessary: smoking cessation, stress management, fitness, media, speaking, or sales skills.
■ Seek media exposure in front of your target groups.
■ Submit articles/research for publication in appropriate journals or at conventions on employee health.
■ Fill up your programs because of your reputation for producing dynamite presentations and effective counseling.
■ Know your niche.

REFERENCES

1. Wellness Councils of America. In: *Health Stats*. Available at: http://preventdisease.com/worksite_wellness/worksite_wellness.html. Accessed February 8, 2008.
2. Anderson D. Wellness Councils of America's Absolute Advantage, 2003. In: *Corporate Wellness Statistics*. Available at: http://www.fitnessworksatwork.com/corporate-wellness-statistics.html. Accessed February 8, 2008.
3. Partnerships for Prevention. In: *Corporate Wellness Statistics*. Available at: http://www.fitnessworksatwork.com/corporate-wellness-statistics.html. Accessed February 8, 2008.
4. *Startling Statistics*. Available at: http://www.wellnesswiz.com/statistics.cfm. Accessed February 8, 2008.
5. Storlie J. Wellness and Disease Prevention. In: King K. *The Competitive Edge*, 2nd Ed. Chicago, IL: The American Dietetic Association; 1995:126–137.
6. Center for Disease Control. In: *Bringing Healthy Choices to the Workplace*. Available at: http://olsencenterforwellness.com/workplace/statistics.asp. Accessed February 8, 2008.
7. Hanes N III. In: *Bringing Healthy Choices to the Workplace*. Available at: http://olsencenterforwellness.com/workplace/statistics.asp. Accessed February 8, 2008.
8. Health and Affairs, 2002. In: *Bringing Healthy Choices to the Workplace*. Available at: http://olsencenterforwellness.com/workplace/statistics.asp. Accessed February 8, 2008.
9. Control Data Corporation. In: *Bringing Healthy Choices to the Workplace*. Available at: http://olsencenterforwellness.com/workplace/statistics.asp. Accessed February 8, 2008.
10. Boston Globe, March 22, 2006. In: *Corporate Wellness Statistics*. Available at: http://www.fitnessworksatwork.com/corporate-wellness-statistics.html. Accessed February 8, 2008.
11. Association for Counseling at Work. In: *Bringing Healthy Choices to the Workplace*. Available at: http://olsencenterforwellness.com/workplace/statistics.asp. Accessed February 8, 2008.
12. Billings Gazette, December 10, 2005. In: *Corporate Wellness Statistics*. Available at: http://www.fitnessworksatwork.com/corporate-wellness-statistics.html. Accessed February 8, 2008.
13. Personal interview. Dallas, Texas, 1998.
14. Employee Benefit News, May 1997. *Health Stats*. Available at: http://preventdisease.com/worksite_wellness/worksite_wellness.html. Accessed February 8, 2008.
15. *Health Stats*. Available at: http://preventdisease.com/worksite_wellness/worksite_wellness.html. Accessed February 8, 2008.
16. American Journal of Preventive Medicine, December 2005. In: *Corporate Wellness Statistics*. Available at: http://www.fitnessworksatwork.com/corporate-wellness-statistics.html. Accessed February 8, 2008.
17. Chapman L. Meta-evaluation of Worksite Health Promotion Economic Return Studies. *American Journal of Health Promotion,* 2003. In: *Corporate Wellness Statistics*. Available at: http://www.fitnessworksatwork.com/corporate-wellness-statistics.html. Accessed February 8, 2008.
18. Benefitnews.com, March 2006. In: *Corporate Wellness Statistics*. Available at: http://www.fitnessworksatwork.com/corporate-wellness-statistics.html. Accessed February 8, 2008.
19. Worksite Health Promotion Economics, 1995. *Health Stats*. Available at: http://preventdisease.com/worksite_wellness/worksite_wellness.html. Accessed February 8, 2008.
20. American Journal of Health Promotion, April–May 1993. *Health Stats*. Available at: http://preventdisease.com/worksite_wellness/worksite_wellness.html. Accessed February 8, 2008.
21. Incentive, June 1995. *Health Stats*. Available at: http://preventdisease.com/worksite_wellness/worksite_wellness.html. Accessed February 8, 2008.
22. Jackson K. Who Said You Shouldn't Play With Food? The Success of FoodPlay. *Today's Dietitian* 7(2):34.
23. Sawyer-Morse MK. What's It All About? *Today's Dietitian,* March 2005.
24. Storlie J, Daly-Gawenda D. Hospital innovation and entrepreneurship. In: Sol N, Wilson PK, eds. *Hospital Health Promotion*. Champaign, IL: Human Kinetics Publishers; 1989:229–262.
25. National Cancer Institute. *Body & Soul: A Celebration of Healthy Eating and Living, a Guide for Your Church*. Bethesda, MD: National Institutes of Health; 2004. Available at: http://www.bodyandsoul.nih.gov/. Accessed February 19, 2008.
26. Peregrin T. Cooking with Soul: A Look into Faith-Based Wellness Programs. *JADA* 2006;106(7):1016–1020.
27. Naisbitt J. *Megatrends: The New Directions Transforming Our Lives*. New York: Warner Books; 1982.

BIBLIOGRAPHY

Hager MH. Medicare Reform Opens Door for Preventive Nutrition Services. *JADA* 2004;104(6):887–889.

Lipscomb R. Health Coaching: A New Opportunity for Dietetics Professionals. *JADA* 2006;106(6):801–803.

A Look at School Wellness Policies. *ADA Times* March/April 2007. Available at: http://www.eatright.org/fnce2007; http://www.eatright.org/development.

Wellman NS. Prevention, Prevention, Prevention: Nutrition for Successful Aging. *JADA* 2007;107(5):741–743.

MARKETING DIETETIC TECHNICIANS

19

Kathy Petersen, DTR, MD

Traditionally, dietetic technicians worked either in acute or extended care facilities. This no longer holds true. A new breed of dietetic technicians is emerging—one that is not content merely to sit in a diet office processing menus as in years past. Today's dietetic technicians wish to be creative in seeking the best ways to utilize their acquired knowledge and skills. Some hunger for one-on-one patient-client interaction in a wellness or disease-prevention setting, where they can provide counseling on proper normal nutrition for optimum health. Others wish to utilize management skills to run a successful and nutritious food service operation. Innovators in the field have even entered the corporate world of food producers. They combine skills in a variety of areas—food science, nutrition, marketing, education, and communication to create a bridge between manufacturer and consumer.

Today's dietetic technicians seek employment opportunities that enhance their abilities while staying within their legal scope of practice as determined by state laws. They work in varied settings with very diverse responsibilities, such as public health nutrition programs, child nutrition, school lunch and elderly feeding programs, and food service management firms, to name only a few.

How did the following dietetic technicians market themselves to obtain their positions? All felt the need to be more challenged in their careers. They were willing to take risks and be persistent. Once they made the decision to further their careers, the next step was to network with other dietetic professionals and community leaders. They pursued their goals by volunteering with different agencies in their communities, such as the American Heart Association, the American Cancer Society, and the AIDS Support Services. Volunteer work can open many doors to opportunity. Interviewees also identified education and involvement in district, state, or national dietetic associations as prime areas for career advancement. Some entrepreneurial DTRs (Dietetic Technician, Registered) have even started their own businesses. This requires ongoing marketing of themselves and their services to build and maintain clientele.

PROFILE 1

Although Alberta Scruggs, DTR, worked as a clinical DTR for over 7 years in long-term care (LTC), teaching people how to eat so their diets "worked for their bodies, not against them" is what she really wanted to do. Working in LTC helped her realize it was better to prevent illness than to try to fix it. Alberta saw many interventions "not work" due to lifelong unhealthy habits. As Alberta says, "the opportunity to do something out of the box does not always jump into our laps. Sometimes we have to make it happen."

In 2003, she left LTC and moved into prevention and wellness. She began working for the Dayton-area YMCA, where she became Director of Wellness. Alberta coordinated the "Young Adult's Healthy Initiative" program, the "Healthy Summer Snack Program," and an "Annual Soul Food Expo."

Now she owns her own business, Nutritional ConCerns in Dayton, Ohio. She is contracted by Faith-based organizations and community centers to educate their client base on how to promote health. She teaches healthy eating and increased physical activity. In addition to her Associate Degree in Applied Sciences of Dietetics and Nutrition, she is a certified Older Adult Fitness Instructor and a Certified Group Aerobic Instructor. She developed a "DancerSize" chair aerobic video. Alberta was recently featured as the nutrition educator for the award-winning Diabetes Obesity Wellness Opportunity Program (DOWOP) in Dayton. This program focuses on children who are at or above the 85th percentile of their BMI. Alberta wrote the nutrition component, which includes a spiritual component to help youngsters understand the difference between God-made and man-made foods.

Alberta is truly an example of how to increase marketability and open doors to a rewarding career. She accomplished this by getting additional complementary certifications in physical fitness and using creativity to include personal interests such as dancing and her faith.

PROFILE 2

Susan Ayres, DTR, began her career in dietetics working as a menu clerk in a local hospital. In just a short period of time, she realized that she wanted more in life and enrolled in a dietetic technician program. Following her graduation, Sue's first position was as a management dietetic technician. Her job included supervising tray-service personnel, developing procedures for in-service training, upholding sanitation standards, and assisting with catering.

After 2 years, Sue moved to the clinical arena, where her main focus was the cardiac patient. For a period of 12 years, Sue educated patients on the Prudent, or low-cholesterol diet, and became an active member of the local American Heart Association Nutrition Task Force Committee and the York County Nutrition Education Committee.

In 1980, a new door opened for Sue. She was appointed to serve on the American Dietetic Association's Council on Practice Quality Assurance Committee, where she assisted with the developing of the Standards of Practice. This was followed by her appointment to the Commission on Dietetic Registration as the first dietetic technician registered member.

By 1989, after 15 years of being employed as a hospital dietetic technician, Sue wanted a new challenge, so she interviewed and won a position as Food Service Director of the Dallastown Area School District in Pennsylvania. In this position, Sue feeds approximately 6,000 students at the elementary and secondary-school levels. She manages a staff of 75 employees at eight different schools. Her knowledge of nutrition and her skills as a manager complement her ability to provide nutritious lunches at minimal cost, while ensuring compliance with both government regulations and dietary guidelines. As director, Sue also purchases all food and supplies needed by the schools and assists in the financial policy planning. She also serves as co-chair of the District Wellness Committee and oversees student nutrition committees in all buildings. Sue implemented Birthday Baskets in the elementary schools for parents to purchase healthy snacks. She is also running a pilot program of after school Food, Fun and Fitness classes with the school nurse. In addition, she is conference chair for the State Board of the School Nutrition Association and a preceptor for dietetic interns from the University of Delaware. As Sue says, "the job is never boring."

Sue feels that she acquired this position simply by doing her homework. She states it is important to "contact someone who has a similar position and be prepared to ask questions; research the history of the facility; know your potential customers and products; and lastly, stage a mock interview to help reduce anxiety and increase self-confidence."

PROFILE 3

Ann Murdock, DTR, has been the Dietary Director at the Texas Masonic Retirement Center in Arlington, Texas for the past 11 years. She manages a kitchen that provides meals for approximately 175 residents and supervises 16 employees. She also develops menus for both the retirement center and the nursing home section of the facility. She does assessments and develops care plans for the nursing home residents. Ann has also assumed the responsibility of maintaining care plan scheduling to assure that regulatory standards are met.

Ann began her career by working as an unskilled relief cook, dishwasher, and stacker in an extended care facility. As she learned about therapeutic diets, her interest in food service and nutrition emerged. To further herself in the field, Ann enrolled in a dietary managers training program. Upon completion of this program, she received a certificate qualifying her to manage a food service department. This, however, did not completely satisfy Ann's thirst for knowledge. She decided that if she were to go any further in the field, she would have to enroll in the dietetic technician program.

During the time Ann pursued her education, she became Food Service Supervisor for an extended care facility that was in the process of enlarging. This immediately thrust Ann into the middle of a construction project. Not only did she have to contend with the retraining of staff to meet the increased needs of the department, but she found herself spending a large part of her day meeting with construction workers, plumbers, and electricians.

After 7 years of employment at this facility, Ann was ready for a new challenge. She took a position as Nutrition Service Supervisor at a newly built hospital, where she assumed the purchasing functions, revised the cafeteria menu to offer more selections, and upgraded internal catering, all while investigating ways to provide outside catering. As time progressed, Ann became Associate Director, with full management responsibility of the department. Unfortunately, the facility's lack of growth forced the downsizing of services and staff, and Ann did not find the position as appealing as it once was.

It was then that she moved to the position of Director of Nutrition Services at HCA Denton Community Hospital in Denton, Texas, a 104-bed acute care facility, for 5 years. Her responsibilities as director of a small hospital were many and varied. Ann oversaw the complete operations of food production, patient tray service, cafeteria, and catering. She was responsible for developing departmental policies and procedures, as well as fiscal and capital budgets; procuring all food and supplies needed in the department; hiring, training, and evaluating all employees; and maintaining the physical environment to meet the required sanitation standards.

Ann feels that the dietetic technician program gave her a good knowledge base on which to build and develop her skills. She says, "The combination of nutrition and management classes was good, but I feel the benefit of classes in personnel management, psychology, and sociology are often not realized until you are out there on the job and find yourself in situations that you can relate directly back to a class."

PROFILE 4

Lynne Hassard, DTR, has been employed for 8 years at Panera Bread Company in Missouri and is now Senior Quality Assurance Manager. She manages all nutrition information provided to customers. She also attends meetings to develop products to satisfy consumer trends. Ensuring food safety is the largest component of her job.

Prior to her position at Panera, Lynne was employed as a Nutrition Consultant for Hazelwood Farms Bakeries for 9 years. She started out there as a part-time, temporary employee. Upon hiring, it was her responsibility to collect nutrition information on all ingredients used in the bakery products. This data, when entered into the computer, produced a nutritional analysis on all Hazelwood Farms products. Lynne also baked and tested products.

As Lynne's term of employment increased, so did her responsibilities. Her position expanded to permanent full-time with the Nutrition Labeling and Education Act to include labeling of products

and ensuring their conformance to governmental regulations. Lynne's other duties included sensory evaluation or taste testing during product development, approval of all raw ingredients used at Hazelwood Farms, and the providing of nutrition information to staff, customers, and consumers. Lynne also helped market products.

Lynne finds her career very challenging and rewarding. She feels that if the local hospital had had a dietetic technician position open when she graduated, her career would have taken the usual path. Says Lynne, "I learned to accept new challenges and overcome the fear that sometimes accompanies them. I have always volunteered to do whatever needs doing, even if it is outside my general job description. I try to give a little more than what is asked for in order to prove myself capable and willing."

PROFILE 5

Bob Wilson is truly a nontraditional DTR. He graduated with honors with a Bachelor of Science degree in biology, then earned a degree as a dietetic technician, and also has extensive personal experience and expertise in weight management. He has worked as a Nutrition Specialist at Kaiser Permanente Northwest, under dietitians' supervision at the Department of Health Education Services for 18 years. He teaches the "Freedom from Diets" program, involving 75 people in four classes per week. Many members are morbidly obese (300 to 700 pounds). He also does community and worksite wellness outreach for Kaiser. Bob offers a telephone coaching weight management service for members. After attending the weight management classes, members can sign up for additional support.

In his own wellness practice, he guides clients toward a discovery of a "healthy eating lifestyle plan" that works for them, while focusing on "self-acceptance and self-love." Bob developed his own holistic free wellness website and does lifestyle and weight management coaching.

What special qualifications does Bob have to be an expert in the field of weight management? Bob's interest in weight management originated out of personal experience. He relates that at an early age he "started using food as a comfort due to family problems," and by age 16, he weighed about 400 pounds. In 1972, Bob started to take control of his life. He joined Weight Watchers and lost 118 pounds in 7 months. To help overcome his compulsive eating, Bob worked with a twelve-step program; and he has maintained his weight around 155 pounds for 35 years.

Through these programs, Bob first experienced the concepts of practical and delicious nutrition. His success in losing weight inspired him so much that he wanted to work in the community helping overweight people to make lifestyle changes. Aware of his goal, but feeling unprepared, he chose to pursue studies in the field of nutrition at a local community college. Upon completion of his degree, he was ready to pursue his dream and offer a more highly educated option to the public than those found at most weight-loss centers.

Bob began to co-instruct the Body Shop Program for overweight children, and developed and taught a series of weight-management classes. His talents did not go unnoticed. In 1987, Bob was offered a position under dietitians' supervision at the West Metro Food Compulsions Clinic and then at the Oregon Dietitians' Clinic. Later, he became a behavioral educator for a medically supervised fasting program. Because of his entertaining speaking skills and empathetic personality, Bob is a big hit with people who want to lose weight.

All of Bob's knowledge and experience culminated in writing for his website and he has plans for a self-help workbook to aid individuals in identifying workable options for permanent lifestyle changes.

PROFILE 6

Jinny Elder, DTR, is President of Energy Enterprises in Carlsbad, California. She holds a BA from San Diego State University in Foods and Nutrition. Jinny began her career path working in a clinical setting as a Dietetic Technician/Food Service Supervisor for 30 employees where, as part of a medical team of dietitians and physicians, she counseled patients on special diets.

After 3 years, Jinny decided to leave the traditional clinical setting to pursue other avenues of interest, which included work in restaurant management and as a food broker in sales and manufacturing. Here she became involved in staff training, product promotions, food show management, demonstration services, marketing, and health care sales. Always interested in expanding her horizons, Jinny also began designing and presenting nutrition-oriented cooking classes together with a professional chef to enlighten and educate receptive audiences on the importance of their daily food choices—for weight management, stress reduction, and overall well being.

In 1998, Energy Enterprises was born. An entrepreneur at heart, Jinny saw an opportunity in the diet/nutrition field that was wide open. Armed with years of experience in all aspects of the diet and nutrition field, she acquired state-of-the-art software capable of analyzing over 27,000 ingredients and 165 nutrients providing detailed and accurate nutritional analyses for recipes. With her marketing and sales background, Jinny soon acquired major clients in the food industry.

As President of Energy Enterprises, Jinny consults with many companies, nationally and internationally, including grocery stores, restaurants, catering companies, food manufacturers, hotels, fitness centers, school lunch programs, and health care facilities. With an eye for detail and a dedication to her clients, Jinny oversees all projects and ensures clients receive excellent service and quality products.

In addition to recipe analysis, it was a natural transition into the food-labeling arena where Energy Enterprises provides full label review following FDA labeling guidelines for both U.S. and international companies. Jinny and her staff create camera-ready nutritional labels, which meet strict FDA guidelines for a variety of retail food products in many formats and in several languages.

Jinny enjoys helping other small companies grow and succeed and attributes her success to an ability to take calculated risks and act—with hard work and persistence. In her own words: "In the end, success is really the sum of small efforts, repeated day in and day out, and excellence is therefore not an act, but a habit."

SUMMARY

The preceding sampling of dietetic technicians is just that—only a sampling. The two-year dietetic technician programs across the country have provided students with a solid knowledge base that can be utilized in the various practice settings. Today's dietetic technician, however, is an innovator, willing to take that knowledge and creatively expand on it, moving from traditional to nontraditional roles.

Dietetic technicians need to take the risks of charting their own courses. Boundless opportunities are available. The challenge is to recognize your talents and skills, have faith in yourself, and, in the words of Henry David Thoreau, "Go confidently in the direction of your dreams."

QUICK "HOW TO" REFERENCE

20

HOW TO SELL

Kathy King, RD, LD

Building a business with traditional advertising is a slow process. Advertising often succeeds in entertaining the public without selling the product. Is there a profitable alternative? (1).

Selling is the alternative that keeps businesses alive and well. Improving your sales negotiation skills can make you more successful in whatever area of dietetics practice you choose. In health care, most of us are not comfortable with "hard sell" tactics—we equate them with time-share and used car selling. Ethically in health care, we are supposed to offer a patient the options of care and therapy, explaining the pros and cons of each, and then allow the patient or his or her family to make the decision whether to purchase.

When selling your nutrition therapy services to individuals in a private practice, ask what their needs are, and listen attentively. Then present the benefits of your service that match those needs. Hard selling is not appropriate because the timing and motivation for behavior change have to come from the patient. The patient's apathy or getting free self-help information on the Internet is sometimes more competition than a clinic or another nutrition professional in the area.

Outside of patient care, in fitness centers, wellness programs, consulting to businesses, food-service management, kitchen equipment sales, pharmaceutical sales, and other management or inventory control positions, it is necessary to be proficient in sales. Everyone, of course, wants to offer products or services that are in such demand that they "sell themselves," but that is a rarity. Also as you surely have heard before, we negotiate and sell everyday in our private lives in one way or another—in order to get what we want from other people. Therefore, it stands to reason that sales are

skills you should know better—if nothing else, you need to know when a salesperson is using sales ploys to manipulate you.

SALES NEGOTIATIONS ARE CHANGING

Roger Dawson, one of America's top experts on sales negotiation, believes the roles of the salesperson are changing because (2):

- Customers are becoming better negotiators—they want better deals and are using sales strategies to improve their bottom lines. With all costs going up, the natural, easiest way to pay less is to negotiate and seek better deals. All of us hate feeling like we were talked into something we did not want or need.
- Customers are better informed—they will go to other sources like the Internet if the product or service is too expensive, or the sale process is too difficult. Nutrition information used to be a unique body of knowledge "owned" by our profession—that is no longer the case, so we have to offer more value or compete on price (the latter is not the best option).

FOUR STAGES OF THE SALES PRESENTATION

Before starting the stages of the presentation, do your homework. Get to know the customer, the market the customer works in, the buyer's organization, and the competing products or services.

"Google" the customer and read his website. Plan your strategies. If you are approaching a business, try to get an appointment with the highest-ranking decision maker possible. If the person or company has real problems like many complaints at the Better Business Bureau or poor Dun & Bradstreet ranking, know that before you set up an appointment. Do not let their problems become yours. If you know that they have a reputation for not paying bills on time, do not begin a contract without half the payment up-front or some other similar safeguard.

STAGE ONE: OPENING OR INTRODUCTION

The purpose of this stage is to establish rapport and common ground. You want to break down the barriers between you and the potential customer and begin differentiating yourself from your competition.

STAGE TWO: INVESTIGATION AND INFORMATION GATHERING

This is one of the most important functions. Qualify the prospect. How interested is he? Is he the decision maker? How soon does he need the product or service? Ask open-ended questions and listen carefully to the answers—never interrupt. Get the buyer to define his or her needs, wants, and expectations. The information obtained in this exchange will help you personalize your presentation and perhaps think of new products or services to offer. Move on and do not waste more time if there is no interest in ever buying your product or service—leave the person with your contact information and some words of wisdom about how your product can save them time, money, health care dollars, or whatever (3).

STAGE THREE: PRESENTATION

During this phase, present facts that you carefully chose for effect on this customer. A good presentation will invoke the prospect to ask questions. Show how his or her needs will be met by what you have to offer. Potential buyers base their decisions on fact and emotion—"This may not be the most expensive product on the market, but it works as well, it offers great customer support, and it will make you *feel* good because you did not pay twice as much." Foremost on every prospect's mind is the question "What's in it for me?" (4). If you can answer this question during your presentation, you are on your way to converting a prospect to a purchaser (4). The presentation stage should

be about 75% of the sales call. That means that you need to know your product or service very well. The outcome of this stage should be a natural progression to the close.

STAGE FOUR: CLOSE

This is the time to bring the sales call to closure, either by asking for a sale or other commitment. One approach is to summarize the client's needs and match them with your solutions. Ask when you can begin, or when he wants to schedule an appointment, or how you can provide more assistance. Your purpose may have been only to introduce yourself and explain your services. Even if the prospect is not interested at this time, leave the session as friends and on a positive note. Do not give up. Look for the next opportunity to present this product or new ones to that prospective client.

After the sales call, write a note thanking the prospect for his or her time.

IMPORTANT POINTS TO REMEMBER

The early moves in negotiations set the tone and may win or lose the sale for you, so consider them carefully. Although we are told to strive for a win-win solution, some experts think that means neither gets what they need instead of both are satisfied (2–4).

- *Figure out what you need to end up with before you start negotiating.* Work your numbers and factor in all your expenses, so that you cover all costs, have a cushion for unexpected overruns, and make a profit with each sale.
- *Ask for more than you expect to get.* In the normal give-and-take of a negotiation, you may have to give up something. Going in on the high side also raises the perceived value of your product or service, provides plenty of "wiggle room" for negotiations, makes it look like you are working with the client as you offer a counter solution to his or her response.
- *Try a flinch.* You might flinch in surprise as a reaction to a proposal from the buyer. They may not expect to get what they are asking for, but if you do not act surprised, they will think their highest offer is a possibility. Seventy percent of the people with whom you deal in a negotiation are visual and will react when they see you flinch. Think about the last time someone wanted to sell you something at a very high price, did you flinch? Did it make a difference? If they could not change the price, they maybe threw in something as a bonus.

- *Seldom say "yes" to the first offer or counteroffer.* They will think they could have done better and be sorry they did not ask for a lower price or more concessions. They may leave unsatisfied, and you will be kicking yourself if you find out that they expected more bells and whistles for that price. Take the time to explore all the included expectations *before* you agree. Consider asking immediately for a concession of similar size when the buyer asks for one. For example, if they want a big reduction in price, that would mean you have to remove some of the services or sell the less expensive product instead—something they may not want.
- *The challenge is to get the buyer to indicate his bottom line first.* You might do this by asking, "If I can get my supervisor down to $____, would that work for you?" or "I can reduce the price to $____ if I took away this extra feature, would that work for you?" You might try adding an attractive feature to the basic product or service, like four revisits or an employee wellness health risk appraisal for a modest price increase and if the buyers show interest, you know they could pay more.

In the middle of negotiations, give-and-take keep the momentum going, but you need to keep them going in your direction (2–4):

- *Differentiate yourself and your product from your competitors.* Knowing how you are unique lets you sell that much more confidently and effectively.
- *Appeal to a higher authority.* Both sides can use this tactic—it takes the pressure off your shoulders and defers making an immediate decision. (Have you bought a car recently? This is where your salesperson says, "Boy, I will have to ask my manager if we can do that.") This can be frustrating too because you find out that there is someone else who has to approve the agreement—and he is not there.
- *Keep the negotiations on the issues, do not take them personally!* Even when the other side makes a negative comment, has flashes of anger, or belittles your new business—keep cool. Take the high road; evaluate whether you want to even work with them, but also consider that this may be deliberate drama to better control the negotiations.
- *Avoid confrontation.* This often makes both sides dig in for the fight or want to walk away—neither option is productive. Add some humor. Return to common ground and remember why you wanted to meet. What can you do to make the buyer's life happier and healthier?

- *Good Guy/Bad Guy strategies really work—either side can use this.* This is where two or more negotiators work together to soften up the other side. One stays tough and plays hard-nosed while the other tries to be friendly and bring about an agreement. This is so obvious sometimes that it may not work. This strategy is diffused when it is pointed out—do not be suckered in.
- *It sometimes helps to show the impressive list of your other clients.* People like to be in good company; they want to feel this is a good decision.

Closing the call takes strategy (2,5):

- *Eliminate distractions.* Keep the client focused and the message on track.
- *Be enthusiastic.* Your happy words and spirit will help the client feel this is the right decision.
- *Emphasize the emotional aspects of the sale.* People make decisions emotionally and then defend them with logic. Get them thinking about how they will feel when they reduce their employees' health care insurance costs by 10% to 20% while improving morale and reducing absenteeism.
- *Be direct.* Do a summary, adding the emotion and then say, "We can start weight loss classes as soon as you can sign people up—hopefully in two weeks—if you agree today."
- *Stop talking.* Stay quiet until the client gives you an answer. They will either give you an answer or give you an objection—then you talk.
- *Watch out for nibbling after the sale.* They want little concessions to be included with the final agreement that were never discussed earlier. Try to counter this by tying up all loose ends and details while making the other party feel like he or she already won.
- *Always remember that you have the option of withdrawing the offer.* Never be so needy that walking away and settling for a bad agreement is your only option.
- *To sweeten the deal at the very end, you might offer a service or concession you had earlier highly valued.* This may be the deal-maker you needed to make the agreement happen.
- *Get it in writing BEFORE you begin and offer to write the agreement.* Do not assume anything. There will always be small points that need clarification. Get them ironed out before any work is done or products are transferred—even when they say they must have them immediately. Bring back the agreement the next day.
- *If the sale did not happen, leave on good terms and call again another day.*

FOUR REASONS PROSPECTS BUY (4)

1. PROFIT

Using your service or product will decrease medical expenses, or sell more food in the cafeteria to increase revenues.

2. PIECE OF MIND

Buyers want a product that saves time, reduces aggravation, protects their interest, or solves their problem.

3. PAIN (OR LACK THEREOF)

Buyers want to be protected from conflict, embarrassment, or loss.

4. PRIDE

Everyone wants to be admired, appreciated, accepted, recognized, and feel good about their decisions.

FOUR REASONS PROSPECTS DO NOT BUY (4)

1. TIME

Most buyers do not have time to research and consider new products and services—so they do not take the time.

2. FEAR

Most buyers fear making the wrong decision, so they do not make any decision—they stay with the familiar status quo.

3. BUDGET

There is no money in the budget to purchase your product at this time—priorities must be set when money is tight.

4. AUTHORITY

Prospect does not have the authority to place an order.

CASE STUDY 20.1

NONTRADITIONAL SALES POSITION

Carolyn Brown, RD, Director, eRecovery, Cardinal Health Supply Chain Services, Pharmaceutical

Every day, I still use the communication and presentation skills that I learned in my college curriculum and dietetic internship. My current position is Director of Marketing in the pharmaceutical supply chain segment of a large global health care company with annual revenue in excess of $87 billion.

I began my career over 30 years ago in the field of dietetics working in hospitals. As family obligations grew, I needed a more flexible work schedule and pursued consulting in long-term care facilities.

When I was ready to go back to work full-time, sales was a logical next step. My first sales position was entry level in a dietetics-related field; however, these skills are transferable to sales in any field. Over the next 15 years, I progressed upward until I reached a plateau in the company where I worked. So, the next step was to move to a larger company with a broader range of products and services, and eventually to an even larger company. Along the way, I took as many seminars in sales, marketing, and presentation as I could, which included a Certification in Marketing from Ohio State University.

The most difficult thing for me was public speaking, especially when presenting to the C-suite (this includes the chief executives, like CEO [Chief Executive Officer], COO [Chief Operating Officer] and CFO [Chief Financial Officer]). It is important to be concise and to present only relevant facts without too much detail due to the time constraints of most executives. Oh, and by the way, your style also must be interesting and engaging.

And finally, a good understanding of business is the foundation of any career. You must be able to answer the following questions for any potential customer. Why do something or change the way it is done? Why now? Why with you or your company? All of the talking points and financial facts in your business presentation must answer these questions.

In summary, the best advice I can give you to prepare for this type of career is to take every opportunity available to market yourself:

- Be active in professional associations—volunteer for committees and run for office.
- Volunteer in your community to do things that promote good nutrition and the dietitian as the nutrition expert.
- Network with your peers in dietetics, as well as other professionals outside of dietetics.
- Look for public speaking opportunities.
- Join a public speaking group such as Toastmasters.
- Keep up to date with technology and become skilled with presentation programs, such as PowerPoint.
- Enroll in sales, marketing, and business seminars or courses.

SUMMARY

Selling does not come easy for many people—that is why you must study the art of the game and practice, practice, practice. This is a game of strategy. Once you know your product or service and you believe it can help other people, create a list of benefits and ways it differs from the competition. Role play to practice the various stages of the sales call. Practice what you would say given different client responses—even what you would do if the prospect became angry. With practice, experience, and adopting the attitude that this is a game you want to win, selling becomes second nature.

REFERENCES

1. Wright GA. *Retail Service & Marketing Support*. Denver, CO; 1998.
2. Dawson R. Secrets of Power Negotiating for Salespeople. In: *Executive Book Summaries*. Concordville, PA; 2000.
3. McGarvey R. Ice Cubes to Eskimos. *Entrepreneur* August 2000.
4. Socrates Media, LLC. *Sell Like a Pro*. Chicago, IL; 2004.
5. Hopkins T. *Sales Closing for Dummies*. New York: John Wiley & Sons; 1998.

HOW TO MARKET NUTRITION IN THE SUPERMARKET

21

Linda McDonald, MS, RD, LD

There has never been a better time or reason for dietetic professionals to market nutrition where most food decisions are made: the supermarket. Advances in biotechnology and medical research have made foods tailored to health needs a reality. There is margarine that helps fight heart disease, orange juice that works to prevent osteoporosis, teas with herbs aimed at calming your nerves and yogurts with probiotics to assist with digestion.

These new options at the supermarket put consumers as well as dietetic professionals in an interesting position. Consumers need help and dietetic professionals are equipped to provide the nutrition education they request.

More Americans are seeking information on food and nutrition, turning to healthful eating messages, and taking action to improve their nutrition and health than at any time in the past decade, according to findings of the American Dietetic Association's nationwide public opinion survey, *Nutrition and You: Trends 2002* (1).

The latest *Shopping for Health Trends Survey* by the Food Marketing Institute (FMI) says that grocery shoppers see the connection between diet and health and are generally dissatisfied with the healthfulness of their diets. More people are trying to move toward healthier diets. This move toward healthier eating is broad based and growing. Shoppers are looking for guidance when putting together food plans to help with both weight loss and specific health concerns. Those retailers who can best assist shoppers will increase the spending and loyalty of these customers (2).

For the most part, the nation's shoppers do not think their eating habits are particularly healthful—52% think their diets could be at least somewhat more healthy, and another 18% figure their diets could be a lot more healthful (3). With two-thirds of Americans overweight or obese, it is not surprising that a total of 86% of shoppers have some level of concern about the nutritional content of their food consumption (3).

Information on fat and cholesterol content are most important to shoppers when reading the nutrition facts panel. In fact, 51% of shoppers consider the fat content very important, supplemented by 46% who have a high interest in trans fat levels. The importance of trans fat jumped 7% as general awareness increased with the introduction of trans fat in the Nutrition Facts Box. With recent media coverage about health implications of trans fats and mandatory labeling in place since January 1, 2006, awareness of trans fat jumped from 84% in 2005 to 91% in 2006. Sugar and whole grains round out the top five ingredients of interest to shoppers (3).

Shopping for Health reports that shoppers are interested in having store staff available to answer questions about nutrition, and half of all shoppers indicate they would be likely to use this service (2). Who is better qualified to answer these questions or train the supermarket staff than the dietetic professional?

SUPERMARKET INDUSTRY BASICS

The supermarket business is highly competitive with retailers often working on a 1% to 2% profit margin. Supermarkets make a profit through volume, which mainly reflects customer loyalty. A lifetime customer may be worth $100,000 to a retailer, which is why retailers make an effort to understand and anticipate the needs and desires of their customers.

FMI's Trends 2006 (3) reports that shoppers make an average of 2.1 visits to a grocery store each week and spend an average of $93.40 on groceries weekly. They also say that while price and location are both powerful drivers behind store and product choices, consumers point at a clean, neat store, and high-quality fruits, vegetables, and meats as the most important factors when choosing a store. They suggest that the focus for improvements be on low prices and faster store environment. Consumers continue to engage in economizing measures, both pre-trip and in the store, ranging from participation in frequent shopper programs, making lists, purchasing store brand products, and clipping coupons.

Although nutrition is not mentioned as a top priority by the FMI consumer survey, it is a service that although only available to 64% of shoppers is utilized at least once a month by a least half of shoppers (3). Nutrition information falls in a value-added category where the service is not highly prized or highly rated but in some stores nutrition programs outperform these statistics because of the competitive edge they provide. Good examples are Whole Foods and Wild Oats, recognized and sought out by shoppers for their nutrition and health information.

In fact, many retailers have increased their efforts to educate consumers about the effects of nutrition on overall health, says *FMI Trends 2006* (3). The supermarket does not appear to be a primary source of information for many shoppers, but it does play a role in the overall information-gathering process.

Almost one in three shoppers (28%) uses nutrition information provided by their grocery store on a regular basis. Slightly less than half (49%) are very or somewhat satisfied with the nutrition information provided at the store. Shoppers who use the store's information on a regular basis are slightly more positive than the general shopper with 57% either very or somewhat satisfied, indicating room for improvement (3).

A nutrition program can increase customer loyalty and enhance the supermarket's position in the community. The *FMI Trends 2006* (3) report concluded that there are three areas that retailers should focus on. They are:

- Quick, easy, and tasty meal time solutions.
- Easy-to-understand and assimilate nutrition education.
- Confidence in the safety of the food.

CAREER OPPORTUNITIES

Dietitians have worked in supermarkets for decades, but only in the past few years has their involvement become more of a standard than an exception. For example, Hy-Vee, a supermarket chain based in Des Moines, Iowa, has recently hired 100 registered dietitians to serve its 199 Midwestern locations. Here are a few of the many career opportunities for dietetic professionals working in supermarkets:

CONSUMER AFFAIRS SPECIALIST

The most common position for a registered dietitian (RD) to hold in a supermarket is as a Consumer Affairs Specialist. Consumer affairs positions typically have numerous responsibilities in addition to nutrition programs that may include consumer boards, corporate donations, customer complaints, consumer information, public affairs, recipe programs, etc.

Example: Shari Steinbach, MS, RD, is Director of Consumer Affairs for Spartan Stores, Inc., in Grand Rapids, Michigan. Her responsibilities include managing all community donations, sponsorships, and events (http://www.spartanstores.com).

CORPORATE NUTRITIONIST

Rather than working in one supermarket, a corporate nutritionist sets corporate policy for all the supermarkets in the system and educates employees or hires dietitians to implement programs on a local level.

Example: Jane Andrews, MS, RD, Corporate Nutritionist for Wegmans Food Markets, advocates for healthful eating at every level of the company, from clerks to executives. In addition, she manages the many facets of consumer nutrition education for the total chain (http://www.wegmans.com).

MARKETING/ADVERTISING DEPARTMENT

The dietetic professional assists these departments by developing health-related and nutrition-related promotions and campaigns. A spokesperson will represent the supermarket to the public via the mass media—newspaper articles, TV commercials, advertisements, supermarket flyers, website, etc. She/he will be asked to speak to community groups such as women's clubs, parent organizations, school classes, etc.

Example: Kim Kirchherr, MS, RD, LDN, CDE, Corporate Dietitian and Spokesperson for Jewel-Osco, worked with ABC News *This Morning Show*'s "Shopping Challenge" to assess the food choices made by four shoppers at the Jewel-Osco supermarket.

PRODUCT DEVELOPMENT

Branded food products by supermarkets are popular. An RD with product development or food technology experience would be a valuable asset to a supermarket. Quality assurance, nutrition and ingredient labeling, regulatory compliance, and sensory testing are all parts of product development.

Example: Janet Tenney, MS, RD, is responsible for the oversight of nutrition programs, consumer food safety information, and labeling concerns for bakery and deli private label products for Giant Food (http://www.giantfood.com).

MEAL SOLUTIONS

Eating more meals together is a challenge for families and you can help by developing quick, delicious, nutritious, and affordable meal solutions. The solutions can be anything from cross-merchandising prepared foods to offering recipes and ingredients in one location for one-stop shopping or developing healthy foods in delis and in store restaurants or meal solutions for takeout.

Example: One of the programs developed by Janet Tenney, MS, RD, at Giant Food is a Meal Solution program entitled "5 in 30." Each recipe can be prepared in 30 minutes or less using no more than 5 ingredients (http://www.giantfood.com).

FOOD SAFETY

Hazard Analysis Critical Control Point (HACCP) is the required USDA program for food safety that must be implemented in all supermarkets. Implementing this program and conducting employee training is needed by all supermarkets. Dietetic professionals who can provide both nutrition and food safety functions for a supermarket are much more marketable.

Example: The SuperSafeMark food safety and sanitation training and certification program was developed by the Food Marketing Institute and is specifically for supermarket employees and covers the typical activities and equipment found in supermarkets (http://www.supersafemark.com).

PHARMACY DEPARTMENT/MEDICAL CLINIC

Many supermarkets are incorporating Pharmacies and Medical Clinics in their facilities as a convenience to consumers. This makes it easier for customers to manage conditions such as diabetes, hyperlipidemia, and hypertension. Creating nutrition programs that tie the pharmacy and/or medical clinic to the supermarket will benefit everyone.

Example: Living Healthy with Diabetes is Ukrop's ADA-approved program that includes private counseling, classes, store tours, and seminars. Ukrop's corporate dietitians and store pharmacists coordinate this program (http://www.ukrops.com/pharmacy/diabetes_03/diabetes_2.asp).

NATURAL FOODS/ORGANICS

The divide between a basic supermarket and a health food store has disappeared with many retailers setting up a "store within a store" concept with an extensive selection of natural products. Dietetic professionals who are educated in this area can help a retailer select and market natural and organic products and help them educate consumers.

Example: Safeway has a branded organic line of processed foods called "O Organics." The line encompasses hundreds of products for adults and recently announced plans to expand the line into foods for babies and children up to age 12. Safeway competes with Whole Foods Markets, the nation's largest seller of natural and organic food products.

RESEARCH

As technology takes over the retail food industry, there are unique ways to tie this technology to research and to tailor nutrition education to specific nutrient needs with precise messages. Supermarket carts with computers, called Smart Carts, could carry targeted nutrition messages along with coupons and recipes for healthy foods.

Example: Researchers from the University of Texas developed a method using marketing research data from a frequent shopper program at HEB and matching it with Universal Product Code numbers to assess food purchase behavior and consequent nutrient availability to evaluate intervention effects (4).

SKILLS NEEDED

Other skills besides nutrition knowledge are required to be successful in the supermarket industry. Not only will you need to market yourself, but you will also need to communicate messages and fit into an extremely competitive business atmosphere.

- Business Skills—Supermarkets are business endeavors working on slim margins. You will need to write proposals, prepare budgets, evaluate results, and demonstrate positive results that impact the bottom line.
- Creativity—Because the supermarket industry is so competitive, you will need to constantly come up with innovative ideas that not only catch the consumers' eye but also set you apart from the competition.

- Communications—Whether it is written or spoken, your words are important. You will need to be an excellent communicator. To communicate effectively, you need to know your audience and relay useful information that they can understand and will retain.
- Networking—Nothing is done independently. You will need a network of professionals both inside and outside the supermarket to help you solve problems and stay current on trends and information.
- Writing—Not only will you need to write proposals that sell your ideas to your bosses, but much of your communication with consumers will be through the written word. Your position may involve writing newsletters, articles, website columns, weekly ads, tip sheets, or other corporate publications.
- Public Speaking—Whether it is pitching an idea to the boss, teaching a class, or representing your supermarket to the media, you had better feel comfortable in front of an audience.

MARKETING YOURSELF AND YOUR SERVICES

Before approaching the supermarket, you need to think about how you will sell yourself and your services. Why will the supermarket want to promote your programs? What sets you and your services apart from what is already being offered either in this supermarket or in competitive stores? You need to think about and answer the following questions:

WHAT EXPERIENCE DO YOU HAVE THAT WILL BENEFIT THE SUPERMARKET?

Have you been a clinical dietitian in a local hospital struggling to educate clients who are not ready to learn while in the hospital? Have you worked with local diabetes, weight control, or cardiovascular rehabilitation programs? Have you developed and delivered nutrition classes that were successful? Do you have examples, newspaper articles, samples of marketing tools, etc.? Anything you have that will showcase your expertise will help sell you.

HOW WILL YOUR SERVICES ATTRACT NEW CUSTOMERS TO THE SUPERMARKET?

First you need to know who the supermarket's customers are and how they are presently attracting customers. Visit the store and observe the present

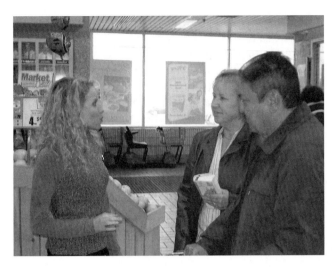

FIGURE 21.1.   ■   Lyssie Lakatos, RD, CDN, CFT—Discussing nutrition with clients at Tops in Buffalo, NY.

customers. Check out the way the store advertises. Where and how are they attracting customers? How can you attract additional customers? Would your diabetes patients follow you to this location for education? Studies show that when a person has attended a tour in a supermarket, they are more likely to come back to that store (Fig. 21.1).

HOW WILL YOUR SERVICES HELP RETAIN PRESENT CUSTOMERS OR KEEP THEM SATISFIED?

Think about what the present customers might need in terms of information. Look at statistics from FMI on what customers are looking for in supermarkets. What new nutrition issues need to be addressed? Have customers been requesting more information?

HOW WILL YOUR SERVICES IMPACT THE SUPERMARKET'S BOTTOM LINE (I.E., SALES/MONEY)?

Nothing will sell you and your services to the supermarket employer more than if you can convince him that you can *bring new dedicated customers into the store or get customers to buy more products.* These are the things that you should focus on in your planning and evaluation.

HOW WILL YOU MEASURE YOUR IMPACT ON THE SUPERMARKET?

Measuring the effectiveness of your services in specific numbers is imperative. Retail foods work on a very slim margin of profits and every aspect of their business must show a profit. Whether you measure the number of customers you impact with your message, the number of new customers you attract to the supermarket, the increase in sales of a particular product or category of products based on your recommendation, or the number of customer questions you have answered. Be sure to include an evaluation component to each project that you provide for the supermarket.

HOW WILL YOUR SERVICES BENEFIT OTHER EMPLOYEES?

Remember that you are part of a team of employees that need to work together to make the supermarket successful. You want to look good, but you cannot do that at the expense of the other employees; and if you all look good, even better. How can you help the other employees? Can you provide in-service training on nutrition issues that will help them answer customer questions? Can you provide HACCP training so that they can be accredited? Can you suggest changes to recipes in the deli that will make their food healthier and therefore more appealing?

WHO PAYS FOR YOUR SERVICES AND PROGRAMS?

There are many ways for a supermarket to fund nutrition and food safety programs. Costs can be included in the supermarket budget under specific departments, depending on the service provided. These funds may be spread around under marketing or advertising or specific departments such as deli or produce. Programs can also have vendor sponsorship where vendors pay a fee to have their logo or foods included in a program's educational materials, tasting, or cooking class.

PROGRAM IDEAS

ASSOCIATE TRAINING PROGRAM

When shoppers focus on their health, they look for help, and 56% of shoppers say that they first seek supermarket staff who can answer nutrition questions. Employee training programs often incorporate general nutrition and food safety topics to better enable employees to answer basic questions. Shoppers are interested in having store staff available to answer questions about nutrition, and half of all shoppers indicate they would be likely to pursue this service.

Example: Sandi Davis, MS, RD, LD, was hired by Wal-Mart to provide nutrition education to employees—more than a million of them. She started by focusing on Wal-Mart's Arkansas home campus, making healthy food recommendations for nine cafeterias that serve over 12,000 employees and teaching classes at Wal-Mart's fitness center.

COOKING CLASSES

Cooking classes are back in vogue and many supermarkets include classrooms with demo areas for classes (Fig. 21.2). Not only should you be able to provide a cooking and nutrition class, but you should also coordinate classes featuring guest chefs, local celebrities, and cookbook authors. Topics might include Vegetarian Cuisine, Cooking with Whole Grains, and Healthy Gourmet Cooking. You could team up with local chefs, hospitals, The American Cancer Association, or the American Cancer Society.

Example: Brookshire Brothers staged a Fresh Harvest Cooking Show with the help of dietitian Amy McLeod, RD, LD. The show featured a local chef with Amy introducing each recipe and providing health tips.

COMMUNITY OUTREACH PROGRAM

Planning events that appeal to the community, such as health screenings, health fairs, and fitness events such as walks, bike races, and marathons, will bring new customers. You may partner with local schools by providing produce tours for elementary school classes, science projects for junior or senior high kids, speakers for career seminars, fundraising opportunities, etc.

Example: Cindy Silver, MS, RD, LDN, Corporate Nutritionist for Lowes Foods, organizes *Be A*

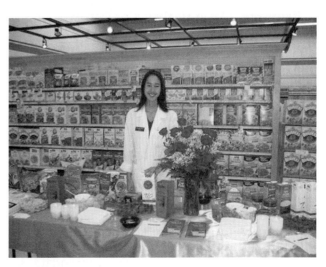

FIGURE 21.2. ■ Courtney Keonin, RD, LD, Hy-Vee Dietitian—In-store healthy cooking demonstrations.

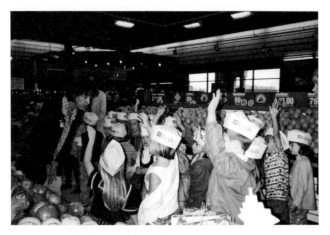

FIGURE 21.3. ■ Cindy Silver interacting with students in Lowes Foods' Be A Smart Shopper Program (BASS). The first graders are learning about different varieties of fruits and vegetables and why they are healthy choices at the supermarket. It is the first of many tour stops these students will make on their 60–minute tour. Our BASS program is in its 11th consecutive year with an expected participation of 25,000 students from preK to 6th grades this year alone. Each year, we offer a new tour theme, healthy sampling and take-home materials to students, and a set of classroom curriculum to teachers.

Smart Shopper!, a hands-on, education-based field trip for children ages 4 to 12 (Fig. 21.3). She reaches 22,000 children through 108 stores a year with this program (http://www.lowesfoods.com).

HEALTH FAIRS

Work with the supermarket Pharmacy or Medical Clinic to provide a health fair that offers health screenings, flu shots, vaccines, and a blood drive. Enhance the event by offering educational materials, coupons for nutritious foods, and healthy food samplings. Team up with local health, fitness, or medical organizations. Be sure to get plenty of publicity.

Example: YMCA Healthy Kids Day is an annual national event that promotes healthy eating and healthy activities for the mind and body. This event, held each April, is a great opportunity to hook up with a local YMCA for a health fair.

NUTRITION AND/OR FOOD SAFETY HOTLINE

Everyone has questions about healthy eating and you are the perfect person to answer those questions. Whether you do this by phone, Internet, or just a box at the check out counter, make sure that you respond to consumers' concerns in a timely manner. Compile customer input and disseminate the questions and answers to the appropriate department in the supermarket.

Example: King Kullen, a New York supermarket chain, provides a toll-free phone number to nutritionist, Layne Lieberman, RD, MS, CDN, who is available to answer questions and offer education as a step toward healthier family nutrition.

NUTRITION LABELING

Knowledge of federal nutrition labeling regulations is important whether you are consulting on supermarket branded products or helping with nutrition information for prepared foods in the deli. See the Resource section of this chapter for information on nutrition labeling references.

Example: Janet Tenney, MS, RD, Manager of Nutrition Programs for Giant Foods, oversees labeling concerns for the bakery and deli private label products.

PHARMACY/MEDICAL CLINIC PROGRAMS

Working with a Pharmacy or Medical Clinic that is actually in your supermarket gives you the opportunity to address clinical issues such as diabetes, heart disease, and hypertension. Programs that integrate nutrition and medical management can make it easier for customers to manage their disease with one-stop shopping for all their food, medical, and pharmacy needs.

Example: Schnucks' Markets in St. Louis provides a certified Diabetes Education Program in cooperation with its pharmacies. The program was developed and is led by a team that includes a nurse, physician sponsor, pharmacist and a dietitian.

POINT OF SALE MATERIALS

Providing nutrition information at the point of sale is effective. This could be a simple nutrition message, a symbol identifying low fat or gluten-free products, or a color-coded system of levels of healthy foods. Several companies have recently come out with small video screens that are activated when a shopper stops in front of them and play a short video advertisement. This would be a perfect venue for a short nutrition message for a healthy food.

Example: Hannaford Supermarkets has a new shelf-label program rating foods throughout the store based on their nutritional content. The Guiding Stars Program assigns from one to three stars, signifying good, better, and best nutritional value, to both packaged goods and fresh items (http://www.hannaford.com).

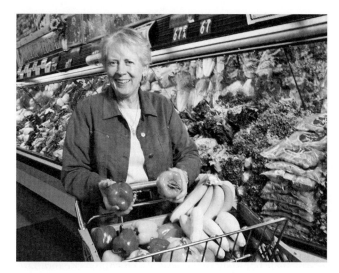

FIGURE 21.4. ■ Linda McDonald in the produce department of a supermarket discussing the importance of getting a variety of colors of vegetables and fruits in the diet.

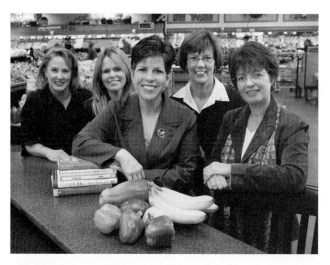

FIGURE 21.5. ■ Ask Wegmans Nutritionists. Pictured on the website are Trish Kazacos, RD, CPT; Jen Felice, RD; Jane Andrews, MS, RD; Janet Flynn, RD; Jean Bauch, RD, CDE.

DEVELOP EDUCATIONAL MATERIALS

Customers enjoy food and nutrition information—everything from flyers and brochures to recipe cards and cookbooks. Topics can range from health needs (diabetes, hypertension, etc.) to nutrient-specific information (fat, cholesterol, sodium, whole grains, etc.) and population specific (seniors, kids, ethnics, etc.). Materials should be easy to read, eye-catching, and targeted to the customer population of the retailer.

Example: Customers at Meijer stores were offered a free menu planner and a diabetes wellness log during National Diabetes month. The materials were developed by Meijer's corporate dietitians, Shari Steinbach, Janine Faber, and Cheryl Bell (http://www.meijer.com).

SUPERMARKET TOURS/IN-STORE SEMINARS

Education events in the supermarket are effective for teaching nutrition (Fig. 21.4). They can be a moving seminar that goes throughout the store looking at foods and labels or a classroom presentation with food samples passed around the class. They can be for general nutrition information or targeted toward a specific population (kids, seniors, vegetarian, weight loss, diabetes, or heart disease).

Example: Linda McDonald, MS, RD, LD, provides a Supermarket Tour Training Kit through her business SUPERMARKET SAVVY Information and Resource Service (5).

WEBSITE

Almost all supermarkets have websites, and this is a great venue to share nutrition information with customers. An "Ask the Dietitian" page can address current nutrition questions and topics (Fig. 21.5). Linking recipes and coupons with food product specials can entice customers into the store and to buy new products.

Example: Kroger has a new website, www.MaketheMost.com, to inform consumers about the benefits of produce. It features recipe suggestions, nutrition information, preparation tips, video demonstrations, and storage guidelines.

CASE STUDY 21.1

MARKETING FOR A GROCERY CHAIN

Melissa Hooper, MS, RD, LD

Presently, I am working as a retail dietitian for a grocery store chain in Southern California called Stater Bros. Markets. There are 164 stores, and I do a variety of work for them. As the chain has plans for growth and adding new stores, I am a part of new store openings by giving store tours, answering questions from shoppers and helping to promote the Healthy Selections program. I also serve as a resource for the media to field questions about the program. Additionally, Stater Bros. has a monthly mailer that is sent to 3.9 million homes. Each month I choose a topic and write a message within the mailer. I also write articles and help put together the quarterly

continued

continued

newsletter that is distributed within the stores. I put together the yearly calendar and write the messages for each month that I record and are aired overhead in all the stores. Since the program is still fairly new, I help find ways to grow the program and extend the reach of nutrition messages to consumers. As a result, we are working on updating the store's website, and we are also looking for ways to connect the pharmacy with nutrition.

Growing a Nontraditional Career

My passion is nutrition, and I love sharing information with people that will help improve the quality of their lives and possibly the length of their lives as well. I also enjoy working with students and interns entering the field of dietetics. When I was studying to become a dietitian, I really did not have much "real world" working experience, as is the case with most 23 year olds. Over time, I have learned, grown, and developed as a professional. This constant learning and improving is a continual process throughout anyone's career—traditional or not.

One critical element that I have done over the years is to create what I call a "career map." Just like you need a map to navigate where you want to go, the same is true in any career path. Knowing where you ultimately want to end up will help you make decisions along the way to ensure you end up at your goal.

Once you know where you ultimately want to end up, here is where you *have* to be open-minded. Think outside of the box. What are some things like programs, classes, other jobs, and volunteer roles that you can do to help prepare you and move you toward your career goal? Many times, you will have to create opportunities for yourself in order to grow in the areas you want to strengthen. And, remember, unless you have already landed your dream job, each job is just a stepping stone to where you want to be.

Although, I have been very thankful for the jobs I have had, I knew I did not want to ultimately make a life-long career out of a couple of them, but I focused on making the most of my time spent in them. And, I strongly suggest getting some form of clinical experience before launching out into nontraditional areas. This will not only make you a well-rounded candidate for positions, but it will also give you a base of working knowledge that may spark ideas for using nutrition therapy in future roles.

Along the way, most of us will experience some disappointments or set-backs for a number of reasons, such as corporate restructuring, loss of funding for positions, competition, misunderstandings, poor communication, jealousy, etc. Actually, the list of possibilities is probably unlimited. You may have to do a job that is not exactly the next step in your career map, but always be on the outlook for ways to continue toward your goals. And never give up. I have now been a dietitian for almost 12 years, and I am glad that I chose this field. Nutrition is a strong area for opportunity, and I am excited to see what develops next.

SUMMARY

The supermarket is no longer just a place to buy food. As the connection between good food and health continues to be confirmed by science, corporate America and food purveyors are finding new ways to educate the buying consumer. Also, as food safety, genetically engineered foods, and sustainable and organic agricultural practices continue to grow in popularity, the public will turn to available experts to help understand the issues. Dietetic professionals need to be the resource of preference.

RESOURCES

1. *Supermarkets and Nutrition Professionals—A Strategic Alliance (2004)*

   Supermarkets and Nutrition Professionals—A Strategic Alliance is a publication of the Food Marketing Institute whose goal is to promote a successful relationship between nutrition professionals and the supermarket industry by educating readers about the industry and the career opportunities it offers. The manual was written by Jeanine Sherry, MS, RD, founder and President of NewWellness, Inc., a nutrition consulting firm, who previously served as Corporate Nutritionist to Ukrop's Super Markets in Virginia for 15 years.

2. *Shopping for Health*

   Shopping for Health is an annual report sponsored by Rodale Inc., *Prevention* magazine, and the Food Marketing Institute. This national survey examines shoppers' interest in and attitudes about health and nutrition, the efforts these consumers make to manage their health, and the ways that these opinions and actions play out in the grocery store. Survey data come from telephone interviews with a nationally representative sample of 1,000 adults who have primary or equally shared responsibility for their households' food shopping and who had shopped for food during the 2 weeks prior the interview.

3. *Trends in the United States*

   Trends in the United States is a consumer attitude survey that was begun in 1973 by the Food Marketing Institute. The survey, conducted each January, tracks the changing needs and priorities of the American consumer. Survey highlights include the general consumer outlook, how consumers view the supermarket, shopping habits, meal solutions, supermarket shopper segments, nutrition, and food safety. Survey data are based on telephone interviews with a representative nationwide sample of 2,000 male and female supermarket shoppers.

4. Van Wave TW. Secondary analysis of a marketing research database reveals patterns in dairy product purchases ever time. *J Am Diet Assoc* 2003;103:445–452.

5. SUPERMARKET SAVVY Information and Resource Service

SUPERMARKET SAVVY Information and Resource Service provides educational products for you to use in educating consumers on shopping for health. Resources include a monthly newsletter, website, Supermarket Tour Training Kit, Brand-Name Shopping List, Power Point Presentation Kits, Tip Sheets, and Food Category Comparison Charts. Visit SUPERMARKET SAVVY at www.supermarketsavvy.com.

6. HAACP—FMI Total Food Safety Management Program. This program developed by the Food Marketing Institute, provides food retailers with a system that is readily adaptable to the wide range of retail operations. It includes a Total Food Safety management Guide (http://www.cfsan.fda.gov/~lrd/haccp.html).

HOW TO ENTER THE FUNCTIONAL MEDICINE NUTRITION MARKET

22

Diana Noland, MPH, RD, CCN

This is an exciting time for expansion in the field of dietetics and nutritional health care practitioners as we sense a shift in the health care needs in industrialized countries. Chronic disease has arrived and is growing exponentially as it challenges the methodologies of conventional western medicine. The conventional medicine model at its best, was, and is, designed for treating acute disease. Studies show that currently 80% of patients being seen in the health care system are for chronic disease complaints (1). In 1998, the *Journal of American Medical Association* published a surprising study showing for the first time more money was being spent out of pocket for Complementary and Alternative Medicine (CAM) than for conventional medicine health care services (2). A new stage has been set for an increasing appreciation for the role that food and diet play in the prevention and treatment of chronic disease. There are presently the demand and opportunity for nutritionists who specialize in nutritional and dietary management of chronic disease. Studies of the American Dietetic Association's (3) members and training program and others (4) recognize the need for this type of nutrition specialist, but admit the training is not adequate and needs to become stronger.

There are many health care groups providing educational opportunities to learn more about this emerging field of Chronic Care Management, but the organization with the most disciplined architecture of how to implement this systems biology approach in a clinical practice setting is the Institute of Functional Medicine (IFM). The IFM is a nonprofit educational institution that coined the term "Functional Medicine" back in 1993. The IFM founders are Jeffrey and Susan Bland. From that beginning, other groups have developed excellent educational programs for health care practitioners. One of the exciting hallmarks of this area of

Chronic Care Management is a fresh embracing of the Chronic Care Team, where all members work together, united in approaching the assessment and treatment methodologies of a patient looking at the whole person.

It is important for all nutritionists to become aware of this nutrition so all nutritionists can contribute and integrate where their specialties intersect. A good example where this is evident is a high-risk care registered dietitian working in the acute setting preparing a patient to discharge and being able to encourage the patient to continue nutritional therapies as an out-patient with a Functional Medicine Nutritionist. Or, this new field of Functional Medicine might entice some of you reading this to consider an interest in this type of nutritional practice.

WHAT ARE THE CRITERIA FOR BEING INVOLVED?

Functional Medicine Nutrition can be taught to any clinician who has an open mind and an eagerness to look at patient care from new angles. It is a matter of acquiring, analyzing, classifying, and prioritizing information in different ways, and then applying therapeutic (or preventive) measures that are aimed at correcting the imbalances that underlie organ-system disease.

Conventional and alternative providers alike are able to integrate Functional Medicine thinking into their existing knowledge base, because underneath the superstructures created by the many professions is an abiding interest in "functionality"—how things work and what to do when they do not—which is a shared terrain (5). When you begin to familiarize yourself with Functional Medicine thinking, become trained, and begin to represent yourself as a practitioner of Functional Medicine, you will attract clients who are looking for its types of therapies. Most important, there is no judgment of the clients' ideas. You will experience unusual thinking and influences from eclectic therapies of which you never dreamed. You provide a safe place for clients to seek professional advice and an opportunity to provide them with sound personalized guidance for their nutritional health.

Information alone is not enough. How practitioners are trained is an extremely powerful predictor of how they will practice. A lot of continuing education (CE) in the health professions is devoted to trying to change and update what was learned in school, and yet even CE that changes health care practitioners' behaviors with some efficacy may not change patient outcomes. Mentoring is an important element in complex change, and follow-up is critical. A personal commitment to change on the part of the clinician is also extremely important (5). As in any attraction one has to a professional path one follows, there is a "spark" that starts to develop a passion to pursue continued learning.

WHERE YOU GET MORE TRAINING

Until recently, one needed to look hard and wide to find a community who taught thinking like Functional Medicine or Integrative Medicine or Complementary Medicine. But as the Functional Medicine paradigm has grown in strength over the last 25 years, and the need for more Chronic Care Health care Management has emerged, the two have been a good match for allowing the field to mature into a discipline worthy of respect. The way those early nutritionists sought training in this field is still a praiseworthy guide to the nutritionist of today who is interested in Functional Medicine.

1. The first is a desire to learn a new way of looking at chronic disease prevention or therapies. Instead of providing an individual nutritional therapy based on studies of a population of thousands of people as a generic treatment for a diagnosis, Functional Medicine considers systems-biology assessment of a client and his or her biochemical individuality to develop the best intervention plan for personalized nutritional therapy. Fortunately, the road is much easier and more opportunities are available today.

2. Find a mentor. Throughout history, the impartation of a profession, or a skill, from one generation to another required a mentor or an apprenticeship for the magic of that

profession to continue at the master proficiency level. That is how any art has survived throughout the ages. The profession of nutritional therapy is not any different. The nuances of a clinician with years of experience bring alive the theory and information learned in school. Find a Functional Medicine Nutritionist to talk with, to intern with, to work with, and you will receive the way of thinking and practicing.

3. READ. Each month, new evidence-based publications become available with information about a Functional Medicine approach to health care. In the age of the Internet, there are excellent websites as sources of credible information in this field. See the references at the end of this chapter for suggested reading to begin learning more about this field.

   a. *Clinical Nutrition: A Functional Approach*, 2nd Ed. Institute for Functional Medicine.
   b. *Textbook of Functional Medicine*, Institute for Functional Medicine.
   c. *Textbook of Natural Medicine*, Joe Pizzorno, ND, Editor.
   d. *Textbook of Natural Medicine Handbook*, Joe Pizzorno, ND, Editor.
   e. *Alternative Therapies for Health and Medicine*, monthly publication (peer reviewed): http://www.alternative-therapies.com/.
   f. *Integrative Medicine: A Clinician's Journal*, monthly publication (peer reviewed): http://www.imjournal.com.

4. Choose continuing education activities in the field of Functional Medicine. There are many different personalities of presenters of educational programs in Functional Medicine. All incorporate clinical nutrition as one of the foundational premises of good medicine. It is important to find the type that you would feel comfortable with and start getting your feet wet. Some are very inexpensive, and some have significant cost. Some good places to start are:

   a. www.jeffreybland.com
   b. www.designsforhealth.com
   c. www.complementarynutrition.org
   d. www.integrativenutrition.com
   e. www.helmpublishing.com

5. Get further training and certification in your field of interest in functional medicine:

   a. "Applied Functional Medicine in Clinical Practice." A week-long course for all members of the Chronic Care Team; http://www.functionalmedicine.org.

b. (2009) Certification in Functional Medicine. A two-year course toward certification by the Institute for Functional Medicine. All professional members of the Chronic Care Team can achieve certification; http://www.functionalmedicine.org.

c. International and American Association of Clinical Nutritionists (IAACN). A post–graduate level course and pathway to Board Certification in Clinical Nutrition; http://www.iaacn.org.

d. "Food As Medicine." Professional Training for the Clinical Nutritionists and other health care professionals; http://www.foodasmedicine.com.

e. Master's Degree (accredited). University of Bridgeport Online; http://www.bridgeport.edu.

f. Master's Degree in Nutrition. Bastyr University, Kenmore, Washington; http://www.bastyr.com.

WHAT IS EXPECTED IN THE JOB

Nutrition is the cornerstone of Functional Medicine. Functional Medicine responds to the advent of personalized medicine, which is a foundation of this approach. To work in a job as a Functional Medicine nutrition practitioner, you need to embrace that paradigm of thinking. If you do not believe in the premises of Functional Medicine, it will be almost impossible to project a practice that comes across with honesty and integrity (5). People that seek out a Functional Medicine practitioner are looking for someone who practices what they preach. Also, employers looking to hire a Functional Medicine practitioner want someone who will represent and be an emissary of their business philosophy. The way a Functional Medicine practitioner practices effects how nutritional assessment is accomplished, the types of foods recommended (tend toward whole organic foods), and the diet and evidence-based application of nutritional supplements (6). The end result is an improved way of addressing the underlying factors of pathologic symptoms and disease. The nutrition professional that practices Functional Medicine has tools to use in chronic disease management, which bring inspiration to one's practice and validation of the power of nutrition in medicine.

WHAT KIND OF JOBS ARE AVAILABLE?

The jobs available in this field are growing from the demand by our population. Each year, more and more people are seeking this kind of health care—from physicians to acupuncturists to nutritionists. The following areas are where most Functional Medicine nutrition jobs are available:

1. natural food businesses (i.e., Whole Foods Market, Nutrition Supplement companies, etc.);
2. private practice;
3. teaching in community colleges, universities, and medical schools;
4. nutritionists working in journalism;
5. integrative hospitals (i.e., Cancer Centers of America);
6. nutritionists teaming with a Functional Medicine doctor;
7. consultants; and
8. fitness centers.

EXAMPLES OF PEOPLE IN THE JOBS

Sheila Dean MS, RD, LD/N, CDE, is a registered and licensed dietitian, certified diabetes educator and exercise physiologist with undergraduate training at Rutgers University, dietetic internship and graduate school with University of Rhode Island and Brown University's teaching hospitals, and postgraduate training in advanced Functional Medicine, nutritional genomics, and medical nutrition therapy from Duke University Medical Center's Endocrinology and Metabolism Disorders Clinic and the Joslin Center for Diabetes as a Certified Diabetes Educator. Currently, Sheila is the owner of a thriving private practice, Integrative Nutrition Solutions, in Palm Harbor, Florida. An educator at heart, she has taught Nutrition Science for nursing students at St. Petersburg College and Nutritional Supplements at the University of Tampa for 10 years. Sheila is the author of *Nutrition & Endurance: Where Do I Begin?*, and is a certified health and fitness instructor with the American College of Sports Medicine (ACSM), the Aerobics and Fitness Association of America (AFAA), and the YMCA of America (http://www.integrativenutritionsolutions.com).

Linda Lizotte, RD, CDN, founded Designs for Health in 1989 with a local team of nutritionists. Managing 22 Northeastern offices, the company's initial focus was to provide nutrition counseling services for the treatment of a variety of health conditions. The success of this endeavor grew, as did the demand for nutritional products to satisfy the specific treatment needs of the company's clinical nutritionists (http://www.designsforhealth.com).

Coco Newton, MPH, RD, CCN, is a registered dietitian, a Certified Clinical Nutritionist (CCN), and the owner of Lifetime Nutrition, LLC, a private practice in downtown Ann Arbor, Michigan. She began her career as a Public Health Nutritionist, focusing on maternal, infant, and child nutrition with the Women Infant Children (WIC) supplemental feeding program. Also, she worked in hospitals, as a clinical dietitian, specializing in critical care and the use of tube feedings and intravenous nutrition support. This is where her interest began in understanding the metabolic management of critically ill patients. She has been in private practice for the past 23 years as a Functional Medicine Nutritionist (http://www.coconewton.com).

Diana Noland, MPH, RD, CCN, is owner of FoodFax, a Functional Medicine Nutrition Services business in Burbank, California. Her patient base includes critically ill clients, and those learning to resolve and prevent chronic disease and achieve optimum health. Her special interests include fatty acid metabolism, nutrition-related issues in dental health, and detoxification. Diana is a frequent lecturer to health professionals and the lay public on various Functional Medicine and CAM nutrition-related topics as an expert in Functional Medicine Nutrition Clinical Application. She was a featured speaker at the 2004 American Dietetic Association FNCE Convention on the topic of CAM Nutrition. She also contracts with the Institute of Functional Medicine to further the integration of Functional Medicine into the professional nutrition community (http://www.nolandnutrition.com).

Kathie Swift, MS, RD, is a registered dietitian and one of the country's foremost Functional Medicine Nutritionists. She is currently the Nutrition Director for The UltraWellness Center in Lenox, Massachusetts, and the co-director of Food as Medicine, a professional training program sponsored by the Center for Mind Body Medicine. She is a nutrition consultant for the Kripalu Center for Yoga and Health in Lenox, Massachusetts. She is also the Chair-Elect of the Nutrition in Complementary Care Dietetic Practice Group of the American Dietetic Association 2008–2009.

REFERENCES

1. "Medicare Looks to Boost Seniors' Use of Preventive Care." *LA Times*, June 19, 2006.
2. Eisenberg D. Trends in alternative medicine use in the United States, 1990–1997. *JAMA* 1998;280:1569–1575.
3. *American Dietetic Association Board of Directors 2007–2008*; 107(6):1045–1049.
4. Knowledge, Attitude, and Self-Reported Practices of Pennsylvania Registered Dietitians Regarding Functional Foods and Herbal Medicine. *Topics in Clinical Nutrition* January–March 2008.
5. *Textbook of Functional Medicine, Instructor's Guide*. Gig Harbor, WA: Institute for Functional Medicine; 2005.
6. Clausen et al. Clinical Decision Support Tools: Focus on Dietary Supplement Databases. *Alt Ther Health Med* 2008; 14(3):36–40.

HOW TO MARKET SPORTS DIETETICS

23

Nancy DiMarco, PhD, RD, CSSD, LD, and Patti Steinmuller, MS, RD, CSSD, LN

Sports dietetics integrates nutrition with physical activity to benefit health and performance. As an emerging specialty for registered dietitians (RDs), sports dietitians work in diverse areas such as in private practice or corporate wellness, with youth, collegiate, and professional sports, or with health, fitness, and athletic performance organizations. Target audiences include physically active individuals and groups across the lifespan from fitness enthusiasts to recreational and highly trained athletes. With many options for employment, the goal of full-time work as a sports dietitian can be a reality.

Nationwide, collegiate and professional sports are growing at a significant rate. Currently, there are 32 National Football League teams, 30 Major League Baseball teams, 30 National Basketball teams, and 30 National Hockey League teams in the United States (1). The fifth most popular sport—soccer—and the fastest growing sport in the United States now has a professional women's team (2). In addition, collegiate teams, especially women's teams, have grown steadily since 1982. In 2000, there were 8,456 NCAA Division I, II, and III women's teams in the United States and 7,908 NCAA Division I, II, and II men's teams (3). As the number of sports teams and organizations has increased, nutrition has become increasingly valued to enhance sport training and performance. Additionally, advancements in sports nutrition research have enabled sports dietitians to develop evidence-based nutrition guidance applicable to specific situations.

WHAT IS THE BOARD CERTIFIED SPECIALIST IN SPORTS DIETETICS CREDENTIAL? WHY IS IT IMPORTANT?

Although sports dietitians are being employed in many settings, sports nutrition remains a highly competitive market where even experienced sports dietitians can find themselves competing for nutrition positions with those who claim the title "sports nutritionist" but are not RDs and possess little or no nutrition education. To set themselves apart from competitors, sports dietitians are encouraged to obtain a strong foundation in clinical dietetics, gain practical experience in sports settings, and earn certification as Board Certified Specialists in Sports Dietetics (CSSD) through the Commission on Dietetic Registration (CDR), the credentialing agency of the American Dietetic Association (ADA).

The CSSD is the premier professional sports nutrition credential and the new standard in the sports nutrition industry. CSSDs are qualified to assess, design, implement, and monitor performance plans that require coordinating the athlete's individualized health and nutrition needs with the demands of physical activity, sport training, and performance. See the sidebar for CSSD eligibility. Successful candidates earn the CSSD credential by meeting eligibility criteria and passing a national specialty examination. To maintain the credential, re-examination is required every 5 years. CSSDs may have advanced degrees in exercise science or have earned exercise or fitness credentials such as those offered by the American College of Sports Medicine, the National Athletic Trainers' Association, or the National Strength and Conditioning Association. To locate CSSDs, use the "Find a SCAN Dietitian" feature on the website of Sports, Cardiovascular, and Wellness Nutritionists (SCAN), a dietetic practice group of the ADA.

WHERE ARE THE JOBS?

Sports dietitians are employed in areas as diverse as:

- athletic performance companies;
- collegiate, professional, and Olympic sports organizations;

BOX 23.1	*Board Certified Specialist in Sports Dietetics (CSSD)*

Eligibility

■ Current RD status by the Commission on Dietetic Registration (CDR)

■ Maintenance of RD status, for a minimum of 2 years from original examination date (by the time of the specialty examination date)

■ Documentation of 1,500 hours of specialty practice experience as an RD within the past 5 years (by the date the application is due)

- health care organizations;
- performance centers;
- corporate wellness;
- military branches;
- academic institutions;
- research facilities;
- government agencies;
- food industry;
- sports nutrition companies;
- high schools;
- the media; and
- in private practice.

Increasingly, employers are requiring the CSSD credential for high-level sports nutrition positions, such as collegiate athletics, professional sports, Olympic training sites, and other situations that require management skills and program development and oversight. In the military, the CSSD credential is required for Army dietitians who work directly with combat troops.

Collegiate sports is an expanding market with approximately 100 sports dietitians currently working part or full time in NCAA colleges and universities. Employment opportunities in professional sports organizations are also increasing. With a burgeoning national interest in health care, corporate wellness is an emerging area for sports dietitians. Opportunities exist in unexpected places such as in clinics that provide services for postbariatric surgery patients and those that treat individuals with eating disorders. Sports dietitians in private practice typically offer diverse services that may include:

- face-to-face and virtual counseling,
- media work,
- writing articles and books,
- academic teaching and research,
- conducting workshops and seminars, and
- consulting with the food industry and health care organizations.

WHAT ARE EMPLOYERS, CLIENTS, AND COLLEAGUES LOOKING FOR OR EXPECTING FROM YOU?

Overall, sports dietitians apply the science of sports nutrition to optimize health, fitness, and performance and to speed recovery from athletic training and competition. Sports dietitians provide safe, effective, evidence-based nutrition services that include assessment, nutrition diagnosis, intervention, counseling, and follow-up evaluation for health and performance for athletes and physically active individuals and groups. Sports dietitians assess and evaluate energy intake and energy expenditure, conduct body composition assessment, and create customized sports nutrition interventions, policies, and programs. They provide weight management services, plan meals and snacks, and develop nutrition strategies for travel and rehabilitation from illness and injury.

Athletes seek the advice of sports dietitians to assess their nutritional status, provide personalized attention, evaluate dietary supplements, and integrate nutrition into their performance plans and schedules. Since many aspects of sports dietetics are individually driven, entrepreneurial skills and experience in communication, public speaking, and teaching are invaluable. Colleagues look to other sports dietitians for networking, sharing, and mentoring. In evolving fields such as sports dietetics, assisting colleagues to succeed expands the market and increases visibility and options for employment.

Expectations vary widely depending on the goals of employers and organizations. Ideally, employers seek sports dietitians who are leaders, self-starters, and team players who possess qualities of decisiveness and creativity. Flexibility is essential since working hours are typically not routine and work environments (training areas, locker rooms, cafeterias) are unlike anything described in a clinical practice. Sports dietitians employed by sports teams are expected to understand the demands of the sport, to integrate nutrition into athletic performance plans, and to evaluate and monitor dietary supplements and sports foods. They must assess problems and offer practical, effective interventions, often within a limited time frame. Designing menus (onsite and travel) and planning snacks and hydration schedules are typical tasks. Sports dietitians may also conduct supermarket tours and teach athletes how to shop, store, and cook foods. Although often operating independently, sports dietitians must also collaborate with other members of athlete performance teams and respect their skills and responsibilities. Frequently, as the sole source of specialized nutrition information, the sports dietitian is relied upon by the entire multidisciplinary sports performance team which may include coaches, athletic trainers, strength coaches, sports psychologists, team physicians, and physical therapists.

Expectations for sports dietitians in corporate wellness may involve nutrition program design, management, and oversight. They may conduct weight management programs, cooking presentations, and supermarket shopping tours. They collaborate with fitness professionals and may be involved in media and marketing campaigns. Sports dietitians in the military or who work for affiliates of the military use their skills to enhance warrior performance, overall health and fitness, weight management, body composition, and to assist in rehabilitation.

Providing sports medical nutrition therapy (MNT) is an essential competency of sports dietitians. Sports MNT is characterized by the ongoing assessment of the nutritional status and developing nutrition intervention(s) for individuals with a condition, illness, or injury that puts them at risk. This includes review and analysis of medical and diet history, laboratory values, and anthropometric measurements. Based on the Nutrition Care Process, nutrition strategies that are most appropriate to manage the condition or treat the illness or injury, while factoring in performance needs, are chosen and include:

- *Diet modification and behavioral interventions* leading to the development of a personal diet plan to achieve nutritional goals and desired outcomes for health, fitness, and athletic performance.
- *Specialized nutrition therapy* counseling for conditions or special needs, such as bone mineral disturbances, cardiovascular conditions, diabetes, disabled athletes, disordered eating, female athlete triad and male body dysmorphia, food allergies, gastrointestinal disorders, high blood pressure, iron depletion, iron-deficiency anemia, hemochromatosis, vegetarian athletes, obesity and other weight related disorders, and assessment of safety and efficacy of dietary supplements and ergogenic aids.

In addition to providing MNT, RDs must comply with the Health Insurance Portability and Accountability Act (HIPAA) in all medical situations.

WHAT MARKETING IDEAS WORK BEST?

A Google search for sports nutrition services yields a plethora of choices. Sports dietitians need to be creative and savvy to differentiate themselves from others and guide clients and perspective employers to their services. Consider the following tips and select those most relevant to your needs. See Table 23.1 for additional resources.

DETERMINE YOUR STRENGTHS AND AMBITIONS

Know who you are and where you want to be in the next 5 years. For example, if you are outgoing and enjoy the limelight, seek opportunities where you can be onstage in public arenas. If you like working in the media, consider applying to become an ADA spokesperson. Use your expertise, personality, and style to your advantage. If you are more introspective, seek ways to position your high-quality work in written form. While you capitalize on current strengths, think ahead for ways to sharpen your skills and add to them. If you need to gain experience or knowledge, volunteer with a local high school or college sports team, maintain an up-to-date library, read journals, seek a mentor, or take an advanced course in sports nutrition. Check the availability of online courses.

DEVELOP YOUR CORE BUSINESS GOALS AND CREATE A BUSINESS PLAN

Goals motivate and guide your efforts. Revise your business plan periodically. Reviewing your business plan on a regular basis and examining how it is working sets the stage to make course corrections and take advantage of new opportunities.

DETERMINE YOUR TARGET MARKET AND SEEK OPPORTUNITIES TO EXPAND THAT MARKET

If your professional presentations are being well received in the marketplace, you might consider developing a book, study guide, e-newsletter, podcast, webinar, DVD, course, or another related product or service.

LOCATE YOUR NICHE IN THE MARKETPLACE

Capitalize on your unique skills in areas of the market where you have expertise. Do you want to write a book or develop a DVD? Do you have experience

TABLE 23.1.   RESOURCES

Professional Boards and Associations	
Organization or Publication	*Website, ISBN*
Commission on Dietetic Registration (CDR)	http://www.cdrnet.org/
Board Certification as a Specialist in Sports Dietetics (CSSD)	http://www.cdrnet.org/whatsnew/Sports.htm
You are the Food and Nutrition Expert: Tips and Tools to Prove It. ADA's PublicRelations Team	http://www.cdrnet.org/pdfs/YouAretheExpertToolkit2005RDversion.pdf
Nutrition Entrepreneurs, a dietetic practice group of the ADA	http://www.nedpg.org
Sports, Cardiovascular, Wellness, and Eating Disorder Nutritionists (SCAN) a dietetic practice group of the ADA	http://www.scandpg.org
Sports Dietetics-USA, a subunit of SCAN with a sports nutrition focus	http://www.scandpg.org

Sports Dietetics	
Books	*ISBNs*
Burke L. *Practical Sports Nutrition*. Human Kinetics; 2007	073604695X
Burke LM, Deakin V, eds. *Clinical Sports Nutrition*, 3rd Ed. McGraw-Hill; 2006.	0074716026
Dunford M, Doyle A. *Nutrition for Sport and Exercise*. Thomson/Wadsworth; 2008	9780495014836
Dunford M, ed. *Sports Nutrition: A Practice Manual for Professionals*, 4th Ed. SCAN dietetic practice group, American Dietetic Association; 2006	0-88091-411-4

Commercial Sites	
Subject or Association	*Website*
E-commerce	http://www.1shoppingcart.com or http://www.paypal.com
E-mail marketing, surveys, newsletters	http://www.constantcontact.com
National Association for the Self-Employed	http://www.nase.org/
Nutrition advisors network	http://www.bitwine.com
Nutrition marketing, Produce for Better Health Foundation	http://www.pbhfoundation.org/
Nutrition marketing, Integrated MarketingWorks	http://www.intgmktg.com/
U.S. Small Business Administration	http://www.sba.gov/
Web hosting site	http://www.lunarpages.com
Website domain names	http://www.godaddy.com

in a specialty area, such as sports nutrition for child, adolescent, or master athletes? Establish your value and stick to it. As you begin, it may be worthwhile to do some work that pays more in experience than in salary, such as volunteering to help a local high school or college sports team. However, as you become more familiar with the market in which you are competing, you will obtain a better sense of your worth and how to market your skills to obtain the level of compensation you deserve.

EARN THE CDR'S CERTIFIED SPECIALIST IN SPORTS DIETETICS (CSSD) CREDENTIAL TO SET YOURSELF APART FROM COMPETITORS

With an ample supply of non-RD "sports nutritionists" vying for employment in the growing sports nutrition market, the CSSD credential provides instant visibility, national recognition, and accountability.

DEVELOP A BRAND OR TAGLINE THAT REPRESENTS WHO YOU ARE AND WHAT YOU DO

SCAN developed this tagline for the new credential, "Demand Experience, Demand Excellence, Demand the CSSD." Create a catchy title, such as "Win with Nutrition" or "Sports Nutrition 4U." Use your name as part of your brand, such as Nancy Clark, MS, RD, CSSD, author of books *Nancy Clark's Sports Nutrition Guidebook*, and *Nancy Clark's Food Guide for Marathoners*. Nancy's name communicates quality in sports nutrition products and services. Use your tagline consistently. When you are asked "what do you do?" offer the benefits of your service rather than your qualifications. Make your message engaging and powerful.

MARKET PRODUCTS AND SERVICES THAT ARE VALUED BY YOUR TARGET MARKET

Enhance success by satisfying unmet needs. Add value to those offerings through multiple revenue streams. Offer a little more than clients may have imagined they needed or wanted, such as related products and services (DVDs, books, virtual counseling).

SEEK ENDORSEMENTS FROM WELL-KNOWN AND RESPECTED INDIVIDUALS

Endorsements from physicians, therapists, business executives, competitive athletes, and athletic directors can enhance your visibility, recognition, and credibility. For example, if you are writing a book or giving a presentation on a medical issue such as athletes with diabetes or food allergies, a physician with whom you work may be willing to write the book foreword or offer a quote to include in your marketing materials. Although endorsements can be very helpful, ensure that you use them in a straightforward and ethical manner.

NETWORK WITH AND REFER TO OTHER SPORTS DIETITIANS AND HEALTH AND FITNESS PROFESSIONALS

Get to know sports physicians, sports psychologists, athletic trainers, exercise physiologists, sport managers, strength and conditioning consultants, and coaches. Learn from established entrepreneurial RDs. Cultivate opportunities to collaborate with other health and fitness professionals.

SEEK OPPORTUNITIES TO CONNECT WITH THE MEDIA TO PROMOTE YOUR EXPERTISE AND SERVICES

Write articles in newspapers, sporting publications, newsletters, and blogs. Present to local groups and sports teams. Conduct interviews for television and radio.

INVEST IN YOURSELF BY EMPLOYING A PROFESSIONAL TO DEVELOP YOUR MARKETING MATERIALS

Unless you possess marketing skills, employ a professional to develop your brochures, business cards, postcard bookmark, or website. Be sure that your photo and tagline are included in each marketing piece.

PARTNER WITH RELATED BUSINESSES AND PROFESSIONAL ORGANIZATIONS

You might develop a business relationship with an athletic trainer or strength coach that you know well. If you each have separate talents and expertise that go well together, your services may be enhanced by a more formal business relationship. Look for opportunities to work together and be seen together such as athlete forums, coaching seminars, or athletic competitions. Solidify your relationship with these professionals in the athletes' minds.

ENHANCE YOUR PROFESSIONAL APPEARANCE—LOOK LIKE THE SPORTS DIETITIAN YOU WOULD EMPLOY

While being an athlete earns a special respect and credibility from other athletes, you do not need to be a competitive athlete to be a sports dietitian. However, you do need to "walk the walk" by incorporating regular physical activity into your lifestyle. Fitness can take on many body shapes and sizes but it is your commitment to a fit, healthful lifestyle that enhances credibility when working with athletes and other physically active people.

DISPLAY PROFESSIONALLY DESIGNED BROCHURES AND BUSINESS CARDS

Display your brochures and cards where prospective clients frequent, such as spas, bike and sports stores, health and fitness clubs, health food stores, and in "goodie bags" for competitive events.

PURCHASE HIGH-QUALITY NUTRITION ANALYSIS SOFTWARE IF NUTRITION COUNSELING IS A MAINSTAY OF YOUR BUSINESS

Choose products that are user-friendly and offer benefits for yourself and your clients. Nutrition softwares that encompass physical activity as well as nutrition are Food Processer, NutriBase, and Nutritionist Pro. Consider purchasing tools for body composition assessment and equipment to estimate resting metabolic rate. Metabolic equipment currently available includes New Leaf, Med Gem, etc.

ADDITIONAL IDEAS

- Consider working in a virtual environment using technology such as online counseling, virtual office calls, podcasts, blogs, and e-newsletters.

- Be willing to mentor others as you become established. In addition to assisting others, mentoring can extend networking opportunities.
- Set aside professional time for charitable work.

SUMMARY

With the growing number of professional and amateur sports teams, increased funding for women's sports and number of recreational athletes, and the mounting research that shows the preventive and rehabilitative benefits of exercise, the field of sports nutrition will be growing for many years to come.

REFERENCES

1. NCAA Sports Participation—Number of Teams 1982–2000. Available at: http://www.ncaa.org/library. Accessed October 24, 2007.
2. Gifford, C. *Soccer: The Ultimate Guide to the Beautiful Game.* Boston: Kingfisher; 2004.
3. Popularity of American Football. Available at: http://www.newsdial.com/sports/football/popularity-football.html. Accessed October 25, 2007.

HOW TO MARKET A WEBSITE

24

Teresa Pangan, PhD, RD, LD

The world has been opened to us in the last 15 years with the use of the Internet and its capabilities: websites, email, store fronts, blogs, telehealth, nutrient calculators, libraries, YouTube, search engines, chat rooms, listservs, video and audio streaming, MySpace, online investing, and gambling, just to name a few options. Dietetic professionals are pursuing all of these avenues of communication and interaction. This chapter will concentrate on marketing using a website.

Attracting thousands of targeted visitors to your website—does that sound tempting? Are you drooling at the thought? It is possible. Visitors can be pulled to your site by careful word choices, networking, and links to optimize search engine placement.

NETWORK, NETWORK, NETWORK

Despite networking being a very simple thing to do, many websites miss out on the traffic that can be gained from networking.

Done right, a well-built network of contacts, friends, and like-minded bloggers can help you get the links you need, both directly and indirectly. Here are a few tips for working your network to increase traffic to your site:

- Include an email signature file on ALL outgoing emails. This can be setup to be automatically entered in all outgoing emails. Include an email signature even to those people concerning non-website related matters. You never know where your next best customer will come from.
- Comment and participate on blogs within your niche. The goal is to became known as the expert in your niche area. Take time to create well thought out blog comments. Include bulleted lists and subheadings in your blog comment if you can. Visitors scan blogs just like they do online content, so if your blog entry stands out—do not write the content in one big long paragraph—instead use lists and how-tos along with resources, and visitors will stop and read it.
- Start a blog yourself. This is an easy way for your visitors to post their mark on your site, and they may come back in the future to check in on it. Include links to other good blogs. Do not worry about sending your visitors to another site, if it is a good blog, visitors will come back to yours to see what else of value you have on your site.
- Find forums, newsletters, and groups in your niche and participate on them. The goal is to be known as an expert and to be respected for creating value for visitors. Take time to formulate your answers. People save listserv replies that catch their eye.
- Be generous. If you respect your network and work hard to be part of the community surrounding your topic, the rewards can really pay off.

SEARCH ENGINES

Your ranking in the results listing of any search query at Google, Yahoo, and other search engines is dependent on the content and labeling of information on your website's pages. The exact components that Google includes in its analysis are top secret. There are no paid positions in the ranking results for Google. However, there are clues that experts use to understand what goes into how the results are calculated for Google and Yahoo.

The goal for site owners is to achieve a top search engine ranking for keywords that relate to the most important content/messages or products and services promoted on their site. This in turn brings visitors to their site. Additionally, when site owners market their site online through other non–search engine avenues, their ranking in search engines will rise.

Next is a how-to guide for marketing on a website and getting your website ranked well in the search engines.

WHY THE BIG SECRECY OVER SEO

SEO stands for Search Engine Optimization; these are services provided by consultants that specialize in helping websites get better rankings. However, what SEO experts do not want you to know is there are no tricks or gimmicks to getting a good listing in a top ranked search engine. Search engine managers are very quick to pick up on any spam tricks (like repetition of keywords to attract a higher ranking) promoters try. What is worse, if you are caught spamming by a search engine, they will blacklist your site. A good search engine ranking and effective marketing campaign are based largely on three key items:

- Write good copy
- Links
- Networking—which has already been discussed

That is not to say these tasks do not require skill, but you can optimize your site for search engines and set in motion an effective online marketing campaign yourself.

AVOIDING SNAKE OIL SALES PITCHES

Not all SEO consultants out there are scam artists—there are many reputable firms in the business. However, anyone promising "guaranteed top results," "submission to 500,000 search engines and directories," "instant results," or "permanent top positions" is most likely a scammer. There is no way anyone can guarantee that your site will be ranked number one.

Also, stay away from services that offer to get your site listed in 300 or 1,000 or 5,000 search engines. The top five search engines account for 99% of the search engine traffic. Search engines ranked below the top 10 are often databases of emails for spammers. In other words, you innocently submit your site to a search engine or search directory that you have never heard of in hopes of drawing more traffic to your site, and their literature says it receives 100,000 views a day. In reality what you did is submit your email into a site collecting emails that will then sell to spammers. If you have not heard of the directory or search engine, your target audience probably has not either.

WRITE BETTER, FOCUSED COPY

Good copy is wording that appeals to your target audience, uses the inverted pyramid writing style (see below), and includes clear headings and a descriptive, thoughtful title.

Content on your site must have interest and value for your target audience. Discover this wording by asking your current clients or customers for ideas on topics they are interested in that are tied closely to the products and services your site offers. There are also online keyword tools that will tell you how many times a certain keyword or keyword phrase was searched for in a given time period. Try out a couple and see which keyword phrases come out on top related to what your site covers and promotes.

Next, do some research and put together interesting and unique facts or advice that provides value to users: "How to select . . .," "The latest trend in . . .," "Be careful of . . .," "How 100 people lowered their . . . ."

INVERTED PYRAMID WRITING STYLE

Do not use the pyramid writing style. The classic academic writing format is like a pyramid. It starts at the bottom by laying the foundations—lots of supporting information from other research and other data. It sorts and summarizes the supporting information into smaller summaries. Finally, it caps the work off with a brief conclusion. The pyramid style educates the reader by making them do lots of work along their way up from ground level to the pinnacle. The pyramid style is ineffective for the vast majority of web content.

Use the inverted pyramid style, which is a deductive writing style that comes from journalism. The inverted pyramid reverses the workflow by putting the essential information first at the start, which is followed with further detail. The quick overview helps the reader get the point and purpose of a page instantly, letting the user make a quick judgment whether to read on for more detail.

BOX 24.1	*Keywords*

Keywords and keyword phrases are the words that a user might type into a search engine to find a topic or person, for example, "nutrition therapist, Detroit, MI" or "cancer prevention foods" or "alternative medicine home study courses." These are specific words that a search engine might find instead of saying something vague like, "professional trained in foods and nutrition."

MAKE YOUR POINT, USE KEYWORDS AND HEADLINES

Remove any paragraphs, sentences, and words that do not directly help get your point across. Can you find ways to say something in fewer words? Fewer words that make your point and integrate keywords, raise a page's keyword density. They also set the stage for visitors to read the entire article once they click to your page off of a search engine listing.

A strong, attractive headline at the top of a page can make the difference between the page being read or ignored. Headlines and lower-order headings benefit from being large and high-contrast, so they attract the eye. Once you have attracted the eye, a headline needs hooks to catch your reader's attention. (Headlines should be programmed as headlines using H1, H2, H3, . . . H6 tags. Emphasize this with whoever is entering or programming the content onto your web pages.) Search engines give higher weighting to words formatted as a heading. If the text goes more than two screens, there should be subheadings using this same formatting principle. Headings give words more weight in search engines and entice visitors to read all the content on a page.

Another tip for writing good copy is to read your content out loud and hear how it sounds. Text that sounds fluid also reads well on the web. Also, look for opportunities to replace pronouns with keywords. Search engines index every keyword and formulate a page's relevancy for subject topics. Words like "it," "she," and "there" will not help your indexing; instead use "diabetes counseling," "Jane Jones, RD," and "Middletown Hospital," respectively. Substitute in the actual descriptive keyword phrases and the times a keyword phrase appears on a page could easily double. Read the passage out loud again to be sure it reads well.

The icing on the cake is writing descriptive page titles. Titles online are not the same as using titles on a printed page. Titles online are the wording at the very top of the browser window screen. It is the text saved if a page is bookmarked. Web pages that do not have a descriptive title will say "Home page" or "Welcome to. . ." Titles can help bring visitors to your site from a search engine results list. Potential visitors will scan the results listing titles for the one that sounds the most interesting. Some experts argue a page's title is one of the most important elements of a web page.

An easy formula for creating a page's title is to start specific and work your way to more general keywords (from left to right), for example:

> "Managing colon disease—nutrition services by Nutrition Now"
>
> "Weight loss results and before and after pictures from clients at Hayden Health"

> "Canola Oil Safety—Frequently asked cancer questions—Cancer RD"

Note: Search engines typically only index the first 40 to 60 characters including spaces. Make sure descriptive and enticing words come first in your page title.

When working well, search engine optimization produces a high ranking for the web page on search engines *and* provides value to a website's target users while convincing them to buy the product or accept the educational message. Well-written copy on topics that interest your target market give you an upper hand when approaching sites to advertise or link on.

LINKS

Links can refer to many things. There are reciprocal links, buying links, linkbaiting, and natural links.

RECIPROCAL LINKS

Reciprocal links are when website A links to website B and website B links back to website A. This link building tactic has been used throughout the web for many years and its main purpose is to help websites increase their search engine rankings. Often, another site will approach you for a reciprocal link. A reciprocal link exchange email generally involves someone trying to solicit you to link to their website, and in return, they will link back to your website. If you decide to go ahead with this offer you will usually get a link on a page that contains a long list of links. These link pages are filled with hundreds and sometimes thousands of links. The reality is your link will probably not get counted by the search engines or if it does get counted it will not hold much weight. The search engines are getting smarter everyday and have caught on to reciprocal linking tactic of posting up pages only for search engine rankings and not for user value.

Agreeing to a reciprocal link on a long page of links is not recommended. Instead, seek links on other sites that satisfy these criteria:

- Sites or pages with content, products, or services related to yours and not on a page with a long list of different topics unrelated to your business.
- The page your link will be posted on should have less than 20 outbound links (links going to external websites) and preferably less than 10.
- For the greatest value, the page your link is posted on should have valuable user content, not a long listing of links.
- Vary the "anchor text" on your links page (anchor text is the underlined wording in the

link—anchored text ranks higher than non-linked text in search engine formulas).

- Anchor text contains keyword(s), not "Click here," or "Visit website" or simply your company name, you want keywords in the anchor text if at all possible.

BUYING LINKS

Buying links involves paying a site or service for link(s) to other prime sites. Typically the purchased links have similar content or products to yours, but their ranking in search engines is much higher. Buying links has become a hot commodity in the last couple of years since website owners have realized they can earn money by selling links and businesses have realized they can increase their search engine rankings by buying good links. The goal is to achieve the optimal criteria listing under reciprocal linking through a purchasing plan. The results can be very effective. Often you will find external links in the sidebar of a site.

If you want to see benefits from purchased links, you need to keep them "live" for a while—do not drop them after a few weeks or months. Search engines know that people purchase links, which is why they take the age of the inbound links into account when determining the ranking of a website. Yes, search engines are very smart nowadays.

If you are going to buy text links, here are some things to consider:

- Buy text links from sites with content, product, services, or goals similar to yours.
- Text links within the content of a website will generally be more effective than a text link within the footer or the sidebar of a website.
- Keep links posted for at least 2 months and closer to 6 months if your budget can afford it.

LINKBAITING

Linkbaiting takes more time than any of the previously mentioned links but the potential for an instant result is much greater. Linkbaiting refers to content, videos, images, or anything on the web that is created with the intention of increasing links to a website in a short period of time. This does cast a wide net. The principle behind linkbaiting is the time-honored tradition of being contrary in order to get attention; done correctly, it is an effective, out-of-the-box way to bring in a rush of traffic to your site.

In order to bait a link, you need a hook. Hooks come in a variety of flavors, some of the more popular include:

- News Hook—debunking a myth in the news, getting the news out first on niche topic, exposing a fraud story.

- Contrary Hook—why a story was wrong, opposite of a story.
- Resource Hook—blog of resources around a niche or a substantial amount of new content around a niche in a short period of time.
- Original Research Hook—offering original analysis on a topic along with properly listed reasoning and methodology.
- Humor Hook—"You know the food is bad when . . ." or "10 things I hate about . . ."
- Photo Hook—photos of an event or unique topic free to visitors.

Linkbaiting is creating lots of great content using a hook to attract a lot of attention (typically the topic is unique and does not cover a broad area). For example, you may post 50 articles in a month's time on nutrition management of celiac disease. Or, you may post photos of harvesting produce in Central California region. It could be recording a unique event and posting it on your own site (e.g., video diary 2 days before seeing dietitian, 1 day before seeing dietitian, day of seeing dietitian, day after seeing dietitian). For many, a visit to the dietitian is very scary.

Last step is for the PR to go out. Visit other prominent blogs related to your linkbait topic and post information on it and link to it. Add links on your own web pages to these blogs to get the attention of others.

Send emails out to people you know in the field. If it is a unique hook, word will spread.

Tips to keep in mind while brainstorming ideas for a linkbait campaign are:

- Create value in whatever you do. If you are going to write content, create videos, tools to calculate a diet, or even images make sure that people can find value in them. If they cannot, you will not get the links you desire as a result of your bait.
- Do your research to leverage the mediums out there. Get to know the respected blogs, the sites that allow video posting, the sites with thorough content and a good ranking in the top search engines. Look to be sure they have not done something close to what you have in mind. This way when you approach them, they will be interested. It will increase your chances of success.
- Make sure that it is easy for all users of all different computer backgrounds to share your blog, your photos, your video, or your content with friends. Setup multiple ways for users to share, different icons and text are highly recommended. If you take all the time to linkbait, you cannot afford to lose out on

visitors sharing your story, photos, or unique content.

NATURAL LINKS

Natural links are simply that—links that naturally happen through content on a site. The focus on this type of site is content and only good content. Links evolve in the content over time, but there is no strategy for links and getting links on a site that pursues natural links. If you plan on going the natural link-building route, make sure you get found by search engines and the top authority sites in your field. Good content is no good to anyone unless it can be found. Be sure at least a couple sites other than your own have links to your site.

BONUS SITES

To learn more and have fun while improving your site's ranking in search engines, try out these online search engine optimization tools. To find more, type in keywords "search engine tools" at any search engine.

We Build Pages—http://www.webuild pages.com/cool-seo-tool/

Enter your site URL and keyword phrase. This tool creates a chart with your site matched against the top sites for that keyword phrase on several different optimization measurements.

This same site also has a backlink checker, which creates a listing of all the sites indexed in Google that have a link to your site and the anchor text in the link (text in the active link).

Market Leap— http://www.marketleap.com/ publinkpop/

This site has tools to make it easy to compare your site against competitors. The link popularity tool calculates the total number of links or "votes" that a search engine has found for you. Additionally, there is a tool that calculates the number of pages a given search engine has in its index for your website domain (search engine saturation) and a keyword tool that quickly returns whether your site is in the top three pages of a search engine result for a specific keyword.

Niche Watcher— http://www.nichewatch.com/index.php

Type a keyword or phrase and get the top 20 competitor pages analyses. You will get technical information to compete for the keyword or phrase in your niche market.

CASE STUDY 24.1

WORKING FROM HOME THROUGH THE WEB—TELEHEALTH

Jan Patenaude, RD, Director of Medical Nutrition, Signet Diagnostic Corporation; http://www.nowleap.com

Eight years ago, I moved to my dream location in the mountains, 30 miles from the nearest grocery store or gas station in a small town.

After doing sales for a couple years, sometimes driving 60+ miles each way, much of it on ice packed mountain roads that drop off 30 feet to the river without guard rails, I decided I did *not* want to commute for any length of time or more than a few days a week. So, I went online looking for work I could do using my RD skills. I did not want to write full time, though that could have been an option.

I "marketed myself" by searching out health-related message boards. I sold my suggestion for an "Eating for Optimal Health" message board to one site and got hired for a pittance, but is was a chance to feel out what "communities" were about; what was going on in bulletin boards, etc., not something I normally did online.

Through my contacts on two of those boards, I "met" the then-VP of Signet Diagnostic Corp. I asked questions. I continued to post what I knew. I caught his attention and developed an online relationship. When the time came for that company to start a pilot project, this VP asked me to see if I wanted to take on some "telephone clients" referred by them.

I did; I studied more; I learned about their company, and it has taken 4 years, but I have developed it into a nearly full-time consultant position. I now consult with patients; train and give in-services to RDs and physician's offices; deal with patient insurance issues; write some on the Internet; plus do marketing and sales. I have done some distance teleconferences with out-of-state RD groups. Occasionally, if I feel like coming down from my mountain, I do some conferences or major presentations to RD groups (Colorado and Montana Dietetic Association Annual meetings); a multidisciplinary PCOS conference in Tucson; the National Kidney Foundation national meeting; and I will occasionally conduct "in office" sales trainings with physician or RD offices.

I never dreamed I would get the variety of work I now have from a home office. No overhead, no advertising costs (I may do my own website someday), no professional dress, no putting face on in the morning, no gas/car expense, and no commute time. (I take that back, from bed to coffee to laptop—heavy commute.)

It works wonderfully for me, except those days I have too much work and sit on my butt all day at the laptop, not getting near the exercise I should. I have had wrens land on my laptop while working; chip-

continued

continued

munks under my feet; deer grazing just a few feet away; my rooster crowing in the background—pretty funny when on the phone with a client, but they love it.

The income was not pretty for the first 2 years, when it was still very part time, but it is getting significantly better all the time.

SUMMARY

Just like any other new technology, those who use it best are the ones who take the time to study how it *really* works. Investing in a website without optimizing its function is a waste of time and resources. Allowing the power and potential of the Internet to pass you by is the loss of a major opportunity.

25

HOW TO MARKET YOURSELF AS A SPEAKER

Becky Dorner, RD, LD

Your marketing efforts have to be ongoing, consistent, and relentless. Hi Tech, Low Tech, No Tech, and sometimes totally shameless. —Patricia Fripp

Professional public speaking as a part-time or full-time career can be extremely rewarding, especially for those who want to make a difference by sharing a message in which they are truly passionate. In addition, the audience feedback coupled with the recognition that public speaking brings can help to increase self-confidence and build professional credibility. As an added bonus, professional public speaking may lead to financial gain. The following suggestions are given for individuals who enjoy the art of speaking, have a talent for speaking, and want to reach their target markets more effectively.

MARKETING YOURSELF AS A PROFESSIONAL SPEAKER

I love this quote from Patricia Fripp, a well-known and loved public speaker and an active member of the National Speaker's Association. As an entrepreneur and a public speaker, self-promotion is a must! To make it in the public speaking world, you have to be comfortable promoting your services and your talents, and take every opportunity you can to promote your services to your target market.

As a professional speaker, you must always be looking for opportunities to market yourself. Writing books or articles for lay and professional publications helps to increase your credibility, build your reputation, and improve your name recognition.

Appearing in the media serves a similar function, and may also offer a little notoriety. Networking with professional groups and becoming an active member of organizations such as the American Dietetic Association (ADA) and the Nutrition Entrepreneurs (NE, a dietetic practice group of ADA), the American Society of Association Executives, the National Speaker's Association, or the National Association of Meeting Planners gets your name in front of people who are influential in selecting speakers.

MARKETING PLAN

In order to create a marketing plan, you must first define the target market that is appropriate for your message and then develop a system for reaching program planners. For example, if your desire is to speak to dietetics-related groups, you might start by sending an introductory letter along with your speaking topics to local, regional, or state dietetic association presidents or program planners. You can also market to home economics, wellness, food service, or clinical organization officers. Include copies of positive letters or quotes from satisfied customers (such as program planners or attendees of past presentations.) You may wish to develop a speaking flier, brochure, or packet (press kit) that includes your topics, your photo, your professional biography, updated resume, quotes from satisfied program planners, etc.

Always include your name and contact information on your handouts and offer business cards or brochures to listeners, if appropriate, at the end of your presentation. Offer your book or other product as a door prize or for the organization's fund raiser. After your presentation, send a gracious letter to your hosts and keep in contact on a regular basis.

JUST STARTING

When you first start your speaking career, expect to do a certain amount of speaking (usually free) to local clubs and organizations. Few of these meetings will result in paid engagements, but they are great arenas for improving your presentation style, building your confidence, and finding out what your audience likes to hear. The old adage still holds true—you must always crawl before you walk, and you will practice walking for some time before you become a desired and well-paid professional speaker. When people enjoy and benefit from your presentations, they will look for opportunities to have you return. Depending on your audience, you may find that it is just as important to entertain as well as to inform your audience. Once you build your resume of professional presentations, it should be easy to market yourself for future paid speaking engagements and obtain referrals from satisfied clients.

USING PROFESSIONAL AGENTS AND SPEAKERS BUREAUS

As a speaker, your time and effort may be spent developing your presentations, pursuing speaking engagements, and/or making money speaking. It can be a full-time job making connections with groups and meeting planners. Negotiations for speaking fees and expenses can also take up a lot of time. There are ways to develop systems for streamlining some of this time; however, it can still be time consuming. Some speakers choose to seek professional speakers' bureaus or an agent to represent them to organizations and conventions. Speakers' bureaus and agents serve that purpose. However, bureaus and agents only represent experienced and recognized speaking experts. Some may also expect their speakers to be published authors of recent well-known books or have some other claim to fame.

SPEAKERS' BUREAUS

Speakers' bureaus are working to promote and place you for speaking engagements and to collect speaking fees. Therefore, their fees for representing you will range from 25% to 30% of your speaking fees. You will want to be sure to price your services accordingly.

Before listing with a speakers' bureau, spend time researching several different ones. Most bureaus will want to interview you or hear you in action before they will agree to represent you. This may be done in the form of live presentations, audio CDs, MP3 files, or DVDs. Many bureaus will handle all topics and all levels of speakers, while others are very selective of topics and speakers' abilities. Check with the local chapter of the meeting planners' association in your area to assess the confidence level and trust they have with the bureaus you are considering. Choosing the right bureau may have an impact on your reputation with meeting planners.

Speakers' bureaus usually promote you only with the materials you give to them and will not assist you in developing more current or exciting promotional materials. Bureaus expect you to provide materials that are "bureau friendly," meaning that your contact information is not on your materials. You either leave room for their contact information or provide materials that include their contact information.

It is the policy of most speakers' bureaus to find the best speaker for an engagement rather than to concentrate solely on promoting you as a speaker, which is understandable. However, this means you may have to sell yourself and your topics to bureau personnel to ensure that they appreciate what you can do. You can help make their job easier if you have clever titles for your presentations and include several distinctive topics that make you stand out from the crowd.

AGENTS

A professional agent will focus on selling you as a speaker at major business and other functions (depending on your topics), while allowing you to do what you do best—speak. However, you must have a certain level of ability and flair as a speaker to attract an agent.

A reputable agent will charge either a set retainer fee to represent you or a percentage of your speaking fees. The agent will represent you and negotiate the highest possible speaking fee with a client, collect from the client, and then pay you, usually within the first week following the engagement.

In most situations, an agent will assist you in designing any brochures or marketing materials you will use for your promotion. He or she will guide you in improving your handouts or slides and creating a mailing list.

Based on past experience, the agent will evaluate you as a package. He or she will look at your strengths in knowledge, presentation, dress, makeup, and many other areas that make you stand out as a great speaker. If you need to build on any of these strengths, the agent might give you names of appropriate specialists or tell you how to find them.

Negotiations on speaking fees and expenses can take hours or even days. Good agents have integrity, confidence, trust in their clients, and a reputation in the industry for promoting quality talent.

Agents can often accomplish things that you yourself could not. For example, when speaker and author Dick Huiras (1) was considering speaking at an annual meeting of a state organization he discovered that the organization was small and had a very limited budget for speakers. The fee they offered was much below Dick's standard fee, which included airfare and, if necessary, one night's lodging. Dick's agent sold them on his ability as a speaker, but told them that Dick would be very reluctant to accept the engagement. Because most organizations have extra money in separate accounts for different activities, they found the additional money required in their lodging and general expense accounts.

A third party will often promote you better and more forcefully than you will promote yourself. If you hate to ask for money or aggressively promote yourself, but are a good speaker with a clever message, an agent may work for you. Look in your *Yellow Pages*, check your library, or call speakers' organizations to find names. The NE Speakers Specialty Group is also a good referral source. Membership is free for NE members and the group provides an electronic listserv, which is extremely helpful for questions and referrals.

PROMOTION PIECES EVERY SPEAKER MUST HAVE

BROCHURES, PRESS KITS, AND WEBSITES

Brochures, press kits, and/or websites are extremely important for marketing your services as a professional speaker. The most important brochure is the *presentation brochure*. The more sophisticated and professional this brochure is, the better it paves the way to a higher speaking fee. First impressions make all the difference. This brochure should include:

1. a recent photograph taken by a professional photographer;
2. a short biography;

3. a complete listing of your speaking topics and a short description of each topic (and objectives if you are speaking to a group that wishes to obtain continuing education credits);
4. a list of groups, organizations, and companies for whom you have presented in the past;
5. testimonials from some of the people who have attended your presentations (your credibility is enhanced when you quote people who have hired you, are well known locally or nationally, or are experts in the topics you present); and
6. your name, address, and phone number.

You may also want to develop a one-page brochure for use with speakers' bureaus that contains information on the topics you present and notable information on you as the speaker.

You should also have electronic versions of all of your materials that may be emailed as attachments or links to your website. Most meeting planners work through a combination of email and phone contacts.

AUDIO

Audio clips on your website can be a great way for meeting planners to hear your presentations. MP3 files of your live presentations can easily be added to a website so that meeting planners may get a sampling of your speaking style.

VIDEO (DVD)

If you plan to market yourself to speakers' bureaus, meeting planners, large companies, or national organizations, you may need a DVD or video to compete in today's market. Your video should be 10 to 15 minutes in length, with four or five segments from different presentations. It is best to hire a professional to record and edit your video. When editing the tape, pick only the footage that shows you at your best, plus enthusiastic reactions from audiences. Eliminate audience members who may be sleeping, yawning, or leaving the room for any reason. The best audience representations are those in which only laughing or applause is heard.

DO'S AND DON'TS

Whether you are marketing yourself or using a bureau or agent, the do's and don'ts remain the same. These are the areas in which most speakers make their biggest mistakes and, consequently, experience some failures in the world of speaking.

DO'S

1. *Homework.* Get to know as much as possible about each group or organization you address. Some good information to know is why and how the organization was formed, its mission statement, its length of time in existence, any outstanding local or national credits, and who the major players are within the organization. Your interest in the organization will set up a positive impression and future recommendations.

2. *Site.* Once you have been hired, ask permission to view the room in which you will be speaking, if it is local, or request a description of the room layout. Identify how large the room is; the configuration of tables and chairs, such as U-shaped, open classroom, or theater, and whether there will be a head table; and if a microphone is required. Find out what audio visual equipment they will provide versus what you need to provide yourself. Find out where the projector, overhead, video player, or screen will be placed, if you need them. This will eliminate any problems or embarrassment on the day of the presentation.

3. *Attendance.* If the group is having a social hour or meeting before you speak, ask if you may attend. This is a great time to get to know the members and find out more about the organization. It will show that you have a real interest in them besides just speaking. Always arrive at least an hour ahead of your presentation to set up your room, take care of last-minute details, and meet and greet your audience as they come in.

4. *Customization and Personalization.* When you know about a group, you can customize your information so that the audience will better relate to your presentation. Nothing is more boring than always hearing about someone else, and nothing is more interesting than hearing about yourself.

5. *Award dinners.* Make an appointment to meet with the organization to discuss the type of award, its reason, and the honoree. During the social hour, spend time with the honored guest to gain personal insight and additional information for use in your presentation.

6. *Themes.* If the organization is using a theme to promote their meeting, find out why they chose the theme and incorporate it into your presentation. For example, if the theme is the "Extreme Sports," you might want to use some graphics in your Power Point presentation or handouts, or draw an analogy between your topic and extreme sports.

7. *Purpose.* If there is a particular purpose for the meeting, such as to provide information, education, or entertainment, it is important to adjust your presentation accordingly. For instance, if the meeting is dealing with governmental regulations, it would not be in your best interest to use examples about basket weaving or cross-country skiing. The success of any meeting depends on the ability of the meeting planner to keep a common theme throughout a program.

DON'TS

1. *Dress code.* This is not the time to make a fashion statement, unless, of course, it is an integral part of your presentation and is expected. In business meetings, you should present yourself as an expert and professional. Men should wear business suits with understated ties. Women should wear something that is acceptable to the audience that is also in good taste and not distracting. Audiences want to hear your words of wisdom, not be dazzled by your wardrobe. Bright, loud, and flamboyant costumes and colors are out, unless required by your topic.

2. *Hygiene.* Look clean and meticulous. Be sure your hair is professionally cut and styled. Your clothing should be neatly pressed and fresh from the cleaners. Do not wear overbearing cologne or aftershave, which can be very offensive to your audience.

3. *Speaking.* Never speak totally off-the-cuff. Have your speech planned and rehearsed ahead of time so that it flows and never becomes confusing to the audience. Speak loudly enough to project to the rear of the audience. Audiences do not want to strain to hear a speaker and risk missing important information. Avoid talking too much about yourself, and never tell off-color or ethnic jokes or make sexist remarks—or you will surely never be invited back or recommended to speak again. Joke telling is an art that should be used very carefully. Instead, learn to use humor in your speeches; it is a favorite of everyone.

THE SELLING GAME

Most professional speakers make it a point to write and publish a book and produce audiotapes or videos for retail sales. When you speak to a group for free, it is almost a foregone conclusion that you will be invited to sell your materials and give yourself a short commercial. However, be sure to clarify this and negotiate it up front.

When you speak for a fee, do not presume that the meeting planner will allow you to sell your materials. You are there to present your topic, not to make a profit on your book. When you contact the meeting planner to discuss the topic and the audience, give him or her a token copy of your book or tape, and offer to donate a copy as a door prize or to raise funds at a silent auction. The planner can then decide if it is appropriate for you to sell materials or even pass out order blanks. Many planners will allow you to set up a table in the back of the meeting room or an adjacent hall after the meeting to give audience members the opportunity to purchase a book or tape. Remember, they are doing this for the members.

If a meeting planner will not allow you to sell your book or tapes, you might give one away as a door prize. Have the audience members put their business cards in a bowl, and at the end of the speech have someone draw one card for the door prize. Keep all the cards and use them to develop a mailing list to promote future tapes, books, and speaking engagements.

Many speakers will, as their last statement, make themselves available for 10 to 15 minutes after their presentation. You will generally get people who have a genuine interest in your materials or wish to hire you for future engagements.

SOME GREAT EXAMPLES TO LEARN FROM

Here are some good examples of dietitian speakers who promote themselves uniquely:

- Zonya Foco sets herself apart with a state-of-the-art website, top notch media kit, video presentations, books, and CD-ROMs. Her message is "making good intentions come true." She speaks on good health, and she is an expert at using photos and testimonials to promote her uniqueness. At trade shows such as the ADA convention, Zonya puts on a great show at her booth providing cooking demonstrations and promoting her books, products, and her speaking. She is truly unique, and she lives her message—she is high energy, positive, enthusiastic, and passionate about good health! And audiences love her! Check out http://www.zonya.com.
- Maye Musk promotes herself as a wellness and image expert. Her book, *Feeling Fantastic* sets

her apart from other dietitians. Her speaking topics are divided into different categories for different audiences: lifestyle topics, image topics, and topics for dietitians. All you have to do is meet Maye to know she is an incredibly positive person. She truly lives her message— she looks fantastic! She feels fantastic! She is fantastic! See http://www.MayeMusk.com.

- Becky Dorner created a niche for herself in the long-term care and geriatric specialty areas. Becky started speaking as a way to promote her consulting practice. After 12 years of "free" CEU presentations, Becky discovered that speaking was an aspect of her practice that she truly loved. She began marketing herself as a speaker and has been a popular and well-paid professional speaker since 1995. Becky presents on nutrition for the older adult, business, and wellness topics. (Her marketing efforts really paid off: She celebrated 25 years in practice in January 2008 with her staff of 25!). Visit http://www. BeckyDorner.com.

SUMMARY

These professional speakers are truly great examples of people who know how to position themselves and to promote their speaking in a very positive way! Follow their lead: Promote yourself "shamelessly" all the way to incredible success! Now that you have the marketing tools, success can be yours in the world of public speaking.

REFERENCE

1. Huiras D. How to Market Yourself as a Public Speaker. In: King Helm K. *The Competitive Edge*, 2nd Ed. Chicago, IL: ADA; 1995.

BIBLIOGRAPHY

American Speakers Association, Houston, Texas. Phone interview, August 1993. Available at: http://www.american speakers.com/ASpk/.

Nutrition Entrepreneurs (a dietetic practice group of the American Dietetic Association), Speaker's Specialty Group. Available at: http://www.nedpg.org.

Speaker's Roundtable. *Speaking Secrets of the Masters: The Personal Techniques used by 22 of the World's Top Professional Speakers.* Mechanicsburg, PA: Executive Books/Life Management Services; 1995.

Walters D. *Dottie Walters Speak and Grow Rich.* New York: Penguin Putnam, 1997.

Walters L. *Secrets of Successful Speakers.* New York: McGraw-Hill; 1993.

Walters L. *Secrets of Superstar Speakers.* New York: McGraw-Hill; 2000.

HOW TO USE A BOOK TO GROW YOUR CAREER

26

Nancy Clark, MS, RD, CSSD

If you believe you have a book in you, what do you do? First of all, you need to define your niche and figure out how your book will be better than any of the other competitive titles. Visit bookstores and scrutinize other books that are already in your niche. Find out who published the books, and look in the acknowledgement page to learn if an agent was involved. This information can help you find a potential publisher and agent. With luck, they will help you through the process.

In this day and age where book authors are a dime a dozen, finding an agent and a publisher is difficult at best (unless you happen to be a high-profile politician or celebrity!). An alternate route is to self-publish your book. You will have to learn a whole new business in the process, but many RDs have taken this route. Some have attended Publishing University, sponsored by the Publishers Marketing Association (http://www.pma-online.org), and held each year in May. Others have read "how to" manuals, such as *The Self-Publishing Manual* by Dan Poynter, and have used John Kremer's resources at www.bookmarket.com. They have joined the Nutrition Entrepreneur's dietetic practice group of ADA (http://www.NEdpg.org) and have used NE's Author Specialty Group listserv. With more than 300 supportive and encouraging RD authors on the Author's email list, you can find the answer to any and all of your publishing questions!

MY STORY

After I had landed my dream job as a sports nutritionist at a sports medicine clinic, I fretfully asked a wise friend, "Now how do I fill my office with clients?" As we walked, talked, and brainstormed ideas, my friend suggested I gather recipes from members of the numerous running clubs in the Boston area and then write *The Boston Runners' Cookbook*. By reaching out to the runners, I could let them know that I, a sports nutritionist, existed and they would then come clamoring to my office (wishful thinking!).

That sounded like a brilliant idea to me. I contacted the local running clubs and started marketing my nutrition services as well as collecting recipes. Meanwhile, a neighbor, who happened to work for a cookbook publisher, arranged for me to meet her boss. By the end of that meeting, I had agreed to write what was now titled *The Athlete's Kitchen*, with a publishing date of April—in time for the Boston Marathon. Mind you, the marathon was only 6 months away and I needed to get busy!

After seemingly endless hours, *The Athlete's Kitchen* was "born"—and, to my surprise, the harder part started: marketing the book and keeping it alive. To market *The Athlete's Kitchen* both locally and nationally, I welcomed the help of students in Boston University's Nutrition & Communications graduate school program. The professor assigned a group of students to use my book for a "real life" marketing project. To this day, I am grateful to them for putting *The Athlete's Kitchen* and "sports nutritionist Nancy Clark" on the map.

Locally, I arranged to give talks (and sell books) to running, cycling, and other sports clubs. I submitted articles and book excerpts with timely topics to the *Boston Globe*, such as how to carb-load for the Boston Marathon, or how to lose weight healthily for wrestling. Each article included a credit line that mentioned my book and my nutrition counseling services.

As a result of authoring *The Athlete's Kitchen*, I became established as the sports nutrition expert in the Boston area. My speaking career flourished, and clients started coming for individual consultations. The book expanded my career growth far beyond my wildest dreams. Health professionals now saw me as "the expert" and invited me to give keynote talks, be a website sports nutrition expert, write articles for major magazines, appear on TV and radio talk shows, and be a spokesperson for the food industry. I never would have guessed my efforts to grow my counseling business—my book—would have such a big impact on my professional portfolio!

SUCCESS STORIES OF OTHER NUTRITION AUTHORS

Other nutrition authors have experienced similar successes with growing their careers. By being an author, you get elevated to the status of "expert in your field." This opens doors to speaking at professional meetings, appearing on TV talk and news shows, and writing for websites and magazines. Here are just a few examples of how other RDs have used their books to grow their businesses.

PROFILE 1

Shelley Case, BSc RD, author of *Gluten-Free Diet*, specializes in nutrition counseling for celiac disease, food allergies and intolerances. Initially, Shelley worked as a teaching dietitian at the Diabetes Education Centre in the Regina General Hospital. Because she herself has many allergies and food sensitivities, the physicians sent her their clients with those problems. She began researching and compiling scientific and practical information into her *Gluten-Free Diet* book. She marketed her book to local and national celiac groups, dietitians, gastroenterologists, health food and gluten-free specialty stores and others. Before she knew it, she was the gluten-free food expert and has even appeared on The Today Show! Shelley is now a sought-after speaker for professional and celiac organizations.

Becoming a best-selling author/expert in a growing niche market has resulted in numerous opportunities for speaking and media interviews, a magazine column, consultant work with gluten-free companies, private patient counseling, as well as the opportunity to develop spin-off products from her book, including a home-study course for continuing professional education and a DVD. So to all aspiring authors, Shelley recommends you dream big and work hard; you never know where you may end up!

PROFILE 2

Elisa Zied, MS, RD, CDN, author of *So What Can I Eat?!* and *Feed Your Family Right!*, hired a publicist to help her work with her publisher to market and promote her books. This helped expand her career. Elisa has appeared on several high-profile TV shows, including CBS's *The Early Show* and *The Maury Show*, as well as in high-profile newspapers, including the *Washington Post*, the *Chicago Tribune*, and the *Miami Herald*. Elisa hopes her books will help her strengthen her healthy-eating platform and pave the path to hosting her own TV show. This would enable her to follow her passion for getting positive food and fitness messages out to the public.

Elisa originally wrote the books because she loves to write and she saw a need for science-based tools that she (and other RDs, physicians, etc.) could use with clients and with the lay public. Her books have certainly added to her professional credibility and that, along with her freelance writing for msnbc.com and other magazines, has added to her platform as a food and nutrition expert. Being an author had certainly opened doors to many professional opportunities.

PROFILE 3

Marlene Koch, MS, RD, culinary nutritionist and author of *Unbelievable Desserts with Splenda*, specializes in delicious food for healthy lifestyles. Marlene has sold over 500,000 books—as well as helped many people with diabetes along the way. Marlene started as a cooking instructor at a culinary academy. When she was asked to teach a class on low-sugar desserts, she struggled to find recipes, especially for baked goods. Having a family member with diabetes (and a sweet tooth), she was keenly aware of the need for healthy, low-sugar recipes. She began developing recipes with Splenda. Today, Marlene is known as the expert on how to make low-sugar foods and is well known in diabetes circles.

PROFILE 4

Janice Newell Bissex, MS, RD, and Liz Weiss, MS, RD, co-authored *The Moms' Guide to Meal Makeovers*. Although they got a nice advance from the publisher, they were disappointed in the lack of promotion the publisher gave their book. They picked up the slack and have worked feverishly to promote their book. As a result, Janice and Liz have become known as the experts in fast, healthy cooking and recipe makeovers for favorite family foods.

Being published authors has opened the doors to many media and speaking opportunities for Janice and Liz. Because they use products such as canola oil and canned foods (such as beans, pumpkin, and tomatoes) in their recipes, a variety of food companies—including CanolaInfo and the Canned Food Alliance—have hired them as spokespersons. They are also the online experts at www.aboutseafood.com, where they answer consumer questions and create seafood recipes for the website.

Liz and Janice continue to market their book (and their careers) by writing magazine articles, hosting a blog, sending a bi-monthly newsletter to their 8,000 Meal Makeover Moms' Club members, and offering video tips on cooking and mealtime suggestions via their website, www.MealMakeover-Moms.com. They are gearing up to launch a weekly podcast and redesign their website. They are also working on their second book. Having a book has enabled them to expand their career into a virtual business. (For more on the Meal Makeover Moms, see Chapter 14.)

PROFILE 5

Madhu Gadia, MS RD CDE, author of *Lite and Luscious Cuisine of India* (1997) and *New Indian Home Cooking* (2000) wrote her books as a spin-off from having taught Indian cooking classes. She had wanted to share her passion about the art of cooking Indian foods, so she started teaching a class at an adult education center. The class was very popular, and inspired her to write her book. As a result of promoting her book, Madhu has been invited to teach at cooking schools, such as Kendall College in Chicago, Peter Kumpís Cooking School in New York, and Cambridge School of Culinary Arts in

Boston. As an author, she has also been invited to speak at organizations like the American Association of Physicians of Indian Origin and Culinary Collector's Society.

Today, Madhu is a health editor at *Better Homes & Gardens*. She contributes to magazines such as *Diabetic Living* and *Heart Healthy Living*, and is the editor of *Diet* magazine (annual). Being an author of a book established her as a writer, recipe developer, and a food expert along with being a nutrition expert. After having been a consulting dietitian for over 20 years, Madhu was able to revamp her career using her book as the springboard. "It is hard to believe that writing a book—a hobby, a passion—would change my path and open doors I never envisioned," says Madhu. "The culinarians, health professionals, and journalists now see me as the health and Indian food expert. That they request interviews and quotes still boggles my mind."

SUMMARY

Writing a book is only a small fraction of your job as an author. Marketing the book consumes the most time! But by effectively using the media to market your book (using the ideas that worked in the above case studies), you also market yourself and grow your career. I have yet to meet an RD author who has regrets about writing a book. I can assure you, you will never look back. Go for it!

HOW TO SELF-PUBLISH AND MARKET YOUR BOOK

27

Linda Hachfeld, MPH, RD

You have written a book (actually a manuscript), and you are not sure where to go from here. You could send the manuscript to a publisher, but you have enjoyed writing it and have other title ideas. You are excited about how the book could be designed and have a good idea of where it could be sold and who will buy it. Currently, you are wondering, "Why not do it myself?" You may be on the threshold of becoming a self-publisher, but there are many considerations before you make that decision.

No "recipe" exists to create a successful self-publishing undertaking. This chapter explains what self-publishing is all about and describes some of the marketing challenges, risks, and rewards. In the end, only you can decide if this is the best route for you.

WHO DOES IT?

Self-publishing has brought us great works, many considered classics! This well-worn path has been traveled by such notable authors as John Grisham, Irma Rombauer, and Vicky Lansky. That is right, these well-known individuals put such titles as *A Time to Kill*, *The Joy of Cooking*, and *Feed Me I'm Yours* into print themselves. Few people know that John Grisham sold his first work out of the trunk of his car or that Irma Rombauer self-published her cookbook in 1931 as a project of the First Unitarian Women's Alliance in St. Louis. Today, Scribner's sells more than 100,000 copies each year of *The Joy of Cooking*. Forty-nine publishers rejected Vicky Lansky's work, then she self-published her book, and sold 300,000 copies. Bantam bought the publishing rights and *Feed Me I'm Yours* has gone on to sell 8 million more!

It is clear that a number of authors can publish their own work, some with great financial success.

Indeed, some, as cited above, have gone on to have their work, once in print, picked up by major publishing houses, and while these success stories are inspiring, self-publishing is not for everyone, nor should every manuscript be published. In fact, fewer than 10% of the manuscripts written each year are ever published!

Self-publishing often can lead to the formation of a small publishing company, called independent publisher, which are a growing segment of the book industry. According to Michael Healy, Executive Director of the Book Industry Study Group (BISG) there are 192,000 active U.S. publishers (defined as having published 1 or more books in the past 12 months) that contribute to today's book industry.

Today, registered dietitians are using self-publishing as an avenue to get their message into the marketplace. Here are just a few who have self-published and created their own publishing companies with very respectable book sales to date:

- Diana Dyer (Swan Press) authored *A Dietitian's Cancer Story* in 1997 and has sold about 50,000 copies.
- Rachel Rudel (Apple-A-Day) authored *Cooking Healthy & Fast* in 1994 and has sold about 10,000 copies.
- Shelly Case (Case Nutrition Consulting) authored *The Gluten-Free Diet* in 2001 and has sold about 50,000 copies.
- Ann Litt (Tulip Hill Press) authored *The College Student's Guide to Eating Well* in 2000 and has sold about 18,000 copies.
- Kathy King self-published *The Entrepreneurial Nutritionist* and *Nutrition Therapy* and recently sold the rights to Lippincott Williams & Wilkins for a textbook series.
- My own experience (Appletree Press) is that my first-born title, *Cooking A La Heart*, has sold over 100,000 copies since its first publication in 1988.

HOW HARD CAN IT BE?

THE GOOD NEWS!

Books continue to sell and sell well. According to Simba Information, an RR Bowker Co., books on health & fitness and cookbooks are enjoying decent growth and are expected to stay strong. The Book Industry Study Group (BISG) projects net revenues for all books to top $40 billion by 2010. The printed word is still in demand.

THE BAD NEWS!

It is crowded out there; about 200,000 new books are published each year. According to *Books in Print*, there are 1.4 million active titles in print in the United States today. There is lots of competition.

THE INSPIRING NEWS!

The average life expectancy of a nonfiction book is about 6 to 8 months with a New York–style publisher; but can be in print for years with an independent or self-publisher. (Note the number of years the registered dietitians mentioned above have kept their titles current and still on the market.)

THE SOBERING NEWS!

Out of every 10 new books published, 3 will sell well, 4 will break even, and 3 will lose money.

You may decide that you have spent a lot of time and effort already in writing your book, and feel your reputation is at stake if you publish under your name. Furthermore, selling to an established book (commercial) publisher means *the publisher will pay* the cost to have your manuscript edited, illustrated, reviewed by professionals, printed, bound, distributed, and marketed. The publisher takes the full financial risk. You could hire a literary agent and negotiate the best advance and contract you can, then go on with your life and wait for the royalties to come in.

If only it were that easy. One major trend in the large publishing houses today is that fewer titles are being published. Given a choice, publishers would rather release a new title from a best-selling author with a proven customer base than take a chance on a title written by an unknown author. The reasons are purely economic; in 2004, 9 authors wrote 27 of the *USA Today* top titles. If you recall, fewer than 10% of the manuscripts written each year are ever published.

With these realities in mind, self-publishing becomes a plausible option. For a great many people, the primary reason for self-publication is *control*. If you sell the publishing rights of your manuscript to a commercial publisher, others will control the details of your book—the title, color, size, design, and finished content (although you may have contracted for overall approval; your wishes still may not be the final decision in the end). More importantly, someone else will also determine the time and amount of money dedicated to promoting your work. But are you willing to undertake the responsibility of publishing on your own?

WHAT ARE YOUR GOALS?

Before venturing into self-publication, you must consider your goals. You need to answer the question, "What do I want to achieve from the publication of my book?"

Hopefully your book is a vehicle for a meaningful message from your heart or your mind. You are expanding a reader's world, introducing a voice society needs to hear, or offering practical knowledge where none existed before. So, success may be just seeing the book that you wrote in print.

How do you expect to spend your time? If you self-publish, be prepared to devote a great deal of time to the promotion and marketing of your work. In publishing, your books are your business. A list of various duties that will demand your time is provided later in the section entitled, "What is Self-Publishing?"

Was your goal to make more profit if you self-published rather than sell to a commercial publisher? If you have a clear sense of who your audience is and how you can reach them, you might be able to generate more income from your book by doing it yourself. Let us look at the trade-off here. Typically, for a paperback, an author will receive a royalty of 7% to 9% of the net receipts for the first 30,000 to 50,000 copies and 10% to 12% of the net receipts thereafter. The standard hardcover royalty ranges between 10% to 15%. If your paperback book is published at a retail price of $15.00, your expected royalties can be figured as follows:

TABLE 27.1. YOUR PROJECTED INCOME FOR YOUR BOOK IF PUBLISHED BY A COMMERCIAL PUBLISHER	
1,000 copies @ 7% royalty at full retail price	$1,050
3,000 copies @ 7% royalty with a 55% discount to distributor*	$1,064
1,000 copies @ 7% royalty with a 42% discount to retailer	$609
Projected royalty income total on 5,000 copies	$2,723

*With 25% returns from the distributor

If you self-published, you can print a 250-page, soft cover, 6-inch × 9-inch, one-color text with a four-color cover in quantities of 5,000 for about $2 to $3 per copy. Your projected profit can be figured as follows:

TABLE 27.2.	YOUR PROJECTED INCOME FOR YOUR BOOK IF SELF-PUBLISHING	
Expenses		
Development Costs		
Graphic Artist and Editor		$4,000
Paper, printing and binding (PPB)		$12,000
Marketing Costs		
Postcards, brochures		$1,500
Mailing List Rental		$1,000
Postage		$1,500
Operating Costs		
Phone, rent, utilities, software, website, ISBN registration, etc.		$12,000
Fulfillment costs (amount not recouped from charging shipping)		$1,000
Total Expenses		$33,500
Sales Income		
3,000 book sales to a distributor @ 55% discount (each book would sell for $7.18 w/ 25% returns)		$16,200
1,000 sales to mail promotion @ $10/each (your special Introductory offer!)		$10,000
1,000 sales on your website @ full price		$15,000
Total Income		$41,200
Net Profit		$7,700

Remember, you have not paid yourself, which comes with employment taxes (FICA, SS, and Federal and State tax). Will it be worth it to you? How much time did you devote to accomplishing the sales? Variables abound! Will your book sell 5,000 copies in a year, in 6 months, or will it take 5 years? Maybe you are operating from your home and your operating costs are far less than calculated in Table 27.2. Perhaps the book you published has launched a speaking career for you or you kept your day job and your income is not dependent on the sales of the book.

You can see why very few independent publishers remain single-book publishers. So, what does it mean to become a self-publisher?

WHAT IS SELF-PUBLISHING?

Becoming a self-publisher means taking ultimate responsibility for the whole process of preparing, producing, selling, physically distributing, and collecting money for your work, as well as for all the business functions that inevitably relate to the funding of your business. The decision to publish your own work is a decision to undertake everything any other publisher might do on your behalf. And, yes, you are fully responsible for the financial risk.

The desired goal is to produce a well-edited, well-designed book that can compete with similar books and develop marketing and promotion plans for distribution to both trade and consumer markets through wholesalers, distributors, and/or the Internet.

You are embarking on an entrepreneurial venture, which means you are entering a new industry and will need to run it as a business. If you are the entire staff of your new company you will find that you will perform many jobs, some of which you will welcome and enjoy, others of which may be tedious and objectionable, yet necessary to your success. Here is a list of how you will spend your time as a self-publisher or independent publisher. You will assume each of the following positions.

WRITER/ACQUISITIONS EDITOR

Develop and write the books to be published or, perhaps, acquire other writers' works for publication.

MANAGING EDITOR

Oversee preparation of manuscript: determine the exterior and interior design elements, hire the talent for artwork and illustrations or determine if a book designer is necessary.

PRODUCTION MANAGER

Prepare specification sheets for obtaining bids from printers; analyze and compare bids assuring the printer you select can do the job at the level of quality you expect. Determine the print run for your book and where you will store your inventory.

FULFILLMENT MANAGER

Assure books are delivered when ordered; establish freight company accounts, keep records of all sales and shipments; pack books for shipping; prepare invoices, shipping labels, and billings; establish a system in which all the "little details" are accounted for, from having the right size box and the right amount of packing material to completing an order on a timely basis.

FINANCIAL/BUSINESS MANAGER

Obtain the funds to finance the publishing operation, develop a budget for the book, secure the software program that will help you prepare budgets with projected income and expenses, keep financial records, establish accounts, deal with vendors, track and monitor all expenses and revenues; in short, establish the management information system that will enable you to take the financial pulse of your company. You will need this information to determine whether your company is self-sustaining, losing money, or making money.

MARKETING/PROMOTION/ SALES DIRECTOR

Develop a marketing plan for your book, make decisions about where to sell your book, set the retail price and plan how you will make sales happen. Write press releases to garner publicity; write ad copy for different markets; meet with book-industry folks, such as sales representatives, bookstore managers, and distributors; and spend a great deal of time by phone or email making contacts and promoting your book to news, food, and health editors of magazines, radio programs, and television shows. At last count, this could potentially include 296 special-interest magazines, newsletters, and newspaper columns on cooking alone, as well as more than 560 on health.

PUBLISHER

You chart the course of your business; you write the mission statement. Staying proactive and determining the constant creation of new products means looking through a number of book proposals and fielding a lot of "I have an idea" phone calls. For long-term success, you need to define your own vision of your product line and develop a business plan, determine long-range plans for keeping titles on the active list, write contracts and negotiate terms with other authors or collaborative partners who will help market your books. Be visible, attend trade shows, and belong to appropriate associations and organizations. Stay up-to-date with printing technologies; uphold rigorous publishing standards to ensure your books stay competitive in the market. You will bear full responsibility for all functions to your investors, authors, vendors, suppliers, and customers.

The list of self-publishing activities may look overwhelming, but no one does everything at once. What is important to realize is the scope and range of activities in which you will become engaged.

THE REALITIES OF TAKING YOUR BOOK TO MARKET

Marketing never begins *after* the book is printed. It begins at the very inception of your book idea. Surely, the content, style, wording, illustrations, and cover were based on what appeals to your market and it is priced according to what that market will bear. Writing the book was the easy part, now comes the challenge—finding your audience and persuading them to buy your book.

ISBN

Before the book goes to press, every publisher needs to secure an ISBN (International Standardized Book Number) for his or her book, which is printed on the back cover and the title page verso (copyright page) inside the book. The 13-digit ISBN is required on every book sold in bookstores or on Amazon.com. If you want your title listed in *Books in Print*, you must have an ISBN. This unique identifier is assigned to each edition of every published book. It provides identity to the country in which the ISBN is assigned, to the publisher to whom the ISBN was originally allocated, and to the title of your book. The ISBN then is translated into a worldwide compatible barcode to allow for barcode scanning by major bookstore chains.

In the United States, ISBNs are available only from RR Bowker, the official U.S. ISBN agency (accessible at http://www.isbn.org). They are allocated in batches of 10; 100; 1,000; and 10,000; you cannot buy just one. A batch of 10 ISBNs costs $270 for a 15-business day turnaround; $370 for a 48-hour turnaround and $395 for a 24-hour turnaround. The price range for a batch of 100 ISBN numbers is $915 to $1,040. It is important that you own your own ISBN number if you are self-publishing your book. Without it, you are shut out of taking your book to market yourself.

SALES OUTLETS

Many venues exist for you to bring your book to market. I have grouped them into three major categories: brick-and-mortar, specialty sales, and cyberspace (Internet).

TRADITIONAL MARKETING: BRICK-AND-MORTAR BOOKSTORES & LIBRARIES

As a self-publisher, you will need to work to get your book into bookstores. The average bookstore carries 100,000 different titles (recall, there are 1.4 million books in print—they will not all fit on the shelf) and 70% of all book sales are in bookstores. So, you do not want to leave them out. Major trade retailers include Barnes & Noble, Waldenbooks, B. Dalton, and Books-A-Million. You will need to submit your title to their corporate headquarters for pre-approval. Once accepted, they will ask which wholesaler or distributor you work with and record that as the "vendor on record;" they will not buy directly from you—they do not want to deal with lots of small vendors. Libraries use library wholesalers, so you will want to approach them independently, two such library distributors/wholesalers are Quality Books and Baker & Taylor.

To sell your book to a wholesaler, who warehouses your books and fills orders only, the industry standard is a discount of 50% to 55% of the retail price for their services, they in turn, sell to stores at a 40% to 45% discount, which leaves them 10% to 15% for warehousing your book. Distributors will market your book to retail stores through their catalogues and sales staff. They usually sell books for 45% off the retail price to a bookstore and expect a 60% discount from you. On a book that retails for $10, that would mean $4 back to you, a little more than the cost of printing, paper, and binding (PPB). Both work on consignment—that is, they do not buy the books; they pay as the books are sold, and generally you pay to ship the books to them. They pay you for books they have sold after 90 days, and have return privileges. A return rate of 25% is not uncommon. No independent publisher wants to accept these terms; but that is the trade-off to having your book available in bookstores, where your market can find your book.

Local bookstores (including gift shops, museums and hospital gift shops) will consider buying your book from you because they are interested in promoting regional authors or sell similar merchandise. They will expect a 40% to 45% discount based upon the quantity they buy. College bookstores will ask for a 30% discount on orders of 1 to 15 copies and 40% to 45% on larger orders, but it is all negotiable. Many stores may ask for the right to return unsold copies, but the returns are often in poor shape because price tags or careless handling ruin the covers.

NONTRADITIONAL MARKETING OR SPECIALTY SALES

This is a broad area and depends upon what niche your book fits. This is a much more profitable area because you can negotiate the price for special markets, such as incentive or motivational sales, professional or organizational group sales, direct mail sales, book clubs, your back-of-the-room sales at every presentation you give, catalogue sales, schools, commercial organizations such as TOPS, Curves, YMCA . . . the sky is the limit. And, do not forget to include FNCE's Product Marketplace at the ADA annual meeting and consider other annual conventions sponsored by professional groups. Explore every nontraditional avenue and be relentless in book promotion.

I am happy to report this has worked well for my company. One of the books Appletree Press publishes titled *The Essential Arthritis Cookbook* has sold more than 30,000 copies to specialty pharmaceutical companies, who, in turn, provide the books to physicians to place in their waiting rooms. When *Cooking A La Heart* was first published, 10,000 copies were purchased by Harvard Medical School; when elementary schools in California discovered children were coming to school without breakfast, the Los Angeles School District purchased 10,000 copies of *What's for Breakfast?*; and we have made bulk sales to NIH-sponsored research projects, the military, hospitals, and to various HMOs. This year we made a subsidiary rights (a licensing fee) sale of the Spanish version of *Healthy Mexican Cooking*, allowing a cookware company (that is targeting the Latino market) to use recipes for booklets that will be placed into each cookware set they sell.

CYBERSPACE—THE INTERNET

A core challenge for many publishers is increasing the visibility of their titles, so they can reach people looking for books on specific subjects. Setting up your own website to make your book available is important. It allows your market to "Google" your subject and have your website pop up. Here your audience can check out your title(s) at their convenience and, hopefully, either call you to place an order or, if you have an online shopping cart, place their orders immediately. It also allows you to post book reviews, your press release, and timely book events; market your services as a speaker on the topic; provide recipes from your book; and give the viewer a peek into the book— all without leaving the comforts of their home! It is easy and painless, and more and more people prefer to buy online. And, it is important to let search engines know that you exist. Your web provider should be able to steer you in the direction of what search engines are the most viable.

TABLE 27.3.   IMPORTANT INDUSTRY REFERENCES

Resource	Comment	Where to Find
Book Industry Trends 2006, from Book Industry Study Group (BISG)	This is the industry's leading trade association for policy, standards and research. The mission of BISG is to create a more informed, empowered, and efficient book industry.	http://www.bisg.org
Books in Print by R. R. Bowker	Subject guide lists 1.4 million active titles by subject headings. The absolutely essential starting place when evaluating the uniqueness of a prospective new title.	Library or http://www.bowker.org.
Literary Market Place (LMP) by R. R. Bowker.	The who's who in American publishing today. It provides address sections for reviewers, subsidiary rights buyers, wholesalers, printers, fulfillment houses, artists, and publishing houses; and it identifies subject interests of over 5,000 publishers.	Reference section of public library
PMA Independent	A monthly newsletter by the Independent Book Publishers Association; this is a nonprofit, trade association of independent publishers whose mission is to provide cooperative marketing programs, education, and advocacy within the publishing industry.	http://www.pma-online.org.

*Also see books listed in Bibliography of this chapter.

Amazon.com is another cyberspace avenue. This site is frequently trafficked and garners book sales for independent publishers, like *Live Like You Mean It* by Ellyn Luros-Elson, RD, and Ken Wasco, published by Helm Publishing. Amazon will expect a 55% discount with you paying for shipping. They do an automatic deposit into your bank account every 30 days for books sold that month; earning them a reputation as being a very reliable outlet for book sales.

For more information, be sure to check the list of industry resources shown in Table 27.3.

RISKS OF SELF-PUBLISHING

The risks of self-publishing can be captured in two words: time and money. As you can tell from the list of activities a self-publisher performs, the job is enormously time consuming. Only you can answer the question, "Do I really have the time to devote to the promotion of my book?"

Another valid question to ask yourself is, "Can I, or do I want to, wear all the hats of a self-publisher?" If writing is your love and you truly want to do more of it, will you have enough time to write and run a business?

Perhaps your book will do so well that you will have the means to hire support staff or pay someone else for the tasks you are willing to give up. It can happen, as it did for me in starting and operating Appletree Press, which is approaching its 18th anniversary. I added full-time staff after 18 months of operation and now hire necessary talent by the project.

This brings us to the other risky part of becoming a self-publisher—money. You will need money to produce and launch your book. In this industry, you will spend a great deal of money up front in the hope of earning it back through sales of a finished product. It is risky, and it is a key factor that prevents many from self-publishing.

SUMMARY

If you were to ask a number of self-publishers what they gain from self-publishing or if they would do it again, you would get responses similar to the following:

"Absolutely!"

"It is an unending learning experience. It is so exhilarating to make decisions that will make or break your business. What a great feeling to know you are important to the existence of a business!"

"I enjoyed it at the time, but I do not ever want to spend that much effort again on so many chores I do not enjoy. I will let a publisher do it next time."

"The recognition. People see me as an expert, and it has opened doors for speaking engagements and even writing another book."

"My book is my baby. I would not dream of letting someone else 'raise' it!"

It is obvious that on a personal level, realizing your book in print is a reward in and of itself. Books are irresistible to many people, and the author is one of the first to marvel at how the blank page has been transformed into something that has lasting presence.

The book you have produced is also of value to other people, and they are willing to spend money to get it. The financial rewards may be a means of building your own company, realizing a dream, or launching you into something more lucrative. As with any business, the more attention and effort you invest, the more effective you are likely to be.

In conclusion, I would like to share the following references, which I use in my day-to-day operations. I referred to them in writing this chapter, and I heartily recommend them as balanced views of what you need to consider in self-publishing.

An anonymous saying best fits the decision to self-publish, "One good wish changes nothing; one good decision changes everything." As you decide what to do, may you enjoy the journey and may your book bring you success!

BIBLIOGRAPHY

Poynter D. *The Self-Publishing Manual*, 15th Ed. Santa Barbara, CA: Para Publishing; 2006.

Ross T, Ross M. *The Complete Guide to Self-Publishing*, 4th Ed. Cincinnati, OH: Writers Digest Books; 2002.

HOW TO WRITE A MARKETING BROCHURE

28

Tara Liskov, MS, RD

The objectives of a marketing brochure are four-fold (1): it must capture the attention of the target audience (2), it must be informative and factual (3), it must present the information as beneficial to the client from the client's point of view, and, finally (4), it must call the reader to action. In other words, instead of having a brochure that states, "Our services include low-fat diets and grocery shopping tours," it might say, "Are low-fat diets ruining your social life? They do not have to! Call now to sign up for our next culinary class!"

STEP ONE

The first step in preparing a great brochure is to determine the message you want to convey to your chosen target audience. Physicians and other health care professionals, sports teams, business and industry, fitness centers, speakers' bureaus, and prospective patients are examples of audiences you might be interested in targeting for possible business.

If physicians and other health care providers are your targets, emphasize your role in helping them provide excellent care for their patients. You should present your scope of service and areas of expertise. This target group wants to know that you are qualified and trustworthy, so a paragraph on your credentials and experience is useful here. When possible, use quotes from physicians who have expressed satisfaction with your work.

In a brochure directed to sports teams, discuss how your handling of sports nutrition problems can help players and teams win. Possible services include body-fat analysis, nutrition and exercise profiles, nutrition traveling tips, individualized counseling, and group lectures. Give sport-specific examples of how you have helped others. End with a call to action.

If business and industry are your target audiences, clearly identify the benefits you could offer (or the problems you could solve), such as calculating food labels, reducing health care costs through nutrition lectures and weight-loss programs, or acting as a spokesperson for food products. Explain your credentials for doing the work by giving examples of work for other clients, listing other satisfied business clients by name, and offering several quotes from satisfied customers.

For a patient brochure, clearly convey that you are competent and skilled in personal counseling. Readers need to be convinced that you can help them with their specific problem.

Write the tone of the text to fit the target audience. Consider hiring a professional public relations expert or other person skilled in such writing to edit your work. You want your reader to be sold on your practice just from reading your brochure (see Fig. 28.1).

STEP TWO

Once you have determined your target audience, you must establish your credibility. If your brochure focuses on you as an individual, highlight personal achievements and accomplishments. A brief description of your academic credentials and a summary of work experience will help establish your credibility. Also consider listing any highlights from your experience that will be of interest to your target market.

If your brochure is intended to highlight a program that employs several individuals, highlight the successes of the program and briefly describe each speaker and his or her credentials. If the speakers will vary each time the program is given, generically describe the credentials of all the individuals (for example, "all counselors are registered dietitians and hold advanced degrees in nutrition or related fields").

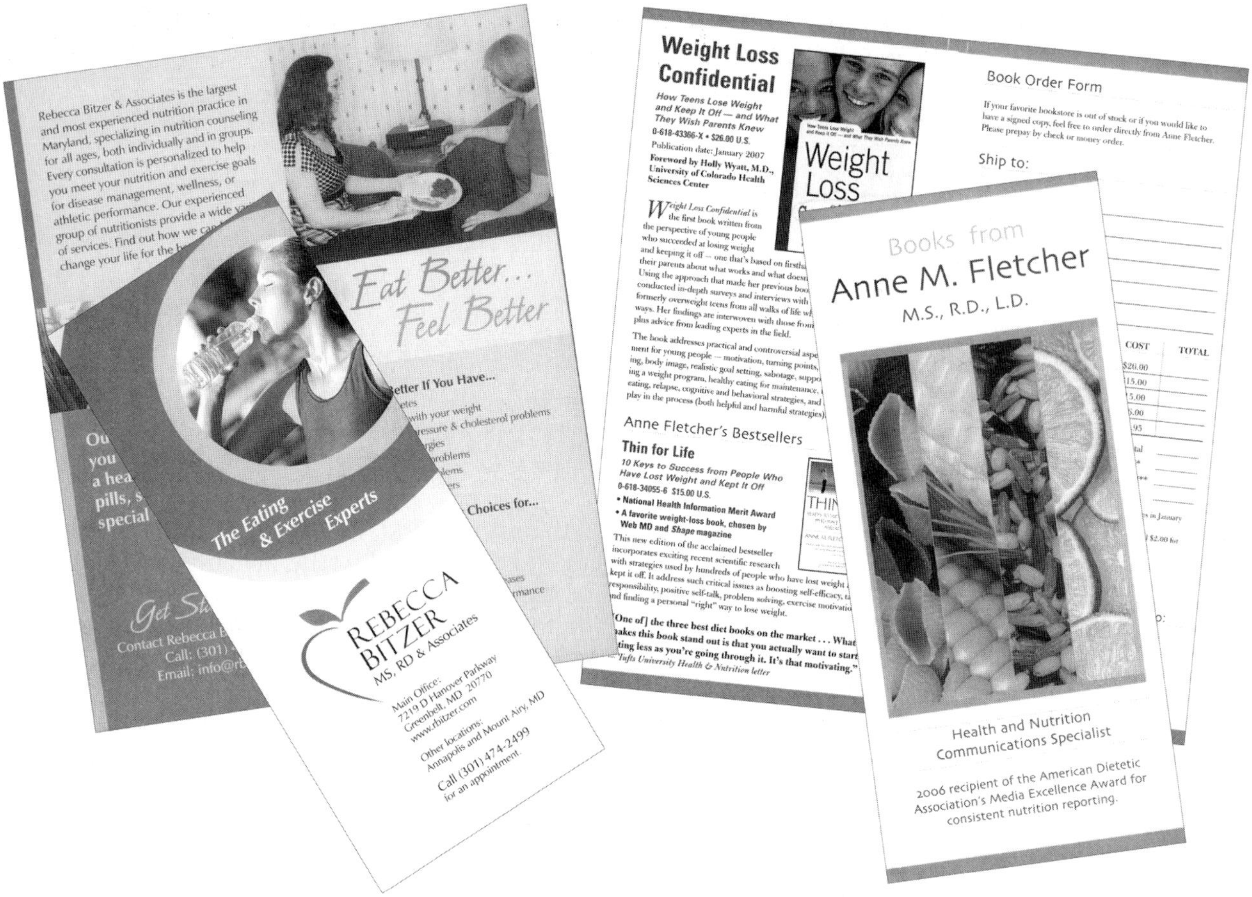

FIGURE 28.1. ■ Sample brochures.

STEP THREE

Convince the reader that you and your services or programs are successful. As mentioned above, present testimonials and quotes (with written permission from the authors). Cite your success rate or rate of business growth. List satisfied business customers. State how many clients have been seen in the last year or since the business began. Be tasteful and tactful, but do not over-sell, as you may risk sounding desperate.

STEP FOUR

A great brochure must show that you are available and convenient to reach. List your telephone number, fax number, e-mail address, website, and office hours. Many prospective clients like to review websites or have the option to e-mail you with preliminary questions. If your location is hard to find, include a small map. If there are specifics about parking or building entrances, list that information in the brochure. This will put a new client at ease and make the first visit less stressful.

STEP FIVE

Once you have developed the text of your brochure, you must choose the format, style, and paper quality. Again, consider hiring a consultant for graphic art ideas, or if a print shop is available at your employer, consult them. You could also use the Internet to get graphic ideas. Keep samples of your favorite brochures from other businesses so you can decide on the kind of layout, colors, or style you like or want.

If you are marketing primarily to an audience that will refer business to you or may hire you as a business consultant, add a perforated Rolodex card at the bottom of one brochure panel. A detachable card increases the probability that prospects will file your business information with other important telephone numbers for present or future reference, as opposed to discarding it.

Your brochure can take any number of forms, but it should reflect to some degree your personality and style or that of your institution. Consider using bullets and different typefaces, shading, or boxes to emphasize various kinds of information. Err on the side of brevity instead of wordy paragraphs and long explanations. Leave open spaces to highlight your message. Choose words that interest and excite readers and encourage them to want more.

Some dietitians use a photograph of themselves in their brochures with good success. The quality and attractiveness of the photo are very important. You should look alert, intelligent, well groomed, and professional. Very dark photos do not reproduce well, and home snapshots may not look professional enough for your target market. Consider using a professional photographer (or an artist for a line drawing) and work with that person until you get what you want.

Choose the highest-quality paper stock you can afford that fits your purposes. Good paper can add richness and subtly imply high-quality services. There is often a volume discount for printing, so inquire about prices for different quantities. Try to avoid dating a brochure by including exact class times or other information that may change. You could leave an empty space that could be used to apply laser-printed labels with up-to-date information. Alternately, you could print the information, but cover it with a label if it changes. It can be an effective marketing tool to leave your brochures in physicians' offices, fitness centers, corporate wellness offices, and anywhere else prospective clients may see it.

CASE STUDY 28.1

MARKETING A BROCHURE SERIES

Jessica Setnick, MS, RD/LD, Dallas, Texas, http://www.UnderstandingNutrition.com

The Problem

People would tell me, "I referred so and so to you, I do not know if they ever called," and so often I had not heard from the person. I was pondering why there is so much attrition between the referral and the appointment with the dietitian, and also, what could be done about it. I received a lovely brochure in the mail from a local psychotherapist I worked with, and studied it to find why it was so compelling, compared with other brochures I had seen. It was on heavy card stock and professionally printed; information on her specialty area was presented, along with photos of people who I assume were not her clients but could have been; and finally, a photo of the therapist, her credentials, and contact information. This was very different than the typical brochures I had seen, which use a lot of space telling about the professional and not so much about WIFM—What is in it for me?—from the potential client's perspective.

I had read an excellent book, *The Little Red Book of Selling*, by Jeffrey Gitomer, which hammered home the point that to "make a sale," you must show VALUE, that is, the benefits of what you do for the client, NOT just explain who you are, why they should choose you, and why your price is the best. With all this background info mulling around in my head, I came up with the idea of an informational brochure that referring professionals could give out to their patients, rather than just a business card or, worse, the dietitian's name and number on a scrap of paper.

The Product

Using a paradigm from eating disorders treatment, along with Jeffrey Gitomer's philosophy, I chose a benefits and fears approach. I thought about what people might be afraid of that would keep them from making the call for an appointment. I decided to caption the brochure, "I do not want to see the dietitian!" to try to relate to that fear-based thinking. The idea was to show that lots of people feel that way . . . to face and normalize the fear and then to neutralize it.

Only one person has expressed concern that the brochure title gives a negative tone, and that person was not a dietitian. I do not think they realize the negative connotations that people subliminally associate with having their favorite foods restricted, and, therefore, I do not think he really "got" the brochure. In order to make the brochure something people could relate to, I used stock photos of "average" people, and wrote storylines for them based on patients I have seen in my practice. I tried to include a variety of "types."

For the flap of the brochure, I used a photo of a woman with no food on her plate and the caption "Confused about what to eat?" This was the entrée for the nuts and bolts of dietitian credentials. I feel that most info sheets on dietitians capture this dry information, but there is no counterpoint of anything a potential patient can grab on to. In my brochure, the basic info is almost incidental, as I do not believe people make their choice of dietitian based on who has the most credentials, but rather on who their doctor recommends, who they match personality-wise, and who is convenient to their home. But I also wanted to support dietetics as a profession and promote registered dietitians as the nutrition experts.

On the back of the brochure is copyright and ordering information. The space for the business card was

continued

continued

moved to the lower right of the main panel. This way the potential client will have the dietitian's contact information right there when they finish reading and are less anxious and more positive about making that call.

Marketing Strategies

Although the storylines and clients represented are not clients of that dietitian, the message is that a dietitian will listen and teach what is important to YOU. To promote the brochure, I gave out a sample copy to each dietitian who attended my workshop, Eating Disorders Boot Camp, and to everyone who stopped by my booth at Product Marketplace or the Sports Cardiovascular Nutrition (SCAN) symposium. I also sent a sample with my card inside to all of my current referral sources, explaining that I would be happy to provide more at no charge if they would use them.

Response from dietitians and other professionals was very positive. Most dietitians expressed that this would be a huge time savings for them versus designing their own brochure. Other comments included feeling pride in being a dietitian, and that this would avoid misinformation that well-meaning referral sources might give while recommending a dietitian to a client.

Evolution of the Idea

I produce the brochure in batches of 1000, and they are for sale in batches of 50. This way the commitment on the part of the purchaser is small, but most who have bought one pack come back for more. With the purchase of 100 brochures, a free Lucite brochure holder is included for a professional presentation.

After the success of the initial "I do not want to see the dietitian!" brochure, a colleague, Tracy Siravo, identified a need for a different version of the brochure, targeted toward sports dietitians. We worked together to choose photos and storylines that would ring true to a health club and athletic audience, including vignettes from all ranges of the sports spectrum—from competitive athlete to weekend warrior. We chose language and photos that we felt this audience would relate to, and again we tried to choose a variety of "types." We kept the same "Confused about what to eat?" panel, but modified the wording and the photo slightly to match the theme, and we changed the back panel to be sports nutrition–specific. We changed the color scheme but left the style and layout almost the same. We named the brochure, "I do not need to see a dietitian!" expressing less that the reader might be worried or hesitant and more that the target audience might be overconfident in their own nutrition knowledge or perhaps unclear on the benefits of seeing a dietitian.

Once Tracy and I had developed the sports nutrition brochure, we brainstormed other possible versions. We came up with several specialty areas that dietitians work in, including pediatrics, women's health, diabetes, cardiology, and so on. Although certainly dietitians may work in more than one such area, the use of the brochure is in the hands of the referring professional, so we used medical specialties as our topics. We kept the layout and style consistent, changing only the colors of the basic template. We chose photos and created storylines in keeping with each practice area, and modified the flap, title page, and back cover to match the theme. Then we proofread over and over and made small changes until we were satisfied that the brochures read well and were attractive.

To market the brochures, we created an info sheet with testimonials, small photos of the brochures, and ordering information. We are now poised to market the brochures on a wider scale.

SUMMARY

In summary, your brochure should: (a) emphasize benefits to the client as the most important information, (b) establish your credibility, (c) highlight your successes, (d) show your convenience and availability, and (e) use the best and most effective wording, format, and style to attract customers to your door. Then you will be well on your way to having a great brochure!

HOW TO WRITE A RESUME, CV, AND BIO

29

Michele M. Fairchild, MA, RD, LDN, FADA

Whether you are in the market for a conventional job or you are entering the arena of private practice as an entrepreneur, you are about to find yourself in the business of selling yourself and your abilities! Promoting yourself through your resume, curriculum vitae (CV), or personal biography is a form of sales, packaged uniquely for your targeted audience with the primary objective of promoting your abilities. You use these tools for visibility, to rise above the mass of competition. They distinguish you from all others who profess to offer services like yours.

Remember that promotion should create a positive image for you and your service. It should make your chosen clients and prospects aware that you exist and stand ready and willing to perform your service for their benefit.

YOUR CAREER: THE FOUNDATION

Good, successful careers do not just happen. They take careful exploration, assessment of options and opportunities, trial and error, and dedication to produce a product that is in demand—you. If you seek a future as a sports nutritionist to the pros, clinical director at the hospital, culinary chef, or entrepreneur in your own private practice, consider what you wish to do, then determine what you will need in the way of documented and proven experience. Pursue those opportunities or assignments that will provide the most desirable personal experience. Be active in professional and trade association activities for they will enable you to develop key business skills while expanding your sphere of influence. Consider preparing articles for publication and papers for presentation at professional meetings. Consider pursuing high-profile jobs at major medical centers, at cutting-edge wellness programs, for Olympic teams, at culinary schools, or with well-known health organizations or food companies.

YOUR RESUME: A GIFT-WRAPPED PACKAGE

The style, composition, content, and appearance of your resume will change to suit different purposes and audiences. Experts suggest you use action verbs to add more interest. Also, with more and more businesses posting job openings on the Internet and requiring candidates to post their resumes, employment experts highly suggest using keywords on your skills and abilities in an introductory paragraph just in case resumes are scanned and ranked by a search engine. Most experts suggest that new graduates keep their resumes to one page to avoid looking like they are padded—unless of course, the person has extensive experience.

If you are targeting a job in business and industry, you would probably focus on:

- career objectives,
- what you can offer toward those objectives,
- past experience in business, and
- numbers that show you made a difference (i.e., increased sales, profit, or satisfaction, met budget or doubled return on investment, produced 35 training workshops per year, and so on).

If you are pursuing academic employment, you would focus on:

- past academic work,
- areas of research,
- teaching awards,
- advanced degree work,

217

- published papers and books,
- presentations, and lectures.

If you are an independent contractor, you must place yourself in the position of the person to whom you will send your resume, and give them what you think they will want.

The recipient of your resume will be making a serious business decision based upon your resume. Therefore, first impressions will be lasting impressions! If your resume fails to pass the first-glance test, it may never be read, or, if it is read, its poor initial presentation may seriously detract from its content. See Figure 29.1 for a sample of a well-presented resume.

Ask yourself a few important questions: Is your resume visually appealing? Is it neat? Is it readable? Are there typos? Is it labeled and categorized to guide the reader through its content? A great way to answer these questions is to send your resume to some trusted critical-thinkers who will read it over and give you honest feedback.

Impact is the secret—clearly stated, briefly presented, and quickly noted impact! Start your resume with an impact statement, one that epitomizes the service you offer and delineates the benefits a user of your service can expect. Make it a statement or promise of direct and immediate interest to the reader. Be careful not to over-sell, and do not over-promise. Too much hype will detract from your credibility.

It is important to keep the momentum going when addressing your capabilities. Present your areas of capability in short, concise, but clear statements, either in narrative paragraph form or as a list of bulleted items. Remember to concentrate only on the items that are directly relevant to the service you are offering.

If your readers were attracted by your impact statement and capabilities, they will look for evidence to support your claims, so present your educational training and employment history, complete with dates, places, company names, job titles, and, when appropriate, areas of responsibility, accomplishments, recognitions, and awards. As part of this section, you should insert your key professional affiliations and activities.

If you are re-entering the workforce after years of not working, or your age might be an issue, take the dates off your resume and highlight your skills and years of experience. Be sure to add any awards or recognitions you have collected over the years.

The challenge for anyone writing a resume is to keep it within two typewritten pages, for readers have very limited attention spans, and a thick document is all too often laid aside. Once you have met this initial challenge, the next critical element is the printing of your resume. No expense should be spared in this area. Good-quality bond paper with clear black lettering will put the finishing touches on your resume and communicate a sophistication and style that will distinguish your resume from the rest.

In summary, whether you are using a traditional resume or a broadcast letter format (a narrative letter with descriptors of successes strategically positioned by paragraph), you should cover the standard categories of information. Include your:

- name,
- address,
- telephone number,
- email address,
- professional experience,
- education,
- proficiency in computer skills and programs,
- awards,
- professional affiliations, and
- activities.

YOUR CURRICULUM VITAE

A curriculum vitae (CV) is a comprehensive listing of your education, job experience, awards, professional memberships, leadership activities, grants, publications, speeches, honors, and the like. As shown in Figure 29.2, it presents a more complete listing than a resume does, and may entail many pages. The format usually follows reverse chronological order, with the most recent additions listed first under each category. The CV is used primarily in academia, in government, in securing grants, and whenever very extensive, detailed information about a person's career is needed. Keep your CV on your word processor and update it as new additions occur. Glean information for your resume from your CV.

YOUR PROFESSIONAL BIOGRAPHY

A professional bio is a promotional vehicle that carries your business message, tells of your experience or qualifications, and, most importantly, announces to the recipient what benefits can be derived from dealing with you. A bio is a substitute for a conventional resume whose format requires you to be more inventive, more attentive to details, more determined, and bolder than ever before. Because a professional bio generally does not

SAVANNAH HELM

Seeking Professional Position

Self-motivated, passionate person devoted to doing my best. Extremely organized and detail oriented. Fast learner. Works well with others. Strong work ethic.

Experience in:

- Customer Service
- Organizational Skills
- Event Production
- Team Work

EDUCATION

Texas A&M University College Station, TX ~ August 2002-May 2006
- Bachelor of Business Administration in Marketing.

WORK EXPERIENCE

Helm Publishing Lake Dallas, TX ~ 1996-Present (Publisher of nutrition titles and continuing education for dietitians, nurses, CDEs, PFCS, and CDMs)

Marketing and Product Development 2001-Present
- Contributing author for continuing education courses.
- Proofing of book manuscripts.
- Consultant on design decisions and appearance of website, as well as data entry.
- Order fulfillment, customer service and inventory.
- Proficient in QuickBooks Pro.

Operations Manager and Customer Service 1996-2001
- Customer service representative, filled orders, maintained inventory of over 150 products.
- Worked in company booth at speaking engagements in the United States, Germany, South Africa, and the Philippines.

Material Marketing & Communications Glasgow, UK ~ Summer 2007 (Public relations and production for Scottish music festivals and events)

Production Assistant
- Organized, ordered and managed promotion materials and teams, as well production elements for events and festivals.
- Assisted in branding and production for T In The Park festival, which is Scotland's largest outdoor and green festival.
- Managed branding for four indoor venues at T On The Fringe (the music component of Edinburgh's Fringe Festival) and assisted an outdoor stadium totaling 44 gigs in August with 105,000 tickets sold.
- Collaborated on design decisions for dressing venues: floor stickers, posters, bar decals, stage backdrops, banners, etc.
- Secured the venue and negotiated the contracts for the first annual T On The Fringe After Party, which drew a crowd of 500 contestant winners.
- Aided in production for the Bank Of Scotland's Fireworks Concert with the Scottish Chamber Orchestra in Princess Street Gardens.

FIGURE 29.1. ■ Sample resume.

Experience

Memorial Student Council (MSC) Town Hall College Station, TX ~ 2002-2006 (Texas A&M Concert & Entertainment Committee)

President of MSC Town Hall 2005-2006

- Managed a 17-member executive team and 75 general committee members.
- Oversaw 70-80 concerts that promoted diversity and provided entertainment on campus.
- Developed the budget for the organization and 12 sub-committees.
- Wrote grant proposals for outside funding, securing 25% more for programming and music education.
- Texas A&M delegate to 2004-2006 South by Southwest Music Conferences in Austin, TX.
- Served on the MSC Council for Arts and Entertainment, which oversaw art exhibits, concerts, entertainment and a film series in 2005-2006, its most productive year.
- Received the J. Wayne Stark Award for excellence in service, innovation, motivation, and involvement in the MSC.
- Town Hall received Outstanding Co-Programming Event and Distinguished Committee during this time.

Executive Vice President of Special Events 2004-2005

- Developed and managed a 13-member sub-committee.
- Produced 45+ small-scale concert events including direct responsibility for advertising, booking performers and venues, negotiating contracts, organizing volunteers and sound setup and maintenance.
- Directed bi-weekly sub-committee meetings.

Executive Vice President of Co-Programming 2003-2004

- Developed and managed a 6-member sub-committee.
- Produced 15+ concert or entertainment events working with other Texas A&M organizations and creating several annual concerts.
- Student director of Showtime at the Apollo on Tour (National Touring Company).

Northgate Music Festival College Station, TX ~ 2003-2004 and 2005-2006

Assistant Event Coordinator 2005-2006

- Assisted with band selection from over 300 applicants.
- Assisted with advertising decisions and ordering of promotional materials.
- Assisted with running weekly coordinator meetings.
- Oversaw operations during festival: vendors, volunteers, artist assistance, sponsors, and community relationships.

Assistant Community Events Coordinator 2003-2004

- Assisted with band selection from over 250 applicants.
- Assisted with outdoor "Artist Market" area including 20+ vendors and artists.
- Assisted with Poetry Reading and Artisan Displays during festival.

102.1 The Edge Dallas, TX ~ Summer 2004 (Clear Channel Radio Station)

Intern

- Member of promotions Street Team.
- Participated in radio remotes at businesses and concerts.
- Worked the largest concert event of the year for this radio station, Edgefest 13.
- Worked in station office to assist promotions department.

FIGURE 29.1. ■ Sample resume *(continued)*.

APPLETREE PRESS, INC.

PROFESSIONAL PROFILE—LINDA J. HACHFELD   Email: eatwell@hickorytech.net

PROFESSIONAL EXPERIENCE	**Founder/Owner,** 1989-current Appletree Press, Inc.

Nutrition Consultant 1981-1999, 2007
Minnesota Dept of Health, Golden Heart Daycare and
Minnesota Valley Action Council, Region IX.

Acting Director, 1992-93, Wellness Center of Minnesota

Community Organization Specialist/Consultant, OSAP
(Office of Substance Abuse Program), Region IX, 1991-1996

Grant Writer & Coordinator, COPC-Kellogg Foundation,
1989-1992, Wellness Center of Minnesota

**Nutrition Coordinator / Allied Health Liaison / Community
Program Specialist,** Division of Epidemiology, School of Public
Health, Univ. of Minnesota—Minnesota Heart Health Program,
1981-1989

Director, Dietetic Services, 1978-1981
Glencoe Hospital and Glenhaven Nursing Home

MILESTONES

Leader in civic and professional organizations:
• Founder, President and Director, *Women Executives in Business*
• Founder and President, *South Central District Dietetic Assoc.*
• President & Director, *Midwest Independent Publishers Assoc.*
• Development Chair, Education Chair & varied positions with the
    Minnesota Dietetic Association
• Volunteer-Environment /Green Infrastructure Plan, *Envision 2020*
• Originator / Writer, Mission Ministries Endowment Fund, *UCC-
    First Congregational Church*

Author, 2 books; *Cooking ala Heart,* (over 100,000 copies sold)
and *Gifts of the Heart* for the nutrition professional & trade markets.

Editor and Publisher of 10 varied nutrition / food books;
3 journaling tools under the *HealthCheques*™ label for the health
professional & trade markets.

FIGURE 29.2. ■ Sample curriculum vitae (CV).

SKILLSET
- Establish vision / mission statement
- Business and marketing plans
- Policy & procedure
- Strategic action planning
- Financial analysis
- Human resources
- Problem solving
- Purchasing
- Grant writing
- Contract negotiation
- Production management
- New product development
- Sales development
- Banking relationship
- Project collaboration
- Customer service

HALLMARKS
- Outstanding Alumna, Minnesota State University, Family & Consumer Science Dept, 1999
- Distinguished Service Award, MIPA, 1999
- Recipient—Benjamin Franklin Award, Best New Voice, 1998
- Recipient—Benjamin Franklin Award, Best Marketing, 1998
- Distinguished Woman Leader, YWCA-Mankato area, 1993
- National Women in Business Advocate Award, SBA, 1993
- Outstanding Services Award, American Heart Assoc., 1991
- Certificate of Commendation for Community Health Promotion Governor of Minnesota, 1989
- Secretary's Award for Excellence for Public Health, U.S. Dept. of Health & Human Services, 1988
- RYDY (Recognized Young Dietitian of the Year) Award, Minnesota Dietetic Assoc., 1981

EDUCATION

Masters of Public Health, Univ. of Minnesota, 1990

B.S. Degree, Dietetics; Minnesota State Univ., 1976

Certificate of Training in Adult Weight Management, American Dietetic Assoc, Commission on Dietetic Registration, 2004

Credential of Advanced Studies in Health Service / Nutrition Administration, Univ. of Minnesota, 1987

American Dietetic Association Active Member, 1981-2011

151 Good Counsel Drive, Suite #125   Mankato, MN   56001   •   www.appletree-press.com

FIGURE 29.2. ■ Sample curriculum vitae (CV) *(continued)*.

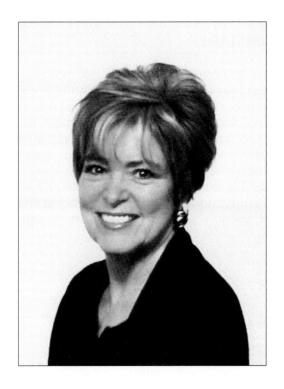

KATHY KING

Kathy King, RD has been an entrepreneurial nutritionist since 1972 when she quit her traditional hospital job to start a private practice in Denver, Colorado. She specialized in weight loss, sports nutrition, and health promotion. She has been a counselor to over 6,000 patients, as well as to the Greenhouse Spa and the Denver Broncos Football team. As a popular speaker, she has given over 800 presentations and 600 media interviews as the Denver NBC TV "NoonDay Nutritionist," host of her own nationally syndicated nutrition radio talk show, and numerous food companies as a media spokesperson. She has been an international speaker in Israel, Germany, South Africa, Australia, and Asia, and a guest on ABC-TV's "Nightline," and NBC's "Connie Chung's 1986" magazine show.

Kathy began Helm Publishing in 1991, to fill a niche in outpatient and complementary nutrition continuing education courses and books. Its courses cover such topics as nutrition counseling, entrepreneurship, marketing, herbs, weight management, eating disorders, and functional and alternative medicine. She has been the author, co-author or publisher of over 50 self-study tests and 17 books.

Kathy is past President of the Colorado Dietetic Association, former ADA Chair of the Council on Practice, and past member of the Board of Directors and House of Delegates for the American Dietetic Association.

Kathy King, RD, Publisher
P.O. Box 2105, 213 Main Street, Lake Dallas, TX 75065
940-497-3558 * Fax 940-497-2927
kathy@helmpublishing.com   www.helmpublishing.com

FIGURE 29.3. ■ Sample professional bio.

exceed one typed page, it can be a challenge to write, design, and lay out. To make it succinct enough, you must also carefully target your audience. The following should be considered in developing your bio:

- Who you are (with examples of prestigious or highly visible career activities)
- What you can do for clients
- How to contact you

If you are in private practice, a professional bio is an important calling card. If you speak professionally, consider attaching a publicity photo. Include your professional bio in marketing packets to perspective clients to reinforce your expertise, and emphasize your accomplishments with a professional publicity photo to complete the upscale presentation of your service. See Figures 29.3 for a sample of a professional bio.

SUMMARY

A resume, curriculum vitae, and professional bio are tactics of selling yourself through past deeds and descriptive words. Their objective is to attract work, whether you are a consultant or an employee. There are numerous very talented people in the world; many of them can do what you do and do it equally well. However, if you create the right documents to present your service where the demand and opportunity are the greatest, you will unequivocally be the person chosen for the job!

HOW TO WRITE A PROPOSAL

30

Linda McDonald, MS, RD, LD

The purpose of a proposal is to sell yourself to a prospective client through a written presentation of facts, financial figures, photos of past projects, if appropriate, and benefits to the client, all while positioning you or your company as the best provider of the product or service. A proposal is a marketing tool, and it had better be a good one because there is just one winner in a proposal competition—the rest are losers.

WHY WRITE A PROPOSAL?

In business you write a proposal for many reasons. For example:

- You may be asked for a proposal because there is a need or problem that cannot be fulfilled or answered by the present staff of a company.
- Clients may request proposals to compare consultants, to verify that a consultant understands the problem, or because they are required to advertise for consultants through RFPs (Request for Proposals). RFPs are often required by government agencies and public companies. Marketing expert Harry Beckwith states that he avoids RFPs because they are used by prospective clients to fish for new ideas and find the lowest bid—not necessarily the best person for the job (1).
- You may write a proposal to document the specifics of a verbal agreement, to explain an idea or unique service that would benefit a particular company, or to agree on specifics as the basis for a contract.
- You may use a proposal to sell yourself—to detail how your services are superior to those of your competitors.
- You may write a proposal to provide private counseling for physicians' patients, weight-control classes for a corporate wellness program, consulting for a nursing home, public relations support for a food company, a book for a publisher, or computerized nutrient analysis of menu items for a restaurant.

KINDS OF PROPOSALS

SOLE-SOURCE PROPOSALS

A sole-source proposal is one for which there is no competition. The client has complete confidence in you and does not wish to consider anyone else, but requests a proposal to make sure you are in agreement on the specifics: expected outcomes, time frame, compensation, tasks, and so on. An example might be a proposal to a physician you know to provide private counseling to patients.

UNSOLICITED PROPOSAL

An unsolicited proposal may result from your insight or knowledge of a client's needs, or as a follow-up to a sales lead or interview. For example, you may send a proposal letter to a restaurant that has nutritious items on their menu and propose providing computer nutrient analysis.

LONG VERSUS SHORT PROPOSALS

Proposals can take several forms, ranging from a formal RFP that is 100 pages long for a major project, like remodeling an institutional kitchen, to a simple letter that is one or two pages long. You can also make a verbal proposal and follow up with a letter. Herman Holtz suggests in *How to Succeed as an Independent Consultant* (2), that small projects in the range of $2,000 to $15,000 dollars usually require only simple, informal proposals or a letter proposal.

Above $15,000, a formal proposal of 25 to 50 pages is suggested. Proposals take valuable time and effort, so whether you respond at all and how much time you put into the project will depend on the benefits to your business, both financial and image-building, and your chances for winning. Winning will depend on preparing a successful proposal.

HOW TO PREPARE A SUCCESSFUL PROPOSAL

DO YOUR HOMEWORK

The secret of writing a winning proposal is to give the impression of being supportive without being overbearing. You want to show that you are knowledgeable, efficient, professional, and empathetic to the potential client's needs and position. *Focus on what you can do for the client* and not just on your credentials and experience.

Before you write a proposal, it is essential that you do your homework and assess some basic issues. These include knowing your client, the problem, and the solution. Next, select the type of proposal that is appropriate, draft a tentative outline, develop a plan of action, and do the necessary research. Questions to ask include:

- Exactly what is the need or problem?
- Has the assignment previously been attempted?
- Who will you be reporting to?
- Who will be making the decision on the proposal?
- Who needs to be interviewed?
- What kind of personality and culture does the company have?
- Have you been involved in similar situations in the past?
- Who are your competitors? What are their strengths and weaknesses?
- Is there a planned budget?
- Will you be expected to do this work, or can it be done by staff or a subcontractor?

Many sources are available for collecting information for your proposal. Interview senior management and employees of the company; ask for an annual report, company brochures, and sales literature; talk to other suppliers, consultants, and vendors; and visit your local library and newspaper.

Herman Holtz states that a proposal must have great impact if it is to do its job well. To provide that necessary impact, he contends that the following qualities must be apparent to the client (2):

- *Competence.* The client must sense your power as a consultant who brings complete technical and professional competence to the job.

- *Dependable.* The client must feel that you are completely reliable and will never fail to carry the job through to a successful conclusion.
- *Accurate.* The proposal must convey the sense that you are careful to be absolutely precise and accurate in every action and in every step you take.

Following are the keys to accomplishing this effect (2–4):

- *Details.* A presentation that cites specific facts and details, particularly quantified data, is much more likely to impress a reader and be credible. Anyone can generalize.
- *Interesting statistics.* Study your facts to see what impressive numbers you can develop (such as total number of contracts you have fulfilled or total dollar amount of contracts resulting from similar proposals). If your numbers are startling enough, see if you can work them into the introduction.
- *Clear language.* Be direct; leave no doubt about your meaning.
- *Quiet confidence.* Hype sounds defensive, as though you are trying to compensate for weaknesses. Avoid adjectives and superlatives that convey this weakness; instead use a quiet, confident tone that conveys strength (2).
- *In Control.* Clients want a consultant who seems to know exactly what to do. They want you to relieve them of worry and tedious, time-consuming involvement. Be sure to reflect confidence in what you propose to do. However, make it clear that you know the client is still in control.
- *Thoroughness.* Carelessness and lack of attention to detail can lose you the contract.

You do not have to tell the client how you are going to accomplish your job—that is your competitive edge. Ron Tepper (3) states that one of the most difficult decisions is how creative to get in a presentation without fearing that someone will steal your ideas. He continues by saying that a consultant should present unique, curiosity-stirring ideas that the client knows will meet the company's objectives, but that implementation should not be detailed.

In *Writing Business Proposals and Reports* (4), Susan Brock suggests testing for the "I" perspective. She states that proposals will be more effective if you use "you" more than "I." To test for the "I" perspective, compare the number of times you use the words: me, us, I, and we versus the words you, your, and yours. The more often you use the latter words, the more likely your writing will convey your concern for your reader's needs. Compare the first statement with the following one:

"I can provide the best nutrition counseling by using my unique experience and skills."

- Your patients will benefit from knowledgeable and unique nutrition counseling services in the convenience of your office.

"Our calculator is the best buy and most complete on the market for calculating nutrient intakes and exchanges."

- You will have more time to spend with your patients when you use our time-saving, user-friendly calculator.

Do not make the proposal an intimidating legal document; make it reader-friendly. Do not ramble. Do not confuse readers who are not used to dietetic jargon or acronyms. Use colorful terms, and write in a practical, how-to manner so that everyone understands what you mean.

STRUCTURE OF A PROPOSAL

A proposal should contain the following elements (3):

1. *Overview or summary*. Provide an overview in a cover letter, an abstract, or the first paragraph of a letter proposal. A cover letter should state the purpose of your proposal, offer to answer questions either by phone or in person, request the assignment, and express thanks for the opportunity to submit the proposal.
2. *Objectives*. Describe your understanding of the client's problems or needs.
3. *Solutions*. Describe your unique approach to solving the problem or serving the client's needs. What strategies will you use, and how will you implement the strategies and approach you are promising? Keep strategies general rather than specific so that you maintain your competitive edge.
4. *Information about you*. Explain why the client should select you. What are your experiences and qualifications? In a formal proposal, include resumes of the individuals you are proposing to staff the project. Do not put down the competition, just play up your strengths in areas where competitors are weak.

5. *Fees*. Tell what the client can expect to pay, including your fees and all expenses. There may already be a proposed budget for the project, but you must explain how you will allocate funds.
6. *Summary*. Present the key selling points of your proposal at the beginning. Then use this portion to summarize the important information so that managers can quickly get a good idea of what your approach will be.
7. *Appendix*. Include any other relevant or supporting materials that will enhance your proposal: timelines, references, sample literature, news articles, research papers, copy of the Ethics Code of ADA, and the like.

Robert Kelley (5) suggests that before the proposal is due, and while it is still in rough-draft form, you call your client to go over your work so far and ask for advice. This makes the client a working collaborator in the proposal. Incorporating some of the client's advice and suggestions into the formal proposal makes the client feel that you are truly trying to address his or her problems and want to collaborate to find solutions.

Ask to present your proposal in person. Remember that your proposal is a marketing tool, so structure its physical appearance and your presentation accordingly. Proposals need not be dry or boring. Your proposal will provide an initial impression of your professional work and of your ability to communicate. A well-written and well-presented proposal can give you the competitive edge.

SUMMARY

A proposal is another way to market yourself. It opens doors, introduces you to prospective clients, formulates your ideas and forces you to think like a business owner. The experience is invaluable to your growth as a businessperson.

REFERENCES

1. Beckwith H, Beckwith CC. *You, Inc.* New York: Warner Business Books; 2007.
2. Holtz H. *How to Succeed as an Independent Consultant*, 2nd Ed. New York: John Wiley &. Sons; 1988.
3. Tepper R. *Consultant's Proposal, Fee and Contract Problem-Solver.* New York: John Wiley & Sons; 1993.
4. Brock SL. *Writing Business Proposals and Reports.* Menlo Park, CA: Crisp Publications; 1992.
5. Kelly RE. *Consulting, the Complete Guide to a Profitable Career.* New York: Charles Scribner's Sons; 1986.

HOW TO OBTAIN PUBLICITY FOR YOUR SPECIAL EVENT

31

Sue Goodin, MS

Part of my job description as Special Projects Manager for Swedish Hospital Wellness Program was to create community events that would help educate the public about our hospital services. Our philosophy held that if we took care of people when they were well, they would come to us when they were sick. In the 1970s and early 1980s, this was not standard thinking for any hospital. We were considered a forerunner in the field of wellness and preventive care.

CREATING A SPECIAL EVENT THAT "WORKS"

One of the most successful events I helped create was the "Go for Gold Race." It was sponsored in part by the hospital, a local television station, a national athletic shoe and clothing company, the local professional basketball team, and a race event company. We also gave a percentage of the profit to a local charity. We could not be sure of how many runners would turn out for a race sponsored by a hospital, so we invited the Denver Nuggets basketball team to be involved, and their presence attracted the media. An athletic company, in turn, was attracted to the potential for exposure to the runners and the media.

We wanted to create an event that would appeal to local corporations as well as the community. To attract local corporations and the public, we provided free running shorts and a free ticket to the opening-night professional basketball game, as well as free food, music, and entertainment. There were also special drawings for merchandise, special guest appearances by the professional basketball players, and the local "runner" TV weather forecaster.

PRESS RELEASE

We publicized our event through a press release—an informational document that usually runs no more than a page. They can be used for general news about a special event or program. The release should include the five W's: who, what, when, where, and why. If you do not think you can write an adequate release, substitute a fact sheet that simply lists your major points. Both a press release and a fact sheet should include:

1. the announcement of the event: what it is, when it will take place, where, and who will be participating;
2. ticket prices and where to get tickets;
3. names of sponsors as they become available; and
4. facts and figures on the event.

We called first and then sent a press release to the local media (not directly competing with our sponsor). Press releases are the staple of the public relations business. However, Fox News Dallas reporter, Jeff Crilley, relates that the media get hundreds of emailed press releases each day, so first make a phone call to get the correct reporter's attention (1). See Chapter 32 for information.

Press releases can be used for various purposes:

1. to announce a new appointment or the opening of a practice,
2. to give details of a special event or program, and
3. to announce a new product or publication or the release of an association's position paper.

You can also try to get your release on the "wire." A news wire service is a valuable way to gain broad exposure. A release sent over the wire reaches media throughout the country and costs less than a mass mailing.

PRESS KITS

Press kits are used to interest the media in a larger story about your event (see Chapter 34). Press kits should be descriptive, attractive, and to the point. They should provide solid information and explain why the public would be interested in the event. The kit should include the following:

1. A press release or a pitch letter describing the event you want to publicize;
2. Samples of promotional giveaways and copies of related articles, advertisements, and critical reviews; and
3. Resumes or short biographical sketches of noteworthy organizers and participants.

Press Briefings

Press briefings are one-on-one desk-side interviews or more formal editorial board briefings that are used to provide the media with in-depth, background information about your event.

SPONSORSHIP

Event marketing and sponsorship have grown into a billion-dollar industry. Virtually every major special event or program held today requires at least some financial support from commercial sponsors.

Three types of sponsorship opportunities are available at each special event or program:

- financial,
- media, and
- in-kind.

All are important and worth pursuing. Financial sponsorship includes grants, donations, and corporate contributions. Media sponsorship includes radio, television, magazine, and newspaper support. And in-kind sponsorship is the donation of services or products in lieu of cash. These are services or products that you would normally have to buy to conduct the event anyway.

It is often best to secure your media sponsorships first. When print and broadcast sponsors commit their support and agree to promote your major financial sponsors, it becomes easier to secure cash-giving sponsorships. Media sponsors may contribute radio, TV, or newspaper advertising to promote the event. When my company does a national program, we target sponsorships with specific magazines. Both *Shape* and *Harper's Bazaar* magazines have provided ad space to help promote our women's sports programs.

Corporate sponsors are often in a position to help promote an event at little or no cost to themselves. Printing on grocery bags, adding bill stuffers, and tagging existing radio ads are a few examples. In-kind sponsors save you money by donating items that would otherwise have to be purchased. For example, a print shop may agree to print your brochures, signs, posters, or fliers at no charge. We also use a bulk mail company to help defray some of our bulk mailing and sorting costs. We get the service for free, and they get exposure in our promotional materials.

What are some of the benefits to the sponsor? Meaningful business returns can come in many forms:

- *Publicity.* Sponsors often benefit from the publicity generated by a community-wide or national event.
- *Enhanced image or public awareness.* Association with a popular or respected event can enhance a company's public image and is a good way for a new company in the community to get exposure.
- *Improved customer relations.* Special events allow sponsors to make their existing and potential customers feel very appreciated. Sponsors can show their appreciation by offering free tickets or underwriting a free special event for the entire community.
- *Sale of products or services at the event.* Certain types of companies will find that a community-wide special event enables them to sell large quantities of a product or service in a short period of time.
- *Increased employee morale.* Sponsorship of an event can include an opportunity for a company to provide perks for employees.
- *Opportunity to be a good corporate citizen.* More and more companies are realizing the long-term benefits of giving to the community in which their employees reside, and they are taking the responsibility seriously.
- *Economic development.* A special event can contribute to the quality of life in a community and provide monetary benefits as well.

Securing corporate sponsors for a worthwhile event need not be a difficult task since potential sponsors usually recognize a good investment. When soliciting a corporate sponsor, allocate sufficient time and follow a systematic process, which should include the following steps:

- *Define the sponsors' opportunities.* Describe the event in detail, including the date, day, time, location, past attendance figures, and target audience. State your goals and any experience from past events to substantiate your position.

- *Identify potential sponsors.* Potential sponsors are looking for exposure to their identified market. They are also looking for event exposure. Propose that brochures, ads, T-shirts, banners, signs, posters, fliers, and other printed materials include sponsors' logos. It is important that sponsors' names and logos be involved in the program or event, and that the nature of their business match the needs of the event.

- *Research potential sponsors.* Learn as much as you can from your potential sponsors. What is the company philosophy? Do they budget for sponsorships? What type of events have they sponsored in the past? Who buys and uses their product? What is their advertising strategy? What are their corporate goals for image enhancement, publicity, customer relations, employee relations, community relations, and economic development? Who makes sponsorship decisions? The event organizer who has taken the time to gather specific information about potential sponsors may have an advantage over others competing for a limited amount of sponsorship resources.

- *Develop the sponsorship proposal.* Develop a sponsorship package for each desired sponsor and write a formal sponsorship proposal. Each proposal should include a description of the event, information from past events, and a description of sponsorship levels that details what you are requesting of sponsors. Also include a list of benefits the sponsor will receive from the event, a market profile, the names of past sponsors, any promotional materials from past events or testimonials, and a clearly stated deadline for responses.

- *Follow up on the proposal.* Be sure to include a cover letter in your proposal specifying the date you will follow up. It is helpful to allow companies a week to 10 days of discussion time after the proposal has been received.

- *Sign a formal agreement with the sponsor(s).* Once you have an agreement with the sponsor, put the terms in writing. This can be done informally by a letter of agreement or formally by a contract. Either format should be signed by both parties.

- *Send a follow-up highlight report.* After the event's conclusion, put together a highlight report for your sponsors. The report should include the results of the event, photographs and stories from the event, copies of promotional materials focusing on the sponsors, and any other pertinent information.

OTHER MARKETING TOOLS

Celebrities attract attention and bring in the media and the crowds. When we held the "Go for Gold Race," we used several celebrities. Some were members of the local professional basketball team. We also invited top runners and race walkers as well as local media celebrities. The local news taped and narrated the entire event. The event was filmed and shown on cable in its entirety, and clips were shown during the 5 PM and 10 PM newscasts on the local TV station.

Posters, *signs*, and *banners* are potentially effective promotional tools if they are used appropriately. It is an important part of your master plan to determine the use of signs, banners, and posters. Make sure that they are eye-catching, provide pertinent information, and call your reader to respond. With signs and posters, you may want to include a tear-off, mail-in card. Banners draw attention. At a large outdoor event, such as a bike or foot race, banners can assist in directing and educating the crowd. State-of-the-art sign shops now use computerized equipment. Your message is put into the computer by keyboarding or scanning. The computer then sends the information to a plotter, which cuts the letters or symbols from a vinyl material. The vinyl is then transferred to a sign, banner, or poster. There are several levels of quality to choose from. This approach is not only cost-effective, but also time-saving.

Giveaways are always popular, whether they are T-shirts, shorts, notebooks, mugs, bumper stickers, gym bags, sweatbands, or posters. For our 4-day walking wellness getaway, every participant received a free pair of name-brand walking shoes from our sponsor. We worked out an agreement with our sponsor to sell us the shoes wholesale, and we allocated a very small amount of our per-person budget to cover the cost. The sponsor gets the name-brand exposure in all our promotions plus its normal wholesale cost for the shoes, and we get a very attractive perk for our program that the participants value at full retail price.

There are various opportunities for promotional tie-ins with every program or special event, but they are not always obvious. It may call for the promoter to use some imagination. A health or sports event may want a tie-in with a talk radio station. Not only is the exposure free, but it can be ten times more effective than any advertisement because of its direct relationship with the media. Without the proper promotions, your event or program may never get off the ground.

CASE STUDY 31.1

EXPERIENCE OF SMALL TOWN SPECIAL EVENTS COORDINATOR

Holly Deitrick, Events Coordinator, City of Lake Dallas, Texas

I have found that what works in some areas does not work in a small town. Recruiting celebrities and securing free media sponsorships are *very* difficult in our area. Radio and TV stations and newspapers in the metroplex are more focused on partnering with events that are occurring in Dallas and Fort Worth. However, our local newspaper and the one in Denton have been very good to us by printing articles to promote our events. Maybe when our events grow to 100,000+ in attendance, I will be able to secure one of the big media sponsors.

One method of publicity that seems to work no matter where you are located is the press release followed by a phone call. I have had great luck with numerous media outlets picking up one of my press releases on an event and publishing something about it either online or in print. So, although I cannot get most media outlets as "official sponsors," they do come through many times by just publishing (for free) something about the event.

I also create sponsorship packets to recruit corporate sponsors and this works well. I add one more thing to this. *After* the event, I send a report to show them how their sponsorship dollars were used (I always show that we gave them far *more* exposure than what they paid in sponsorship dollars through event advertising, promotions, etc.). This follow-up report is important because it allows your sponsor contact person to show their corporate "top dogs" how beneficial their sponsorship was and makes them more likely to sponsor future events. It has to be a win-win situation, so the sponsors need to be able to prove that their investment was worthwhile and beneficial to their companies.

SUMMARY

In summary, there are several key steps to gaining publicity for your program or event:

- Make a written plan for your event and set deadlines for completing tasks.
- Develop a budget and determine sponsorship contributions based on levels of exposure.
- Research and identify the appropriate sponsors for your event. Make sure to offer a win-win proposition to all sponsors.
- Work out a written agreement with each sponsor that includes a break-down of who is responsible for each task.
- Involve the media as sponsors to generate credibility in the eyes of potential participants in the event. Promotional tie-ins generate inexpensive or free media coverage.
- Bring your event to the media. The press release is a great way to introduce your program or event to the media.

REFERENCE

1. Crilley J. *Free Publicity*. Dallas, TX: Crilley; 2003.

HOW TO WRITE A PRESS RELEASE

32

Mona Boyd Browne, MS, RD

A press release, also called a news release, is used to generate publicity, and is the cornerstone of a successful public relations program. A press release is a newsy announcement from or about an organization that is written in journalistic style, follows a standard format, and is intended for publication or broadcast. Releases can be sent to print and broadcast media outlets, such as newspapers; magazines and newsletters; and radio, television, and cable stations. Press releases are used by editors, writers, reporters, and other members of the media to tell worthwhile stories and report news. Many published news and feature stories originate from press releases. The most important part of a press release is information. A good release provides a newsworthy story or announcement, stated clearly and simply. Press releases that are poorly written, contain misspelled words, or present sketchy or inaccurate information will likely end up in the trash. This quick how-to reference section shows you how to write a professional press release. It also contains several sample releases.

NEWSWORTHY TOPICS

Releases are used by dietetics professionals, public relations firms, and media experts to communicate newsworthy information and gain publicity. Press releases will help keep a company name and its products in the public spotlight. However, editors receive hundreds of press releases a day. Quick judgments are made based on a release's headline, first few paragraphs, and format. If it does not look like news or there is not an interesting title that grabs the editor's attention, he or she will not even read it, according to Jeff Crilley (1). This process is less hit-and-miss when you have ongoing relationships with people in the media and can pick up the phone to call a reporter or editor that you know.

A writer who knows what is newsworthy is more likely to create a press release that will be picked up by the media. How can you determine what is newsworthy? Start by identifying things that interest others. A good release will use a "hook," or story angle, to make a topic relevant, timely, and interesting. To grab an editor's attention, a press release might be written to:

- introduce a new or improved product;
- describe a new service or new merchandising;
- react to other late-breaking news;
- counter negative problems;
- offer an educational brochure or publication;
- publicize a campaign kickoff or completion;
- report research or survey results;
- present new information;
- promote a public appearance, media interview, speech, or trade show activities;
- announce meetings, anniversaries, special events, or awards;
- disclose staff changes, such as promotions and appointments, or employee activities; and
- announce the formation of a private practice or relocation to a new or improved facility.

TYPES OF RELEASES

There are two basic types of releases: straight news and feature. A *straight news release* reports a serious subject in a serious manner—it gets right to the point. The lead, or first paragraph, contains a summary of the essentials: the who, what, when, where, why, and how of the story. The remainder of the release uses facts and other details to expand the lead. Announcements of the results of a scientific study, campaign kickoff or conclusion, new product or service, or personnel changes are examples of straight news releases.

A *feature news release* may deal with either a serious or a light topic. It is written in a relaxed, informal style; its tone may be light and entertaining. The feature news release lead teases the reader instead of summarizing the main points; it reaches its point in the third or fourth paragraph. Feature press releases use the human interest factor to draw attention to a product, service, or company. See the sample press release in Figure 32.1.

FORMAT GUIDELINES

A professional press release follows a standard format, although many writers take liberty with certain components. Use the following guidelines to write a professional press release:

1. *Paper.* Use 8.5- by 11-inch, 16- to 20-pound white bond paper or company letterhead. Use only one side of the paper. Type neatly.
2. *Length.* Keep the release as short as possible—usually one page.
3. *Spacing.* Double-space all copy.
4. *Margins.* Leave a one-inch margin on each side of the page and at the bottom. Leave three to four inches at the top of the first page. Indent the first line of each paragraph 5 or 10 spaces.
5. *Release date.* Type FOR IMMEDIATE RELEASE or FOR RELEASE plus a specific date a few spaces above the first paragraph in the upper left corner. A release may also be embargoed, or held, until a certain date or time, if you have a good reason for asking an editor to do so. In such a case, the heading might read FOR RELEASE AFTER 10 AM, MAY 18, 2009. A dateline—a first line telling where the story originated—may also be used. For example: New York, October 1, 2009—The art of writing a press release.
6. *Identification.* Place the name and telephone number (including area code) of the person to contact for more information in the upper right corner of the first page.
7. *Photographs.* If there are pictures with your release, use the phrase "With Art" and include a brief description of each photo.
8. *Headline.* Headlines are optional, and many editors compose their own. Nonetheless, use a headline on your release unless you know an editor dislikes headlines. A short headline that tells the whole story can capture an editor's attention. Center and underline the release headline, leaving at least one or two inches between the headline and the start of the text.
9. *Style.* A straight news release follows the inverted pyramid style. The lead, or first paragraph, contains key facts: the who, what, when, where, why, and how of the story. Subsequent paragraphs back up the lead with facts, placing less-important details last. A feature release uses the lead to tease the reader rather than summarizing the main points, and reaches the point in the third or fourth paragraph.
10. *Technical words.* Translate jargon and technical words into everyday language. If technical terms are necessary, define them. Use simple words as often as possible.
11. *Quote.* Quotes are used to lend personal authority to a statement made in the release. If a quote is used, identify the spokesperson by name and title. Quotes must be taken directly from a person or approved by the source.
12. *Sentences and paragraphs.* Keep sentences short and simple, twenty words or less. End lines with complete words to prevent typesetting errors. Paragraphs should also be short and limited to four or five lines.
13. *Active voice.* Every word counts. Use the active voice to make a stronger statement with fewer words. Cut out extra words and phrases to clarify the message.
14. *Page numbers.* If the release is more than one page, place the page number in the upper left corner (excluding the first page). Also use a header of one or two words so pages can be easily identified. Try to end each page with a completed paragraph, or at least a completed sentence. For press releases longer than one page, type "more" at the bottom of each page, except the last page. Always end the release with the symbols # # # or the digits -30-or -0-.
15. *Editing.* Always edit the release. If possible, let the draft sit overnight. Review it the next day from a fresh perspective.
16. *Proofreading.* Accuracy is critical. Check for spelling errors and grammatical mistakes. Use a word processor spell checker and check by eye. A publicist who makes mistakes will be considered unreliable by editors and reporters.
17. *Correcting errors.* If an error is discovered after the release has gone out, issue a correction immediately to every recipient.

COMPUTRITION
HOSPITALITY SOFTWARE SOLUTIONS

19808 Nordhoff Place
Chatsworth, CA 91311
Phone: 800-222-4488
Fax: 818-701-1702
www.computrition.com

Media Contact:
Stephanie Luros
Director of Marketing
Computrition, Inc.
800-222-4488 x 250
sluros@computrition.com

FOR IMMEDIATE RELEASE

Live Like You Mean It Tackles the Quintessential Boomer Question

"Now that I've done everything I was supposed to do, what do I really want to do?"

Chatsworth, Calif., June 26, 2006—Most people don't know the answer to this question – and don't know how to find it. In fact, say *Live Like You Mean It* authors Ken Wasco and Ellyn Luros-Elson, RD, most people bring more soul-searching, focus, determination, action and self-evaluation to planning their vacations than they bring to discovering and planning what to do with their lives.

Live Like You Mean It (hardcover $22.00), released in late August by Helm Publishing, uses a travel metaphor – R.O.A.D. – to coach the reader through the process of **R**ecognizing a goal or dream; **O**ptimizing the environment to promote success; **A**cting with vigor and determination; and **D**elivering results worthy of legacy building. Throughout the book, the concepts of choice and attitude act as a compass, keeping the reader on track toward self-fulfillment.

Although inspired by the needs of their fellow boomers, Wasco and Luros-Elson's model for personal fulfillment is a meaningful tool for people of all ages. The authors use their own triumphs and occasional "bumps in the road" as examples in this motivational book-meets-instructional manual on savoring life's journey.

Ken Wasco, a marketing executive with Gordon Food Service (www.gfs.com), the largest privately held food distributor in North America, is a sought-after motivational speaker and facilitator.

Ellyn Luros-Elson, a registered dietitian, is the founder of Computrition, Inc., a multimillion-dollar international software systems company specializing in foodservice and nutrition management software. In 2005, she became the first woman to be honored with the International Food Service Industry Executives Association's "Food Service Industry Award of Excellence."

For more information, or to schedule an interview with either author, please visit www.computrition.com, or contact sluros@computrition.com.

#

FIGURE 32.1. ■ Sample press release.

18. *More information.* If the story has more information than will fit in a release, enclose a fact sheet or backgrounder. A fact sheet or backgrounder supplements a press release with additional information and is used when the release alone cannot tell the whole story. For example, a press release from The New York State Dietetic Association announced its Hunger Alert Day with a fact sheet detailing local area activities and participating organizations.

SUMMARY

A press release is the standard communication tool in public relations and working with the media. Write your rough draft and then let other people read it for impact and clarity. Consider hiring a person with marketing or public relations background who has experience writing press releases to write or review your work. With the clutter that editors and reporters now receive daily, it is time to return to personal phone calls (that avoid being too close to newspaper deadlines and going on the air), along with emailed or faxed press releases.

REFERENCE

1. Crilley J. *Free Publicity*. Dallas, Texas: Crilley; 2003.

BIBLIOGRAPHY

Aronson M, Spetner D, Ames C. *The Public Relations Writer's Handbook*. San Francisco, CA: Jossey-Bass; 2007.

Doty DI, Pincus M. *Publicity and Public Relations*. Hauppauge, NY: Barron's Educational Series; 2001.

Yale DR. *The Publicity Handbook: How to Maximize Publicity for Products, Services and Organizations*. Lincolnwood, IL: NTC Business Books; 1991.

HOW TO WRITE A QUERY OR PITCH LETTER

33

Neva Hudiburgh Cochran, MS, RD, LD

Seeing your great nutrition story idea in print, or on the radio or TV requires having the right story and delivery, and using the right tools. In the case of the media or a book publisher, this tool is called a query or pitch letter. While the two are similar, they have somewhat different purposes. A *query letter* is used when you want to write your own story, article, or book, usually for a fee or royalty. In contrast, *a pitch letter* sells an idea to the print and broadcast media with someone else writing the article or producing the story with you quoted as an expert. The latter option is typically used when you do not have the time, skills, or money to write the article or produce the radio or TV story, or when you want the credibility of the media producing your story for their audiences.

Since editors formulate their impressions of you and your idea from this letter, it is important that it looks and sounds professional. Ideally, your letter should be one to two single-spaced typed pages on good-quality stationery. It should be long enough to develop your idea but short enough to be read quickly.

SIX STEPS TO A BEST-SELLING LETTER

1. Begin a query or pitch letter with an attention-grabbing opening sentence. For example, "Kids are nuts about peanut butter," or "Of the nearly 80% of U.S. women who have tried a fad diet, 64% considered it a failure."
2. Next, summarize your idea in one paragraph to pique the editor's interest so he or she will want to know more.
3. Follow with an explanation of why the editor's audience would be interested in the story. Show that you have done your homework by mentioning other recent stories in their publication or on the air. According to Jeff Crilley, Fox News in Dallas, Texas, "We all want compliments on our past work—show us that you have seen our work. Then tell me why I cannot live without your story! Do not waste my time and yours on stories that do not fit my kind of show. Do not call me and pitch an idea that I had on last week!"
4. Once the groundwork is laid, give a few colorful details about the story and include a photo or visual ideas, if you have them. The art possibilities alone will often sell an idea.
5. Include information about yourself and why you are qualified to write or be interviewed about the topic. If you plan to write the story yourself, include names of experts you would interview as well as one or two samples of previously published articles.
6. Conclude your letter by telling the editor how to reach you if he or she is interested in the idea and whether or not you plan to follow up by telephone. Always include your telephone number and a business card.

It is acceptable to send simultaneous query or pitch letters to several editors, producers, or reporters. However, if more than one expresses interest in your idea, you will need to use different angles for the articles or interviews, particularly if the publications or broadcast outlets are in direct competition. For example, a pitch about healthy eating for children could focus on ideas for nutritious sack lunches for one story and getting kids involved in planning and preparing meals at home for another. If more than one book publisher is interested, you can choose the one that appears to be most capable or the one that gives the best offer.

The following is an example of a successful letter (see Fig. 33.1) used by this author to pitch a

Neva Cochran, M.S., R.D., L.D.
Nutrition Consultant

11840 Brookhill Lane • Dallas, TX 75230 • (972) 386-9035
FAX (972) 386-5593 • nevacoch@aol.com

Caroline Tredway
Nutrition Editor
First for Women Magazine
270 Sylvan Avenue
Englewood Cliffs, NJ 07632

Dear Caroline:

Is it really possible to avoid feeling as stuffed as your turkey without taking the cheer out of holiday fare? Absolutely! According to the American Dietetic Association, healthy eating doesn't mean giving up your favorite holiday foods.

I'm sure your readers would be interested in an article with tips on slimming down holiday favorites without sacrificing flavor and fun. Interviews with registered dietitians would reveal their secrets for slashing fat and calories while maintaining taste and tradition for holiday meals and parties. Topics could include:

- preparation tips to cut fat and calories in traditional holiday dishes
- makeover of a typical holiday meal to slash 1200 calories and 70 grams of fat
- clever suggestions to avoid overindulging at holiday meals and parties
- ideas for food gifts that are easy on the waistline

As a registered dietitian with over twenty years of experience, I have a wealth of knowledge on nutrition and diet topics of interest to women. I have been quoted in over 500 media interviews about nutrition and diet including many in national magazines and served as a spokesperson for the American Dietetic Association for the seven years. In addition, I currently write the **Diet Club** column for **Woman's World** magazine and have had three feature stories published in that magazine during the past two years.

I look forward to hearing from you about this or any other ideas for nutrition and diet articles I might write for **First**. You may call me at 972-386-9035.

Sincerely,

Neva Cochran, M.S., RD, LD

FIGURE 33.1.   ■   Sample successful query letter.

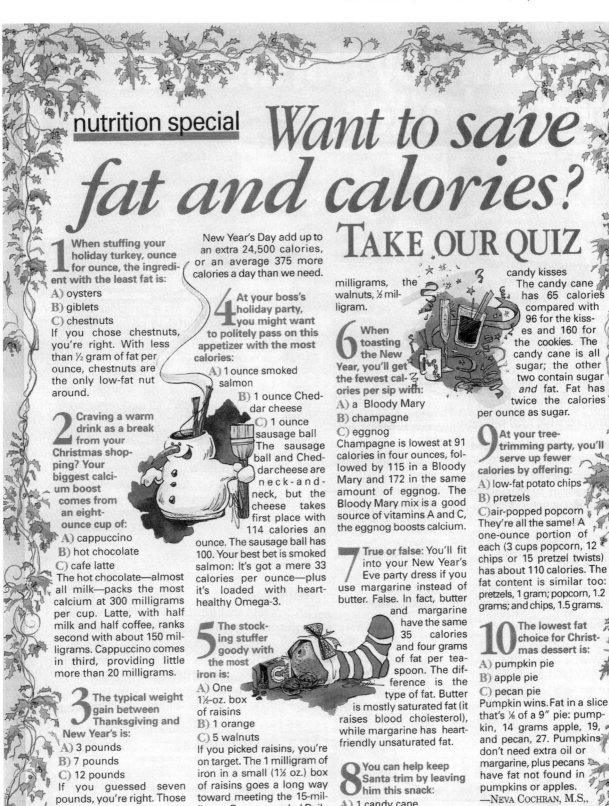

nutrition special

Want to save fat and calories?

TAKE OUR QUIZ

1 When stuffing your holiday turkey, ounce for ounce, the ingredient with the least fat is:

A) oysters
B) giblets
C) chestnuts

If you chose chestnuts, you're right. With less than ½ gram of fat per ounce, chestnuts are the only low-fat nut around.

2 Craving a warm drink as a break from your Christmas shopping? Your biggest calcium boost comes from an eight-ounce cup of:

A) cappuccino
B) hot chocolate
C) cafe latte

The hot chocolate—almost all milk—packs the most calcium at 300 milligrams per cup. Latte, with half milk and half coffee, ranks second with about 150 milligrams. Cappuccino comes in third, providing little more than 20 milligrams.

3 The typical weight gain between Thanksgiving and New Year's is:

A) 3 pounds
B) 7 pounds
C) 12 pounds

If you guessed seven pounds, you're right. Those holiday treats we eat between Thanksgiving Day and New Year's Day add up to an extra 24,500 calories, or an average 375 more calories a day than we need.

4 At your boss's holiday party, you might want to politely pass on this appetizer with the most calories:

A) 1 ounce smoked salmon
B) 1 ounce Cheddar cheese
C) 1 ounce sausage ball

The sausage ball and Cheddar cheese are neck-and-neck, but the cheese takes first place with 114 calories an ounce. The sausage ball has 100. Your best bet is smoked salmon: It's got a mere 33 calories per ounce—plus it's loaded with heart-healthy Omega-3.

5 The stocking stuffer goody with the most iron is:

A) One 1½-oz. box of raisins
B) 1 orange
C) 5 walnuts

If you picked raisins, you're on target. The 1 milligram of iron in a small (1½ oz.) box of raisins goes a long way toward meeting the 15-milligram Recommended Daily Allowance for this important mineral. The orange has .2 milligrams, the walnuts, ½ milligram.

6 When toasting the New Year, you'll get the fewest calories per sip with:

A) a Bloody Mary
B) champagne
C) eggnog

Champagne is lowest at 91 calories in four ounces, followed by 115 in a Bloody Mary and 172 in the same amount of eggnog. The Bloody Mary mix is a good source of vitamins A and C, the eggnog boosts calcium.

7 True or false: You'll fit into your New Year's Eve party dress if you use margarine instead of butter. False. In fact, butter and margarine have the same 35 calories and four grams of fat per teaspoon. The difference is the type of fat. Butter is mostly saturated fat (it raises blood cholesterol), while margarine has heart-friendly unsaturated fat.

8 You can help keep Santa trim by leaving him this snack:

A) 1 candy cane
B) 2 iced sugar cookies
C) 4 chocolate candy kisses

The candy cane has 65 calories compared with 96 for the kisses and 160 for the cookies. The candy cane is all sugar; the other two contain sugar *and* fat. Fat has twice the calories per ounce as sugar.

9 At your tree-trimming party, you'll serve up fewer calories by offering:

A) low-fat potato chips
B) pretzels
C) air-popped popcorn

They're all the same! A one-ounce portion of each (3 cups popcorn, 12 chips or 15 pretzel twists) has about 110 calories. The fat content is similar too: pretzels, 1 gram; popcorn, 1.2 grams; and chips, 1.5 grams.

10 The lowest fat choice for Christmas dessert is:

A) pumpkin pie
B) apple pie
C) pecan pie

Pumpkin wins. Fat in a slice that's ⅛ of a 9" pie: pumpkin, 14 grams apple, 19, and pecan, 27. Pumpkins don't need extra oil or margarine, plus pecans have fat not found in pumpkins or apples.
—NEVA COCHRAN, M.S., R.D.

28 First for women 12/9/96

FIGURE 33.2. ■ Column resulting from letter shown in Figure 33.1.

story idea about healthy holiday eating to promote the theme of balance, variety, and moderation as the keys. It was sent to the nutrition editor of *First for Women*, who had previously called her several times for quotes for the magazine's nutrition stories. The editor responded with interest in the idea but wanted her to write another article first! When that assignment was completed, the editor asked her to develop a holiday nutrition quiz (see Fig. 33.2). Soon after this, the editor left the magazine for a non–health related publication. When the editor ended up at *The Female Patient*, a magazine for physician waiting rooms, she called again to request a nutrition quiz in each issue and eventually an additional feature, the "10 Tips for Great Nutrition" column. This led to a 5-year tenure with the publication that also included writing several feature articles.

HOW TO START

Before writing a query or pitch letter, familiarize yourself with your target publication or program. Determining its audience, format, style, and choice of topics can give you insight into the types of stories that would have appeal. Also identify the appropriate editor or reporter for your particular idea. Obtain the name from the masthead or by calling the publication or station. It is important that the letter be sent to the right person and that the idea meet the needs and interests of the intended readers, viewers, or listeners.

According to Allison Nemetz, Cover Features Editor for *Woman's World* magazine (a publication for which the author has been a freelance writer, columnist, and researcher since 1993), first-time writers will have the most luck pitching stories that:

- Have a timely topic: new, buzzed-about idea, or the subject of new scientific research.
- Have an angle that precisely suits the publication and department being pitched. Read several issues of a publication and look for commonalities among stories to help deter-

mine what a particular magazine department is looking for. For example, the *Woman's World's* cover department runs inspirational stories on quick or easy weight loss strategies; other publications tend to take a more clinical approach.
- Provide practical information that readers will find helpful, interesting, and important. Essay and opinion pieces are typically assigned to established writers.

Allison also suggests that query letters from first-time writers be mailed, as magazine editors are often deluged with e-mails and may not read those from addresses they do not recognize. And no phone calls, she adds.

Registered dietitian, Tanya Zuckerbrot, a columnist for *Men's Fitness* and author of the recently published book *The F-Factor Diet* learned the hard way that a simple letter is the best approach to get your name in print. "Originally I thought the way to launch my writing career was to submit an article to several magazine editors but discovered that was a mistake when no one got back to me," she says. So next she sent out a letter with her bio, photo, and list of topics she could address, inviting editors to call her if they thought she could help them with a story. "I got several calls and was quoted in a few articles." Over time, being quoted in numerous magazines helped build her resume, identified her as a credible source of nutrition information, and led to an invitation to write the nutrition column for *Men's Fitness*.

SUMMARY

While not all query or pitch letters will result in an immediate assignment or interview, a well-written letter may prompt an editor to call about another story idea or an opportunity to do an interview. Letters are often filed for future reference, and a request may come months later. By continuing to send your best ideas to the media or publishers, you begin to establish rapport, which one day may lead to a good working relationship.

34

HOW TO DEVELOP A PRESS KIT

Amelia Catakis, MBA, RD

You just wrote an exciting, informative press release. But there is more information that needs to be shared. What should you do? You need a press kit! Besides the press release, what else should you include? Whatever it takes to grab the attention of the recipients! The press kit is used to interest the media in doing an interview or article on the subject or person being promoted.

THE OUTSIDE FOLDER

First, you need a distinctive, quality folder that has pockets inside and that may or may not have a logo or message on the outside. It should not be too flashy, nor should it look like a term paper. If your resources are limited, a folder made of good paper stock will do nicely.

CONTENTS

The contents must be considered carefully because many media people in larger markets receive hundreds of press releases and press kits per week. (*Time* magazine once reported that it received over 1,500 press kits per week.) The enclosed material should be easy to scan and read, and the purpose for the kit must be obvious.

Materials usually included in a press kit are:

- the press release;
- simple fact sheets;
- any background papers, which give more detail;
- copies of news articles supporting your press release (such as articles substantiating the problem you have identified or showing the

person you are promoting featured in *People* magazine);
- clear reprints of appropriate articles from reputable professional journals, if appropriate; and
- a brief biography and photograph of the main spokesperson.

Always have a contact name and phone numbers. It does not hurt to clip or staple a business card to the press kit. See a sample press kit in Figure 34.1.

GETTING THE KIT TO THE MEDIA AND GETTING A STORY

When press kits are distributed to reporters at a press conference or a media event, the material in the kit should follow the gathering's agenda. Many times, however, press kits are delivered or mailed to reporters and writers who cover the subject of your message, such as a food editor or book reviewer. A properly prepared press kit will grab their attention and interest, which, one hopes, will create the desired follow-up.

Do not leave your marketing to chance. Follow up with phone calls to the kit's recipients, but be sensitive to the possibilities that they may not have much time to talk, especially around deadlines, and that some people do not want phone calls. However, if you do speak to some of them, ask if they plan to do a story or interview. Have a sales pitch ready about how well the children's nutrition campaign is going, how well the book is selling, how the governor has now signed a declaration naming May Blueberry Month, or that you only have one more media interview time slot left for the date you are in that town.

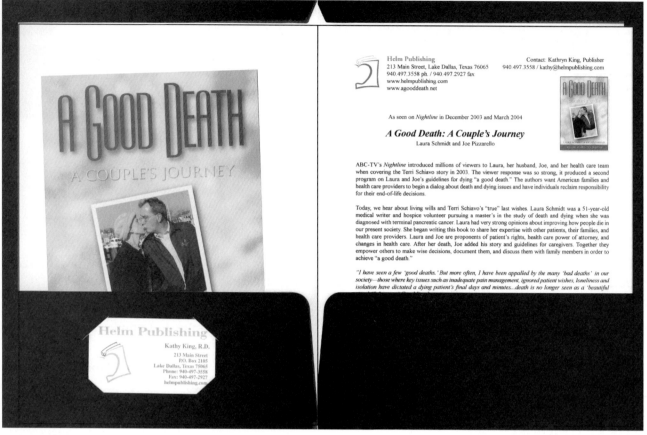

FIGURE 34.1. ■ Sample press kit.

SAMPLE PRESS KIT FOR A CORPORATE PROMOTION

Marriott School Services accounts sent this press kit to their local media to announce their plans for National Nutrition Month.

> Outside: Folder was plain white with the Marriott logo
>
> Inside, right side:

- press release (2 pages) announcing the activities,
- fact sheet (2 pages) with details about the division, and
- sample from implementation guide (4 pages) for food-service managers (typed on appropriate letterhead).

Inside, left side:

- sample materials to be used: lunch bag, USDA Food Pyramid mobile, nutrition trading cards.

SAMPLE PRESS KIT FOR A MEDIA TOUR TO SELL A BOOK

Outside: Folder should be an attractive color with a public relations company logo or your own logo, or plain

Inside, right side (see sample press kit items):

- press release on you, the author, and the book—why is it unique? (1–2 pages),
- your biography (1 page),
- sample news clipping on you and your unique experiences or something else of note (1 page), and
- sample questions the reporter could ask (1 page).

Inside, left side:

- the book, if it is small enough; otherwise, your black-and-white photo or another article of particular interest.

SUMMARY

A press kit is a big step beyond a press release or pitch letter. It holds more information and may include such things as a photo, examples of articles you have written or articles written about you, sample media questions, product specification sheets or sample, or new book.

HOW TO MARKET AT CONVENTIONS AND TRADE SHOWS

35

Ruth B. Fischer, MS

Exhibiting at conventions, trade shows, and health fairs is one of many potentially effective strategies to choose from in marketing your product or service. Since exhibiting is labor-intensive, costly, and time-consuming, it is important to make the most of your exhibit. You must decide why, when or where, and what to exhibit before you decide how to exhibit effectively. Just being in an exhibit hall does not guarantee that your sales or public relations will be improved one bit. Handing out free key chains, pens, toys, etc., may attract many people to the booth, but unless there is interaction and, hopefully, qualifying questions to determine the best prospects for future business, the booth may not produce useful nor valuable results.

WHY TO EXHIBIT

An exhibit is a very visual, dynamic, and interactive way to reach target markets. The reasons for exhibiting are numerous and include both sales and public relations objectives. Purposes for exhibiting at a trade show or convention are:

- introduction of a new product or service,
- increased name recognition for your company and its products,
- selling a product or service,
- demonstration of a product or service, and
- participation in a community event or project.

WHEN OR WHERE TO EXHIBIT

Your product or service, target markets, and marketing objectives help you determine which exhibiting opportunities you should pursue. For example, if you have a catering service in Omaha, is there any reason for you to exhibit at the national ADA

Annual Meeting and Exhibition? Probably not, if you consider only your primary business. However, if you just published a catering cookbook and you want to attract other dietitians or dietetic technicians to your catering regional workshops, it could be a wise choice. Other considerations when deciding whether or not to exhibit at a show are:

- whether it fits into your marketing plan;
- whether it reaches your primary target audience;
- reputation of the show and its management;
- past attendance;
- media or other marketing support;
- number of exhibit hours without competing programs;
- dates and competing events in the region (important if attracting the public);
- location of available booths in relation to flow of traffic;
- types of exhibitors in surrounding booths;
- cost of booth space, rental cost of furnishings, labor costs, whether a percentage of revenues must return to the show, and whether refunds are available if less than the minimum guaranteed number attends (few shows ask for a percentage or guarantee attendance); and
- cost-effectiveness considering all other ways to reach your target markets.

WHAT TO EXHIBIT

When deciding what to include in your exhibit, check your marketing objectives and reasons for exhibiting at the particular convention, trade show, or health fair. To be the most effective, an exhibit needs a focused message; just being represented is not enough to justify the time and expense. Once you determine your central message, it is much easier to develop a dynamic, memorable, and effective exhibit.

THE ANATOMY OF AN EXHIBIT

THE MESSAGE

The message is the core, or heart, of what you want your exhibit to demonstrate. Spend time developing your key message. Make it clear, catchy, and memorable. Your message should be unique to your product or service. It may be that your logo, business name, and descriptive subtitle serve these purposes. It should be used consistently in the heading for the booth, on brochures or flyers, and on your business cards.

KEY DESCRIPTORS

With the heart in place, it is possible to build the skeleton. The parts of the skeleton are the key attributes you want buyers of your service to know and remember. Some examples for a business that sells prepared prenatal nutrition seminars are as follows:

- You as the provider are qualified and experienced.
- The unique benefits as compared to the competition.
- How buyers can use the product or service.
- Why buyers should buy it now (convention discount, etc.).

Choose your key descriptors carefully. For an exhibit, they should be short, like the examples above.

FEATURES

Add other body parts once the frame is in place. For example, bulleted descriptions under your key attributes can explain the features of your program or service and help the target audience understand your message. You could clarify the attribute "How buyers can use the product" mentioned above with its parts or features:

- colorful overheads
- entertaining props
- participant handouts
- practical instructor's guide
- marketing support artwork and sample advertisements

COMPANY IDENTIFICATION

The head of the exhibit is your company identification. Make sure your name and logo are prominent, distinctive, and legible, and still complement the design and character of your exhibit. You want your name and logo to make a statement and become recognizable to your customers.

THE EXHIBIT BOARD/DISPLAY

The exhibit board is like the skin or covering that holds everything together. It serves as the background for your exhibit and helps define your exhibit's shape, size, and texture. The exhibit board plays a large role in determining the professionalism of your exhibit. Remember, a poorly designed exhibit projects a poor image, no matter what the quality of your product or service!

Consider buying or leasing a modular table top exhibit board. Although such displays are not inexpensive, their versatility and durability make them a reasonable investment. For most of us, it is important that the exhibit board be lightweight and constructed with sturdy interlocking joints, and it must be easily transported. Before you buy a large exhibit, make sure that you can afford the shipping, drayage fees in the exhibit halls, set-up and breakdown fees, and added airline fees for extra baggage.

Commercial display boards are two-sided and come in your choice of colors. Select two colors that combine with many colors and accent your logo. Basic, adaptable colors allow you a broader spectrum of options when planning the materials to attach to your board. Many portable, modular exhibits come with a carrying or shipping case that protects them and makes them easier to store. Also, many commercial display boards include optional lighting, shelves, brochure pockets, and other customized features that you can purchase as your budget allows.

DRESSING UP YOUR EXHIBIT

How you design and arrange your exhibit is like choosing what to wear. The style, design, and look of the exhibit should be appropriate for the occasion. Just as you would not wear jeans, a T-shirt, and sneakers to an important interview, your exhibit should not look like just any old thing thrown together. Your exhibit may be your one chance to interest a prospective client in your product or service, so you do not want to give the wrong first impression. When planning your exhibit design, consider these tips:

- Make the artwork, graphic design, and typefaces pleasing, appropriate, and complementary to your overall look.
- Be sure that printing is large and easy to read.
- Keep messages positive and upbeat.
- Avoid clutter.
- Use color to add interest.

- Plan something special about your exhibit to set it apart and make it memorable.
- Consider using photographs, especially colored photographs, to show your product or service in use.

ADDING ACCESSORIES

Although what appears on the exhibit board sets the tone for your exhibit, the handouts and other tabletop accessories are just as important. To tell your story best, a few carefully chosen accessories are often better than too many.

Some tips for a tasteful presentation are as follows:

- Develop or choose no more than four brochures or other pieces of literature to support your exhibit. Have them focus on the product or service you are trying to sell through your exhibit. I am sure you have all been to exhibits that displayed every piece of print material the exhibitor ever produced. You may have picked them up to read later, but probably discarded them or they got lost in the mass of information. The only thing that was memorable was the clutter, not the product. Do not be tempted to over-merchandise.
- Consider developing display notebooks for samples of your program materials or literature that further explains your services. Design the notebook to complement your exhibit and include materials that show and discuss the unique features of your product or service. The notebooks should be compact, easy to handle, and helpful in keeping your exhibit neat and manageable. Mark the notebook "Sample materials. For display only!" The notebook will help stop exhibit attendees from walking away with your precious exhibit-support materials.
- Plan a hook to get people to visit your exhibit. Something action-oriented helps attract potential customers to your booth. Successful exhibits can use one or more techniques. Some examples are to offer a prize or drawing, serve food, conduct a survey, run a computer program, or show a slide series or promotional video.

LAYOUT

Do not set up barriers between your booth and your audience, unless you are selling books or other items that need to be displayed and you want a more secure area for your cash, credit cards, and inventory. If you want to invite attendees into your booth, place the exhibit at the back, allowing easy entry and exit, and consider adding two chairs with a small table or two stools with a high table where discussions can more easily take place. If you need more display space, consider ordering a corner booth.

LOCATION

Many exhibit planners overestimate the number of expected attendees in order to attract more booth sales. Ask how many attended in past years and if the convention moves each year, be sure that you assess the attractiveness of that city as well. Large conventions usually offer huge exhibit areas, but member product booths may be in hallways and side rooms—some locations much better than others—and the same goes for health fairs. Before you sign up, find out the traffic patterns of attendees to and from meetings or major attractions. If the health fair is outside, find out if there are contingency plans for rain, strong wind, or extreme heat.

Studies show that people stop or slow down at every fourth exhibit. Study the floor plan of the exhibit area before you choose your booth location and stay away from anchor exhibits (very large) that will attract a lot of traffic and far back and side booths in a very large room. Instead, choose a more central booth in a high-traffic area on the path going to or away from the anchor. Talk to the exhibit representative to make sure that you will not be next to or across from any other booth that could cause problems with your traffic flow (long lines in front of your booth because people want a photo with a movie star look-alike in the next booth), or a smell is produced that you do not want to handle for 3 days, i.e., deep fried foods, cotton candy, microwave popcorn, and so on.

PEOPLE ARE MOST IMPORTANT

A common mistake by businesses is putting inexperienced or temporary help in a booth instead of their top sales people. All who work at your booth are salespeople for your company and its products and services. They need to communicate the same image and message as the exhibit itself; professionalism, clean appearance, and friendliness are keys to making a positive impression.

If inexperienced people are working at your exhibit, prepare them for what to expect. Exhibiting is a tiring job. With all your other designing and planning, do not forget to train the people who provide that all-important personal representation of your company. Teach everyone how to identify A accounts (top prospects), B, and C ones. Keep the business cards or lead forms in a safe place, not in a bowl on a table. Take the cards or forms back to your room at the end of each day for safekeeping.

When working a booth, train your staff to:

- Know your products and services. Anticipate questions that potential clients may ask. Be prepared.
- Be cheerful, enthusiastic, and outgoing. Make potential clients feel comfortable when talking with you.
- Remember that people attending conventions, trade shows, and health fairs are often looking for new ideas, products, and services. That is what you sell.
- Think of yourself as a professional salesperson. You are there to make contacts and sell your product or service.
- Dress comfortably, but appropriately; you will be on your feet for long periods of time.
- Plan enough staffing to appropriately handle the number of potential visitors. The size of the show, the length of the exhibit hours, and the size of your booth as well as your budget will determine the size staff you need.
- Try to find out the peak times for viewers (when meetings are out of session); this will help you anticipate demand and plan breaks. It is important to stay fresh.
- Enjoy meeting new people and potential customers!

FOLLOW-UP

If you do not sell a product from your booth, use your booth to find qualified decision makers who may buy your product at a later date. These prospects are only as good as your follow-up. Prepare your follow-up materials before you go to the show so they are not delayed. The A group of prospects should be contacted by phone, personal visit, or mailed a packet within a week. The B group should be contacted within two weeks; and the C group should be mailed something, although follow-up can wait until the A and B groups have been contacted. On average, 80% of your business from the show will come from Group A, according to the Small Business Administration.

SUMMARY

After considering all these points, the final thing to do is to ask yourself once again if your company should be participating at this particular convention, trade show, or health fair. To make the best use of your time and marketing budget, be very careful in choosing which exhibiting opportunities you pursue.

36

HOW TO WRITE EFFECTIVELY TO PHYSICIANS

Linda Gay, MS, RD

Written communication to physicians is important when establishing rapport and updating patient-care records. This form of communication is not meant to take the place of face-to-face meetings but to facilitate their occurrence.

FEATURES OF A PROMOTION LETTER

A promotion letter introduces you and your services to a prospective client. This type of letter can help get your foot in the door at physicians' offices when you open a private practice, outpatient office, or any new service that you want to promote. It is well known that physicians refer their patients to people they know and respect. It is important to take the time to get to know physicians in your area and be known. Letters and reports on patients' progress should follow as patients are counseled to strengthen professional relationships.

INDIVIDUALIZATION

The heading and content of one basic letter can be adapted to each prospective physician. Considering the unbelievable amounts of mail people receive today and the fact that 30% of all unsolicited mail goes unopened, letters should not be addressed to "Dear Local Physician" or "Dearborn Clinic Medical Team." Take the time to individualize each letter and address.

Before you compose a promotion letter for physicians, you should first analyze the situation from two points of view, yours and the physician's. Ask yourself these questions:

- what is the physician interested in?
- does he or she have a specialty?
- what can you do for his or her patients?

- why would the physician choose to refer a patient to you rather than to another registered dietitian?

Your letter should target these key points.

CONTENT

A short, well-written introductory letter should briefly describe:

- how the physician can use your services for her or his patients;
- what services you offer specific to that physician's specialty or patients' needs;
- your credentials and experience (or enclose a professional bio or profile); and
- how to schedule an appointment (your brochure with phone number, hours, location, parking, and the like may also be enclosed).

Close your letter by suggesting a face-to-face, five-minute interview in the physician's office or a leisure lunch—your treat. (Box 36.1 shows a sample introductory letter.)

Referral Letters
Private practitioners often use letters from referring physicians along with introductory promotion letters to help open new doors. Even if you move from one state to another, you can become established faster if you use referral letters from former physician colleagues who knew you and respected your work.

Biography
Send a one-page professional biography or profile that outlines your educational background and your experience. This will provide the physician with more detailed information about you and help establish your credibility faster. If you have

BOX 36.1 | *Sample Introductory Letter*

Jane Jones, MS, RD
Ambulatory Nutrition Specialist
828 North Forrest Avenue, New Haven, CT 06504

September 12, 2009

John Smith, MD
Obstetrics and Gynecology
2 Church Street
New Haven, CT 06504

Dear Dr. Smith:

The Yale-New Haven Hospital Centers of Nutrition would like to extend its services to your OB-GYN patients. I have enclosed a package of information that describes our staff and services. Our program emphasizes a medically oriented approach providing in-depth initial nutrition assessment and long-term counseling. Patients are seen either individually or with family members. We welcome clients of all ages, and invite you to send your referrals for individualized nutrition care.

Some problems commonly encountered in our practice include prenatal nutrition, gestational diabetes, diabetes, food intolerance. Our centers are staffed by registered dietitians with advanced degrees in nutrition or public health. We work closely with the referring physician and endeavor to send timely correspondence reporting on patient progress.

I would be pleased to meet with you, your associates, and your staff at your convenience to discuss our program further and answer any questions you may have.

Sincerely,
(Insert signature here)
Jane Jones, MS, RD
Ambulatory Nutrition Specialist

several nutrition counselors in your practice, include a professional profile of each staff member. Do not repeat the same bio information in the promotion letter; it only needs to be explained once.

Brochure with Rolodex or Business Card

As part of your introductory package, you could include a brochure. Since convenience is an important consideration, you might want to provide a brochure with a perforated Rolodex card. The brochure would allow you to describe your facility and its services, while the detachable or enclosed card would help ensure that your phone number is stored in a handy place. You should also include your business card.

TRACK YOUR CONTACTS

Keep a record of when you mailed your promotional letters and plan to call for an interview or lunch within one week.

BUILDING RELATIONSHIPS

Getting to know the office staff is an effective way to increase business as well. Should Dr. Smith tell her staff member to refer a patient to the dietitian, you want to be sure that you are the one who receives that call!

When Yale-New Haven Hospital Centers of Nutrition opened its first satellite office, we needed to increase our visibility with area physicians. After sending a promotion letter and following up with a call, we scheduled luncheons with the office staffs in several of the larger practices. No matter how busy the practice, staff members still need to eat, so we found this a perfect way to get their attention. The office staffs appreciated the meal, and we were able to describe our services in a relaxed environment.

Once you have attracted referrals from physicians, you need to foster the relationships. Physi-

BOX 36.2 | *Follow-up Promotion Letter*

Jane Jones, MS, RD
Ambulatory Nutrition Specialist
828 North Forrest Avenue, New Haven, CT 06504

January 13, 2010

John Smith, MD
Obstetrics and Gynecology
2 Church Street
New Haven, CT 06504

Dear Dr. Smith:

Eating is an integral part of the holidays and weight loss is a challenge for the New Year. With counseling and literature from the Centers of Nutrition, your patients can enjoy traditions, holiday feasts, and celebrations without the extra calories, fat, and sugar.

At the Yale-New Haven Hospital Centers of Nutrition, we would like to concentrate our efforts during the New Year 2010 on reaching patients who, because of obesity, have an increased risk for high blood pressure, diabetes, and heart disease.

I have enclosed copies of our monthly consumer newsletter and would like to make these available to your patients. If you would like additional copies, please give me a call at 555-5555 or 555-3333.

I would also like to thank you for your continued support of the Yale-New Haven Hospital Centers of Nutrition. We remain committed to providing your patients with meaningful dietary counseling, whether it be for existing medical conditions or to promote wellness.

Sincerely,
(Insert signature here)
Jane Jones, MS, RD
Ambulatory Nutrition Specialist

cians appreciate timely feedback that outlines their patients' progress. You could offer a quarterly newsletter or consumer-oriented literature for distribution in their offices. Promotion letters for new services or products can be combined with follow-up communiqués, as illustrated in Box 36.2. In this way you are providing information for the physicians to distribute to their patients while at the same time reminding them of your services. Of course, you will include your name, address, and telephone number on each piece of material. Patients might ask their physicians about your services or refer themselves directly.

SUMMARY

In summary, the important points to remember when writing an effective promotion letter are as follows:

1. Be sure to target your letter to the interests or specialization of the physician.
2. Establish your credibility.
3. Describe the particulars of your practice.
4. Include a business card or personalized Rolodex card.
5. Remember to follow up with a phone call to verify that addressees have received the information.

HOW TO MARKET A NEWSLETTER

37

Betty Goldblatt, MPH, RD

In starting a newsletter, it is important to have a strong idea of what the newsletter is all about. To clarify this to yourself, and eventually to copywriters and prospective subscribers, develop a statement of what the newsletter is—its editorial platform, its special market niche, and what makes it unique. Having a clear concept of what you are all about is a key element in achieving success.

NATIONAL NEWSLETTERS FOR THE PUBLIC THROUGH DIRECT MAIL

This discussion pertains to subscription newsletters that take no advertising. Such newsletters are marketed to a selected population of health-minded consumers. The consumers are identified by list brokers whose business it is to rent subscriber lists to direct marketers.

First of all, there are two sides to selling newsletter subscriptions:

- the actual marketing program, direct mail being the proven best type, and
- the continuing selling of the newsletter through the editorial product.

The editorial product and the direct mail package go together. The promises made in the subscription offer must be fulfilled by the newsletter. Developing a direct mail package that accurately portrays a publication is a job best left for experts in the direct mail copywriting field. The initial expense is high, but a package that works is the key element in gaining initial subscribers who will pay for their subscriptions and renew for years to come. Subscribers who find that the promises of the direct mail package are not met by the product will not pay for their initial subscription and will not renew.

List-marketing firms have two divisions: brokerage and management. List brokers market their client lists to prospective renters and try to keep the lists in use. They charge for names on a per-thousand basis with a minimum number per order. Charges are paid by the list renter.

To find a list broker or list manager in your area or suited to your specific needs, consult Direct Marketing Market Place, National Register Publishing, New Providence, NT, updated annually. It is available at most large public libraries. Another avenue is to search on the Internet for list brokers. Look for ones with multiple years in business, established reputations, and quality control that better assures current addresses.

After reaching a subscription base of approximately 10,000, a newsletter owner can have the subscriber list managed (or rented). The manager offers the list to prospective renters.

FINDING OUTSIDE HELP

If you are thinking of starting a newsletter and have no experience in the newsletter-marketing field, the Newsletter Publishers Association (NPA) is an excellent resource. This is a national not-for-profit trade association of newsletter publishers and suppliers. The association holds an annual international conference that covers all aspects of the industry and publishes the biweekly newsletter, *Hotline*. There are nine chapters located throughout the United States that meet monthly to enable members to network and learn more about the complex newsletter-marketing and publishing field.

WRITING FOR THE PUBLIC MARKET

Writing style for the consumer market is very different from writing for professional journals. When writing for consumers, use a friendly, direct style.

It is best to limit professional jargon, but it is all right to use technical terms because subscribers to nutrition newsletters are quite well read in the nutrition field. Offer readers practical advice. Make an effort to get continuous feedback from readers to determine if you are staying on course and meeting their needs and expectations. Use the feedback to develop a reader profile that will enable you to write with your specific audience in mind.

The design of your newsletter needs to be reader friendly, inviting the reader to continue on to the end. To make the newsletter easy to read:

- use catchy headlines and titles for the articles;
- break up articles with frequent subheadings;
- consider adding summarizing statements in the margins, or highlight key statements in the text with a different typeface;
- use a type size that is appropriate to your audience—larger for children or elderly people, never smaller than 9.5 point nor larger than 11 point; industry standard for the space between letters and lines is 13 point;
- use illustrations or cartoons to add life and human interest to articles;
- stay away from the silly or too cute in a professional newsletter; and
- consider introducing several articles on the front page with continuing text in the following pages.

If you are not a professional writer but think you would like to become one, test your writing skills before going into your own newsletter publishing business. Write some articles and see if you can get them published. Otherwise, seek out experienced professional writers to work with you. A great idea that is poorly written will have less potential for success.

FINANCIAL CONSIDERATIONS

The goal in marketing a newsletter is to earn a profit substantial enough to make all your efforts worthwhile. Newsletter publishing is a challenge and a very expensive undertaking. Marketing expertise and a large commitment of capital are essential. A business plan that includes a comprehensive marketing plan is the first step. Costs include mailing, fulfilling subscription orders, and securing renewals, as well as the monthly costs of editorial salaries and expenses, and overhead. Such costs very quickly mount into the tens of thousands of dollars. Growth from start-up to profit typically takes from 3 to 5 years, so an owner must be able to sustain the extended negative cash flow.

An ideal situation is to combine a nutritionist's expertise with the talents of writers, professional marketers, and copywriters, plus an organization that has funds to invest and is willing to carry the loss during development. This may mean giving up some control to an investor, but it can greatly increase the chances for success.

OTHER MARKETING OPTIONS

Newsletters can be marketed through means other than direct mail. One less expensive option is through a "ride along" in another product's selling package—typically a single sheet of paper with a subscription offer. This method is much less effective than a complete direct mail package, but is much less costly.

Another way to market a newsletter is to offer it as a generic product to organizations such as wellness programs, fitness centers, and medical clinics. The organization prints the newsletter on its own masthead and distributes it through its own means. The same editorial product can thus be sold to many different companies.

Various ways of using print advertising to sell newsletter subscriptions have been tried over the years, but they have never proven to be worthwhile. Advertising in newspapers and magazines is very costly. A more cost-effective way to reach consumers through the print media would be to write an article for a newspaper, get paid for it, and mention the newsletter's name and address in the piece. Interested persons will write in and ask for a sample and how to subscribe.

New competitors that are huge considerations today are the *FREE* online health newsletters. A person with limited funding should think long and hard before starting a new health or nutrition newsletter with such established, well-funded competition. Starting a new website with an online newsletter could still work *if* it has a dynamic concept that attracts so many hits each day that advertisers beg to give you their money. Good luck!

SUMMARY

Newsletters are a communication tool that keeps your name and expertise in front of readers. To attract readers, it requires access to unique information, either created as original work or gleaned from reputable sources. Most successful health-related newsletters are focused on a topic like alternative therapies, a target audience like women who have had breast cancer, or a disease like diabetes or multiple sclerosis, or they summarize the newest research on a broad range of nutrition-related or other topics of interest to their readers. Many free newsletters are positioned to create goodwill and engender loyalty among the readers for the person or business producing it, which helps sell new products or market the owner. Newsletters usually require substantial investment of time and money.

RESOURCES

Brausch, James. *Earn an income by publishing your own printed and mailed newsletter . . . even if you live on a remote island with only internet access to the outside world!* DVD. 2007.

Mathieu J. Tips for publishing a top-notch newsletter. *J Am Diet Assoc* 2007;107(3):384–385.

Woodward, C. *Starting and running a successful newsletter or magazine*, 5th Ed. Berkeley, CA: Academic Sales; 2006.

HOW TO CREATE AND USE FOCUS GROUPS

38

Ruth B. Fischer, MS, and Savannah Helm, BBA

The main idea for a focus group is to bring people together with a moderator to discuss their attitudes toward a product, service, concept, advertisement, idea, or packaging. Over the years, there has been a heated debate on the effectiveness of focus groups as a form of marketing research. The key when conducting your research is to use a variety of methods and not to rely on one form, be it interviews, surveys, or focus groups.

A focus group is a qualitative information-gathering technique that typically brings together 8 to 12 individuals for 1 to 2 hours to discuss a predetermined topic. It is a loosely structured discussion between a facilitator and participants that focuses on psychological characteristics that affect consumer behavior.

Focus groups are a social marketing-research method frequently used by marketers and advertisers to obtain consumer information useful in designing a product or packaging, measuring advertising effectiveness, or determining product pricing. The technique can also be useful in designing, marketing, evaluating, and pricing dietetic and health-education products and services. It is often used before going to a large-scale survey. This chapter will explain the procedure used for focus groups, along with the advantages and limitations of this method.

After many years of observing focus groups in action and then watching the success or failure of their suggestions in action, marketing expert Harry Beckwith has concluded they do not usually work well, especially for intangible service businesses (1). He states that it is human nature to want to please, and so, people tell you in surveys, interviews, and focus groups what they think you want to hear; thus, their actions and buying habits often do not match what they said (1). Focus groups may help you brainstorm ideas and narrow multiple options, but they are not good for creating cutting edge, breakthrough products—the "average" person often stays with what is familiar (1).

WHAT CAN A FOCUS GROUP DO?

Through in-depth interviewing techniques with a small group of people, a focus group examines general concerns about a product or service and can help identify:

- product focus,
- consumer reactions to potential products and services,
- consumer resistance to products and services, and
- potential reasons for buying.

WHY USE A FOCUS GROUP?

Frequently, when designing and marketing nutrition programs and services, we place emphasis on the knowledge or the behavior we want clients to have. Programs and services focus on our message. It concerns, disappoints, and sometimes baffles us when:

- clients drop out of our programs,
- classes fail to fill,
- lack of business forces staff cutbacks,
- people believe our workshops or printed materials are confusing or boring, and
- we feel our programs and services lack administration and colleague support.

Commercial marketers want to know and understand what makes consumers want to buy their products and what contributes to consumer satisfaction. They use focus groups to understand what potential consumers want, why they buy, and what constitutes satisfaction. In other words, they are client-driven.

Unfortunately, too often we train dietetics professionals and other nutrition educators to be content-driven, rather than focusing on what is needed to satisfy the customer and make our sale. Being client-driven does not negate the importance of the content, but merely emphasizes the need for packaging the message appropriately.

WHEN SHOULD YOU USE A FOCUS GROUP?

The focus group is not appropriate for every market research situation. It is important to remember that the data are qualitative rather than quantitative. In some situations, it may be better to do mail or telephone surveys with larger databases.

However, the focus group helps us better understand both our internal (administrator and colleagues) and external (patients or clients) markets. If used effectively, it helps determine:

- the best marketing approach for our programs and services,
- the kinds of instructional materials that might be easiest to use and most helpful for a targeted client group,
- how a program or service might be altered to better meet the needs of a client group,
- the cost of programs and services, and
- the hot buttons for gaining support and referrals from our colleagues.

Focus groups yield a great amount of detail from a small number of consumers. The format of the focus group allows you to understand consumers from their point of view.

STRENGTHS OF USING FOCUS GROUPS

A focus group results in rich and varied data expressed by consumers in their own words. By interviewing several consumers at one time, you save time and money. Another strength is the interactive process of the small group as members respond to questions. The benefits that you can expect to see from the group interaction process are:

- *synergism*—the group's ability to produce results in greater quantity and diversity than the sum of separate individual efforts;
- *snowballing*—the group's ability to take a small point made by one member, add to it, and reveal significant insights;

- *stimulation*—the elements of general excitement, enthusiasm, and even competition created by a group of similar consumers or other members;
- *security*—the feeling of safety in numbers that allows a member to discuss sensitive topics with group support;
- *spontaneity*—the idea that after the moderator asks a question, only interested members respond, making answers more meaningful, less forced, and less conventional;
- powerful tool to get direct input from customers;
- can be used almost anywhere in the world;
- has high apparent validity—easy to understand;
- can increase a sample size; and
- can gain access to various culture and social groups, selecting sites to study, and raising unexpected issues for exploration.

For example, holding a focus group on what type of weight-management program to offer and when to offer it might be very productive before your hospital makes a decision on implementation. The group discussion generates more information than interviewing individuals separately—but not necessarily better information. A point made by one participant might trigger a very important comment from another member of the group, and so on, providing you with additional insight about the type of program to select.

The discussion may excite the participants and make them comfortable about sharing their feelings and needs. You might learn very different perceptions of what participants feel works best for them. Discuss the similarities and allow disagreements. Individuals in the group may feel less pressure to respond to each question than they might in a personal interview.

Give some thought to the strengths of using focus groups and how they provide information to the planning or evaluation stage in your company or organization.

WEAKNESSES OF USING FOCUS GROUPS

The focus group technique is so popular that sometimes we use it when other information-gathering strategies are more valuable or appropriate. It does not replace quantitative data collection. Use it as only one tool in the decision-making process, and not the sole justification for a decision affecting your company's product or services.

Some problems in using focus groups occur when:

- the quality of the facilitator is inadequate, inappropriate, or biased;

- the group is shy and reluctant to participate in the discussion;
- the sample group is too small or not representative of the target market;
- the members are not randomly selected from the target population, thus adding bias to the results;
- the people who participate in the group are only those who can afford to spend 1 to 2 hours at the research location;
- there is no understanding of the principles of psychology;
- the participants provide results that the clients think the moderator wants;
- online focus groups may include repeat participants;
- people who know they are being studied behave differently; and
- participants are too influenced by groupthink—they agree with each other and do not share their individual feelings or thoughts.

Also, it is important to avoid situations that inhibit consumer reaction during the focus group meeting, like looking disapproving or not calling on certain persons who show a desire to speak.

SETTING UP A FOCUS GROUP

Participants of focus groups are usually specifically invited because they represent either the characteristics of the target market or the average consumer of the product or service. Participants may or may not be paid for their time, but if one is paid, all should be paid. Often a gift certificate, product sample, or a meal is given instead of a cash payment.

Look for participants who are willing to speak up and become actively involved in the discussions but will not dominate the group. Imbalance may also occur when group members acquiesce to a more experienced member's opinion instead of offering their own. A good facilitator will help resolve problems at the time of the session, but some problems can be anticipated and avoided.

Dietitians who are affiliated with hospitals or industry probably have people within their organization who can assist in implementing a focus group. If you do not have this luxury, seek help from the business or marketing department of a local college or university. It is not necessary to use expensive market research companies to get a focus group conducted professionally and effectively.

Although a focus group interview is informal and relatively unstructured, the facilitator typically uses a framework to guide the process. Product samples or program materials may be used as props to assist the focus group in reacting and responding to your product or service and your competitors. Frequently, focus groups are audio- or videotaped, but inform participants about either of these procedures and ask for their consent.

A comfortable environment with no outside distractions is important to the success of a focus group. Some people use special rooms with one-way mirrors so that clients can observe the focus group without being seen. This minimizes distraction for participants, but they should still be informed about the observers.

THE ALL-IMPORTANT FACILITATOR

The facilitator is the key person in determining the success of the focus group process. The facilitator should:

- have a pleasant appearance and voice,
- enjoy meeting and interacting with people,
- have a genuine interest in the researched project,
- be sensitive to the needs of both the participants and the client desiring the information, and
- be a quick thinker and a good listener.

Have the facilitator meet with you and other key people in the management group. Clearly define your research questions and what you hope to learn from the focus group. This will greatly assist the facilitator in preparing key open-ended questions to keep the group process flowing and help assure that you meet your goals. You, your staff, the board of directors, the marketing department, etc., may also generate questions.

The facilitator must be skilled in leading the group process. The facilitator needs to do the following:

- *Provide a comfortable environment.* If the participants do not feel at ease, the discussion will not flow and people will not open up to share their thoughts and feelings.
- *Allow participants to do the talking, follow their own train of thought, and use their own words.* Charge the facilitator with the task of keeping the respondents speaking and expressing their feelings about the research topic. The facilitator should not excessively control the environment or prompt speakers to use phrases that are not their own.
- *Summarize the respondents' statements.* Another important function of the facilitator is to summarize the respondents' statements to capture the essence of their thoughts. Restating the

responses may also stimulate others in the group to comment. By videotaping or viewing from a one-sided mirror, the client can better interpret facial expressions, body language, and group dynamics for their meaning.

- *Ask probing or investigative questions.* Well-phrased questions clarify the meaning of what respondents say or allow new topics to be explored. They can also keep the discussion moving when it slows down. However, it should be noted that moments of silence are acceptable. Silence allows respondents to think about what has just been said and to pull their own thoughts together. It is during silent moments that the less-assertive group members may feel more comfortable about speaking up.

- *Have a topic outline available.* An outline makes sure the facilitator covers all topics during the focus group. However, it is important to design the focus group to be free-flowing and spontaneous. Too much structure will impede the flow of useful information.

- *Avoid making evaluative comments.* A focus group discussion is not an evaluative process, but rather an opportunity to brainstorm and gain a wide variety of information. The facilitator should not lead participants to believe that one answer is better than another. Analyze what was said after the meeting is completed and the respondents have left.

SUMMARY

The focus group is a powerful tool that can help dietetic professionals and nutrition educators more effectively position their products and services to meet the needs of their target markets. Although it is a useful tool, it is not a panacea, and should not be misused or overused.

REFERENCES

1. Beckwith H. *Selling the Invisible*. New York: Warner Business Books; 2002.

RESOURCES

Easwaran S, Singh SJ. *Marketing Research: Concepts, Practices and Cases*. UK: Oxford University Press; 2007.

Kurtz DL, Boone LE. *Contemporary Marketing 2006*. New York: Dryden Press; 2006.

HOW TO WRITE A NUTRITION NEWSPAPER COLUMN

39

Celia Topping, MNS, RD, CDE

As owner of a health education and promotion company, I have sought ways to provide visibility for my company. Since September 1991, I have written a biweekly newspaper column called "Nutrition Know-How" in the Rochester, New York, Gannett newspaper. The column has successfully helped me to:

- provide a community service,
- reinforce the role of the registered dietitian (RD) as the nutrition expert,
- increase readers' food and nutrition awareness,
- illustrate my expertise and knowledge, and
- enhance the visibility and image of my company.

As a result of the column, other reporters often contact me for comments on nutrition topics, which provide further opportunities for media visibility.

GETTING STARTED

DO YOUR HOMEWORK!

- Become familiar with local newspapers and reporters and their beats.
- First contact the paper with the greatest potential. Keep trying if the first paper is not interested.
- Know your competition. Generally, editors prefer local sources.
- Consider targeting the health, food, or lifestyle editor. The health column may offer the widest readership.
- Develop and nurture a good working relationship with the editors. Put them on your mailing list, invite them to district nutrition seminars, send monthly clippings and nutrition notes, and send "I liked your article on . . ." letters of congratulation.

- Be current. Be sure you are receiving press releases, new product information, news clippings, the media information from The American Dietetic Association and health news. In addition to the lay press, I use a computer information service.
- Consider taking a journalism course or hiring a professional writer to edit your work until you become more confident and skilled.

SHOWCASE YOUR STYLE

- Prepare three sample columns on timely, seasonal topics. Make them sizzle. Pass them by a colleague for review.
- List 10 other potential topics to show your creativity and range.
- I opted for the question-and-answer format, which seems more personal and connected with the reader.

DO LUNCH

- Over lunch, chat with your prospective editor.
- Explain why the editor's audience would be interested in your column. Do not overly flatter the editor or ask favors.
- Meet the editor's needs, not your needs.
- Suggest a trial period.
- Find out about the editor's budget. Do not be afraid to ask for a fee, but do not be surprised if you are not offered more than $25 to $50 per column, unless you have a well-known reputation. Payment may or may not be offered. Knowing there was no budget, I volunteered to write a column, but requested that a trailer listing my company and credentials be included with each column. The column provides tremendous visibility. That kind of advertising is very expensive. However, when

asked to write a feature article for the paper, I always request and receive payment.

WRITING THE COLUMN

CONTENT

- Choose the topic from the reader's perspective. Then think of the reader as you write. This has been the most valuable tip for me to keep in mind.
- Translate the science of nutrition into real-life activities or behaviors. I write about the art of healthy eating, such as how to select from a school cafeteria menu or pack a picnic cooler.
- Be practical. I often include toll-free 800 numbers, such as the USDA Food and Poultry Hotline or the NCND Consumer Nutrition Hotline, or recommend a free brochure.
- Use bullets to ensure the information is easy to scan.
- Be accurate. I check facts with a product's corporate public relations department, the USDA, and trade associations, and I try to include quotes with my sources' names to add interest and even more credibility.
- Stress the positive—the do's, not the don'ts.
- Make the column easy-to-read, conversational, and entertaining as well as informative. For example, I related the origins of granola cereal to a local health movement that happened over 100 years ago. I also reviewed the nutritional value of all the local pizza and frozen yogurt establishments. Such an approach adds to the uniqueness and appeal of the column.

PROCESS

- Encourage readers' questions, but be prepared to create your own questions. In my column, the questions are typeset in bold and end with the sender's initials and the town in which he or she resides.
- Answer two or three questions per column, choosing one of the topics for expanded treatment.
- Make every word count. Keep your column tight and bright, brief, and easy-to-understand. Do not be afraid to use bullets.
- Keep the column to the editor's specified length. My column is 400 to 450 words.
- My editor rarely changes my column, except to delete a line or two if it runs too long.
- End each column with a trailer about who you are.
- My trailer reads: "Celia Topping, a registered dietitian, is Vice President of Clinical Services

for NutriSmart, Inc., a food and nutrition consulting firm in Rochester. Her column runs every other week."
- With each column appears: "Got a question? Get your nutrition answers by writing to Celia Topping, c/o Eating In, 55 Exchange Blvd., Rochester, NY 14614."
- Submit two or three suggested titles for each column, and let the editor make the final selection or contribute his or her own. This gives the editor some control and input and usually works well.
- Respect deadlines. I set my deadline 24 hours ahead of what is required.
- Check regularly with the editor. Be prepared with fresh ideas and suggestions.

POSTSCRIPTS

- I ask that questions be sent to me in care of the newspaper, rather than to my own business address, so my editor knows how popular the column is.
- I send my column by email directly to the newspaper so it is automatically on their computers. As backup, I send a hard copy in the mail.
- Since I volunteer to write the columns for no charge, the paper does not own them. Therefore, I can offer the same columns, or modified columns, to another newspaper if I choose. Discuss this with your editor. Be alert for publication dates so columns do not appear simultaneously.
- Inquire about liability. In my case, the newspaper is responsible for what appears in print. Insurance for writers is available, but costly. Professional liability insurance does not usually cover writing—but check with the ADA.
- Potentially, any column can be syndicated, which means that other newspapers may reprint the column, usually for a fee to you or to the service that represents your column, which will then pay you.

SUMMARY

Writing a newspaper column in your local market helps establish your reputation and credibility with your readers. If you are published in regional or national publications, it can open the door for speaking engagements and promote sales of your products or services. If you do not mind deadlines and have a knack for communicating through the written word, consider writing a newspaper column.

40

HOW TO BECOME A CONSULTANT

Mary Ann Hodorowicz, RD, LDN, MBA, CDE

Becoming a consultant is often reserved for more experienced persons who have either deeply varied or specialized expertise. Consultants are often called in when the job requires a higher level of knowledge and ability, but the position is not a full time job. For example:

- the job needs a supervisor to oversee chronic care patients and food service sanitation compliance or to write menus (like a long-term care nutritionist),
- the job needs an expert for a short-term project (like a food service dietitian who specializes in kitchen remodeling or a brief research project),
- the job needs a speaker who can energize and mobilize the troops,
- the restaurant menus need a healthy face-lift,
- the food manufacturer wants a dietitian media spokesperson for a two-week media tour, and
- the corporation needs a weekly in-house weight loss program, and so on.

These positions require top-level skill and often years of experience or postgraduate education. Ability is not the only criteria businesses are looking for—they also want someone who has an aura and history of success, as well as great communication skills and reputation. That being said, I want to explore how to become a consultant with you by looking at my own journey and what I teach other dietitians.

HOW CONSULTING BEGINS

One day, my friend Christine called me to say she was going to resign her six-figure position as vice president of sales and marketing in order to spend more time at home with her one-year-old daughter. She had been keeping up with the changes in my career path . . . from full and part-time employee in a variety of positions to the start-up and expansion of a consulting business while working as a part-time certified diabetes educator. Wanting to work from home as a consultant, keep her options open, and be assured of a steady stream of monthly income, Christine asked for my guidance. A tall order, but I was prepared! I had just given a presentation to dietitians on the *A, B, C's of a Dietitian's Successful "Mixed" Consulting Business*. Thus, I had already charted the course of my long and varied career journey, culminating in ownership of my own consulting business.

In the world of professional sports, athletes practice what they are good at every day and tell themselves anything is possible. I like to call this "powering up your mind for success." Reflecting back, I concluded that to conquer the challenges of entrepreneurship and gain the competitive edge, dietitians can look to the first three letters of the alphabet. Just as A leads to B leads to C, the secrets of success also follow a sequence, which culminate in the letter D:

BOX 40.1

A   Positive *Attributes, Abilities, Aspirations*, and *Assurance of Competency* lead to

B   Positive *Behaviors*, which lead to

C   Positive *Consequences*, which lead to

D   *Dreams* coming true . . . SUCCESS!

A SHORT STORY OF MY JOURNEY

The design of my own consulting company did not adhere to the traditional business model wherein the dietitian pinpoints one primary target market and selects one primary service or product niche. For example, in a more traditional paradigm, the owner of a nutrition and wellness dietetics practice might target small to mid-size manufacturing companies and provide in-house weight loss programs for employees. In my business plan, however, I wanted the services of my company to be varied, helping to meet the needs of not one but two different yet synergistic markets: health care and the food industry. You know the saying "variety is the spice of life?" For me, variety *is* my life, my passion! With a marketing-focused MBA under my belt, I knew that if my services were not explicitly defined and somewhat homogenous, my dreams would drown instead of coming true! Knowing I did have the *attributes* required for consulting business success (see Table 40.1 below) and armed with the advice of many successful entrepreneurs spanning several industries, it became clear what needed to be done first:

1. Take an inventory of my *aspirations*. Why did I want to have my own business?
2. Decide on the services I wanted to offer.
3. Determine if I have the expertise or the *abilities* necessary to compete, to gain a competitive advantage.
4. Decide if these services would fulfill the unmet needs of professionals in the health and food industry—professionals I desired to align myself with in my own business.

After taking the inventory of my *aspirations*, I knew consulting was for me (see Table 40.1)!

HOW TO ASSESS YOURSELF FOR CONSULTING

Next came the question, what type of services did I have a passion for? I reviewed my curriculum vitae (CV), and realized that I had a varied mix of career positions from which to draw. In years past, my CV chronicled being a dietetic traineeship coordinator, hospital-based clinical nutrition manager, an assistant food service director, and a university educator for a weight-loss program. There was a mix of responsibilities in each of these roles, which broadens my skills in operations, marketing, clinical nutrition management, food service supervision, quality assurance, finances, insurance reimbursement for medical nutrition therapy and diabetes education, and group weight management. My business and MNT skills were further enhanced after the birth of my second son, when I worked part-time and opened a hospital-based outpatient Nutrition Clinic (the term MNT had not yet been coined). This presented a wonderful opportunity to "start up a new business" without risking my assets and under the hospital's protective veil of security and guidance. With this experience came an invitation to help design and open a new "Diabetes Center," complete with a recognized diabetes self-management education (DSME) program. Once again, another new start-up business was in the making, giving me yet another occasion to enhance my entrepreneurial, organizational, and managerial abilities.

This led me to aspirations of grandeur: offer as many services in my business as my abilities will allow! What seems counterintuitive at first, is now clear to me: a plentiful harvest of skills can actually be a handicap rather than a blessing when trying to narrow down which services to offer! But narrow down I did, while still preserving what I desired—a varied mix of services, my *required* spice of life:

- Provide consumer and professional education and support services in the expanding arena of nutrition in both health promotion and disease, and in diabetes prevention and screening.
- Consult for health care entities on MNT and DSME programs: development, enhancement, standards of care, and related services.
- Sell self-published resources for dietitians and health care professionals in above areas.
- Coach dietitians on all aspects of private practice development.
- Consult for professionals on MNT and DSME insurance reimbursement.
- Provide vendor/manufacturer support services.
- Provide presentations (multimedia) for professionals, including CE events, and for consumers.

After this decision came more soul searching. Did I really have the expertise, the *abilities* required to excel at these services? My father would always tell me "If you cannot do it well, do not do it at all!" The answer was *yes*, due solely to my 28 years of varied and mixed "employee career path."

Now another analysis was required: will these services help fill in the gaps that exist in the health care and food industry markets? It can be argued that the greatest key to success is tapping into an unmet need in the marketplace via your product or service. If the market does not need or want what you are selling, you will not have a viable business. Can I provide services that are unique enough to succeed in the early stages against potential competition? This analysis was actually less complicated

Attributes

- Courageous (courage to take chances, to accomplish tasks on my own terms)
- Attentive to detail
- Aggressive, risk-taker
- Multitasker with good organizational skills
- Open-minded
- Opportunistic
- Passionate about your service/product, but pragmatic
- Not hindered by fear of failure
- Confident and tough-skinned
- Persuasive
- Self-disciplined, determined
- Self-motivated
- Progressive
- Goal-centered, not clock-centered
- Hard worker, tenacious
- Willingness to work non-traditional hours and days
- Creative, innovative, imaginative
- Out-of-the-box thinker
- Telescopic (wide-angle) view of environment, rather than microscopic
- Flexible and negotiable in my thinking, contract agreements, work hours, etc.
- Decisive (dwelling on things too long stalls success)

Abilities (Related to Services I Want to Offer) and Assurance Of Competency

- Expertise in services I want to offer = consulting/writing/coaching/speaking in:
  - Diabetes prevention, diabetes self-management education, DSME program development and recognition certification
  - Medical nutrition therapy and MNT program development
  - Quality assurance, outcomes management and staff training
  - Medicare and private insurance reimbursement for DSME and MNT
  - Nutrition in wellness and weight management
  - Vendor/manufacturer support
- Knowledge of *best* practice/performance/operations
- Licensed dietitian in state of Illinois
- Registered by CDR of ADA
- Member of American Dietetic Association
- Member of professional associations related to services offered
- Specialized certifications related to services offered (e.g., CDE)

Aspirations

- Be my own boss
- Devoid of company hierarchy, office politics, bad bosses
- Work less, make more money
- Freedom to use my creativity
- Flexible schedule
- Recognition (enjoy fruits of my labor, rather than someone else taking credit)
- Feel rush of accomplishment when clients accept proposals or call to retain me
- Feel rush of audience/client adulation after presentations and consulting work
- Do variety of types of work
- Be challenged—push myself into new learning curves, develop competency, and then make money with new abilities
- Responsibility (chance to play bigger role in my chosen field)

Behaviors

- Create comprehensive business plan, which includes: *marketing strategies* to promote recognition of my name, skills and consulting business, and thus help attain new clients and retain existing ones
- Print business cards, brochure, letterhead stationery, envelopes, pocket folders
- Create own website; includes offer to join Mary Ann's mailing list
- Send monthly ezine to mailing list
- Advertise in trade journals
- Obtain free publicity in local newspaper
- Network with everyone, everywhere, all the time!
- Never leave a person empty-handed; always give business card or brochure
- Join national and local professional membership associations. Attend workshops, bi-annual/annual meetings, and social events, and participate in listservs
- Join local membership organizations; e.g., local business owners' association
- Give something away to get something in return, i.e., volunteer regularly for professional membership associations' committees and task forces and for consumer events such as health fairs, blood glucose screening, etc.
- Seek appointed/elected position within professional membership associations
- Write articles at no charge for local newspaper or be quoted as "expert"
- Benchmark against best practices/performance/operations related to consulting
- Know that if you do not ask, the answer is always NO; so, pitch proposals:
  - To be speaker at provider and consumer events, e.g., ADA FNCE, state dietetic associations' and dietetic practice groups' annual meetings, National Kidney Foundation of Illinois' Parent Education Programs, etc.
  - To do work for potential clients via phone calls, emails, meetings
  - To do freelance writing for magazines, websites, etc.
  - To author resource guides for companies and membership associations
  - To do product promotion at industry trade shows and exhibitions
- Keep eyes *wide* open for any opportunity to pitch ideas for work or to speak
- Create win-win scenarios when negotiating contracts and fees
- Make an offer the client cannot refuse in order to get the gig:
  - Discounted fee for multiple presentations, or if invited back second, third years
  - Free copies of own professional resources
  - Free hours of telephone or in-person consultation

Consequences

CONSULTING SUCCESS, defined as
- Obtaining contracts for:
  - Speaking, conducting CE workshops, etc.
  - Writing articles for magazines and websites
  - Writing professional resources, how-to manuals, etc., for other entities
  - Creating/revising presentation slides
- Obtaining contracts for various types of ("mixed") consulting work:
  - Conducting grocery store tours sponsored by product corporations
  - Consulting at hospitals, clinics, physician offices on MNT and DSME: program development, insurance reimbursement, quality management, etc.
  - Coaching dietitians on how to develop/enhance their private practice
  - Acting as dietitian consultant for MNT research studies
  - Doing product promotions at trade shows
  - Conducting consumer education events on diabetes prevention, diabetes management, nutrition in disease states and nutrition in wellness sponsored by product or service corporations and health care associations
- Self-publishing and selling via website two resource manuals for dietitians and electronic forms

for me than it sounds. Why? Because of the many years I spent as an employee. It was during this time that I identified the knowledge gaps in the health and food industry, including the unmet needs of dietitians in many practice settings. These knowledge gaps were all related to the ever-expanding arenas of:

- nutrition for health promotion;
- evidence-based MNT in disease states;
- the development of recognized DSME and diabetes prevention programs to help reduce our country's diabetes epidemic;
- MNT and DSME insurance reimbursement for professionals; and
- dietitians in private practice.

CONSULTING CHECKLIST

Starting a business takes a lot of courage—the first *attribute* in my CHECKLIST! But, as they say, being courageous does not pay the bills! To be successful—to *stay* in business—I knew I needed more than courage. Dietitians need a combination of several *attributes*, expert *abilities* and the *assurance of competence*, all related specifically to the services/products you will market. With these "A's" securely in my back pocket, the next letter I focused on was "B." Replaying the last 5 years of my small business like a DVD, I now realize that the performance of key *behaviors* will put anyone on the fast track toward the "C's"—the positive, wonderful *consequences* of all our hard work, perseverance, and winning attitude.

CASE STUDY 40.1

CONSULTING IN LONG-TERM CARE

Becky Dorner, RD, LD, President, Nutrition Consulting Services, Inc. and Becky Dorner & Associates, Inc.

In January 1983 at the tender age of 24, I made a decision that changed my life! With two young children, I decided to start my nutrition practice. As I write this, my company, Nutrition Consulting Services, Inc. (NCS), is celebrating 25 years of providing nutrition care to the older adults of Ohio and beyond!

NCS began as a sole proprietorship with me as the sole practitioner. I spent almost 4 years doing just about everything you can possibly think of. I counseled people at fitness clubs and pharmacies, in their homes, in restaurants, in physician's offices, etc. I taught classes; I did presentations at health fairs and corporations; and I consulted to a nursing home.

And after 4 years of working mostly 60 hours a week with no guarantee of a steady paycheck and no benefits, I discovered the needs of the long-term care industry. An opportunity presented itself for me to provide services 2 to 3 days a week for a nursing home with a guaranteed 6-month contract. I gradually stopped everything else I was doing and concentrated on learning all there was to know about nursing home consulting. Within 6 months, I had 60 hours a week of nursing home consulting contracts and I hired my first registered dietitian (RD). Within 5 years, I had five full time employees. Here I am after 25 years with 25 employees, mostly RDs along with two DTRs, and three office support staff, plus numerous contractors and on-call staff when I need extra help.

It has been fast-paced and exciting; however, it did have some ups and downs. As the industry began to consolidate, some facilities hired their own corporate RDs and some even went bankrupt, leaving us holding our invoices with nothing to show for our hours of work. We learned the hard way to be more aggressive on our receivables and keep a close eye on the accounting. (Thank goodness my husband is a CPA because this is not my strong point!)

In an effort to market my business and help provide some additional sources of revenue, I began to publish some of the work I was doing for clients. I began with menus and a policy and procedure manual followed by numerous other publications. This eventually grew into a separate corporation, Becky Dorner & Associates, Inc., which provides CEU programs (live, tele-seminar, audio, video, online, and hardcopy) and informational manuals including diet manuals and copy-ready diet instructions. We have evolved through many types of paper brochures to a very extensive website and an email magazine that reaches 20,000 health care professionals all over the United States and other countries.

Along the way, I discovered my strengths and talents and gravitated toward spending more of my time doing the things I loved: writing, speaking, communications, marketing, and networking. I had spent years doing presentations at CEU programs for free—in an effort to market my business, build my credibility, and broaden my reputation for providing excellent service. After 12 years of free speaking, I realized this was something I loved to do, and I began to charge for speaking engagements in other states. I have spoken in 48 states and 5 countries, and I find that presenting continues to provide a sense of personal satisfaction when I feel that I have truly delivered a presentation that makes a difference in the lives of others.

Over the years, I always found time to volunteer for the ADA and take in dietetic students. The benefits of volunteering came back to me in so many ways—all of which I applied to my business to help it grow—and to help me grow as a professional and as a person.

The two most important things I have learned about business ownership in the last 5 years are: (1) *Reach for the stars* and (2) *If you do not ask, the answer is always NO*. Your success can be bigger than you ever imagined *if* you aim high! If you can speak to 20 people at a local consumer event, you *can* speak to one thousand at ADA's annual Food and Nutrition Conference and Exhibition! If you provide one-on-one weight loss MNT to clients, you *can* provide a multi-session group program to 50 people within a well-established organization in your community, such as a health club, manufacturing plant, or university. Allow your self-confidence to support your starry goals. Hope and passion are powerful forces that can provide remarkable motivation and move you to remarkable success—inject them into your action plan. And remember to ASK! Without exaggeration, 50% of my contracts for speaking, writing, coaching, and consulting have come from pitches I made to perspective clients, supported by a strong CV and an upbeat, confident personality. You have everything to gain, and absolutely nothing to lose!

SUMMARY

Deciding to pursue your own business distinguishes you from others. Your clients and colleagues will value your positive mental attitude and support and encourage you to move on to even greater success. Still not convinced? Ask yourself this: "If it does not work, what can I do?" If you have solid qualifications and a good level of work experience, you can always find a salaried job in our industry. Your other option is to "mix it up," that is, work as a part-time employee and a part-time business owner. Life is short. If you have the dream, check your A, B, C's; they may culminate in D—your DREAM coming true!

INDEX

Pages followed by f and t denote tables and figures, respectively; pages in bold denote boxes.

A

Acquisitions editor, in self-publishing, 207
Action plans, 24
Acute care
　dietitians in, 137
　setting of, 136–138
ADA. *See* American Dietetic Association
ADSA. *See* Association for Dietetics in
　　South Africa
Advertising. *See also* Selling
　as defined, 19
　successful, 94
Agents, 196
Agreements
　with corporate health care
　　corporation, 72f
　negotiating, 69–74
　for nutrition consulting service, 71f
American Dietetic Association (ADA),
　　ethics principles of, 83–84
Anger, customer's, 52
Associate training, 173
Association for Dietetics in South Africa
　　(ADSA), 12
Attitude
　developing, 63
　positive, 30
Authors. *See* Books
Ayres, Susan, **158**

B

Badham, Jane, **13**
Bargaining, 69–70
Beauty training, 65–66
Bias
　consulting and, 85
　food companies and, 85
Billable hours, 77
Biography. *See* Professional biography
Bissex, Janice Newell, 202
Bitzer, Rebecca, **151**
Board of advisors, building, 29
Books
　careers grown through, 201–203
　internet sales of, 209–210
　ISBN of, 208
　to market, 208
　marketing, 205–211
　sales outlets for, 208–210
　self-publishing, 205–211
　success stories of nutrition, 202–203
　traditional marketing of, 208–209
　writing, 201–203
Brand, 19
　creating, 89–90
　image, 89

importance of, 90
　selling affected by, 44
Break-even analysis, **119**
Breakthrough, **10**
Broadcast media, 19
Brochures, 99, 214f
　availability shown in, 214
　with business card, 248
　credibility as established in,
　　213–214
　format/style of, 214–215
　marketing, 215–216
　message of, 213
　target audience of, 213
　writing marketing, 213–216
Brown, Carolyn, **166**
Brown, Mona Boyd, **32**
Budget, 119–120
Bundling, as market strategy, 45
Business cards, 97, 248
Business plan, marketing plan v., 113

C

Care. *See* Acute care; Health care; Long-
　　term care
Career(s), 217. *See also* Corporate career
　　coaching
　books used for growing, 201–203
　choosing direction, 27, 29
　coaching, 100–101
　credibility, 31
　equity, 31
　growing, 27
　options for dietitians, 65–66
　plan, 27, 29, 29t
　in product development, 170–171
　shifting path of, 29
　in supermarkets, 170–172
Case, Shelley, 202
Caton, Jean R., **100**
Celebrities, 93
　for special events, 231
Certified Specialist in Sports Dietetics
　　(CSSD) Credential, 186
Change, adapting to, 7
Children, food marketing and, 86
Chung, Susan, **42**
Clients
　ethics and, 86
　marketing to, 32
Communication, 30
　channels, 63
　globalization and, 6
　through marketing, 27
　newsletters as tool in, 252–253
　one-on-one, 90

press release as tool in, 236
　written, 247
Competition
　evaluating, 55–59
　finding, 55–56, 56t
　keeping ahead of, 57, 59
　market research and, 56
　marketing stimulated by, 135
　positioning in environment of,
　　56–57
　price structures of, 57
　worry and, 55
Consultant
　becoming, 261–262, 263t, 264–265
　beginning job of, 261–262
　bias of, 85
　check-list for, 264–265
　dietitian's practice as, 263t
　in long-term care, 264–265
　marketing as, **32**
　self-assessment as, 262, 264
Consumer affairs specialist, 170
Consumption communities, 28
Contacts, tracking, 248
Contracts
　fees and, 70
　negotiating, 70–74
Conventions
　exhibiting at, 243–244
　follow-up after, 246
　marketing during, 243–246
Cooking classes, 173
Copy, for websites, 190–191
Corporate career coaching, 100–101
Cosmetics, 65–66
Cost, of doing business, 77
Cost containment, in health care, 135
Cost plus, 76
Credentials, 11
　requirements, 39
Credibility
　in brochures, 213–214
　career, 31
CSSD Credential. *See* Certified Specialist
　　in Sports Dietetics Credential
Culinary professionals, 123–124
Culinary schools, teaching in,
　　130–131, 130f
Curriculum vitae (CV), 221f
　writing, 218–224
Customer satisfaction, 18
　anger and, 52
Customer service
　defining good, 49–50
　email as used in, 51
　in food industry, 128–131
　interactions, 50

Customers, 18
  identifying, 50
  knowledge of, 49–50
  needs/desires of, 50
CV. *See* Curriculum vitae

D
Deitrick, Holly, **232**
Demand oriented strategies, 76
Demographics, 18
Diabetes, 5
Dietetic professionals. *See also* Dietetic
    technicians
  change adapted to by, 7
  creating opportunities for, 5–6
  employed by food company, 85
  networking by, 63–67
  in South Africa, 12–13
  supermarkets and, 170–172
Dietetic technicians
  foodservice and, 159
  in hospitals, 158
  in long-term care, 157
  marketing, 157–160
  in prevention/wellness, 157–158
Dietetics. *See also* Sports dietetics
  change in, 52
  in Israel, 23–24
  making money in field of, **30**
Dietitians
  in acute care, 137
  career options for, 65–66
  ethnic backgrounds of, 7
  foodservice opportunities for,
    123–128
  in Hong Kong, 42
  in Israel, 23–24
  in Japan, 33–34
  in Lebanon, 58
  as marketed to supermarkets, 172–173
  media success story of, 109–111
  professional development for, 131
  self-publishing by, 205–206
  specialized knowledge of, 39
  in United Kingdom, 52–53
Direct mail, of newsletters, 251
Discharge planning, 140
Discounts, 52
Diversity, 12
Dorner, Becky, **264**

E
EBP. *See* Evidence Based Practice
Economy, changes in America's, 4–5, 4t
Education, 11. *See also* Training
  materials as developed, 175
Elder, Jinny, **160**
Elevator speech, 64
Email, in customer service, 51
Employees, training, 51
Employers, marketing to current, 33
Employment, in services, 35
Endorsements, 187
Estheticians, education for, 66

Ethics, 7
  client considerations and, 86
  dilemmas, 83
  marketing and business, 83–87
  personal/professional, 83–85
  principles of ADA, 83–84
Events. *See also* Special events
  cosponsorship of, 93
  special, 93
Evidence Based Practice (EBP), 139
EVP. *See* Extra-value proposition
Exhibits
  accessories for, 245
  anatomy of, 244
  board/display of, 244
  company identification in, 244
  in conventions/trade shows, 243–244
  dressing up, 244–245
  features of, 244
  follow-up after, 246
  key descriptors of, 244
  layout of, 245
  location of, 245
  people working, 245–246
  purpose of, 243
  when/where of, 243
Extra-value proposition (EVP), 18

F
Fairs, 174
Fees. *See also* Price(s)
  billable hours and, 76
  changing, 78–79
  contingency, 78
  establishing professional, 76–78
  flat rate, 78
  increase, 81
  negotiating/contract, 70
  per-hour, 78
  quoting, 76
  setting, 75–81
  structure of, 78
  for unique expertise, 76
Financial reporting system, 24
Focus groups
  appropriate times for use of, 256
  creating, 255–258
  environment of, 257
  facilitator of, 257–258
  purpose of, 255
  reasons for using, 255–256
  setting up, 257–258
  strengths of using, 256
  as tool, 258
  as used, 255–258
  weaknesses of using, 256–257
Food. *See also* Healthy food
  organic, 12, 171
  outpatient counseling on, 130
  safety, 171
Food industry. *See also* Foodservice;
    Restaurants
  customer service in, 128–131
  dietitians' opportunities in, 124–128
  in healthcare, 129

  marketing, 12, 42, 86, 123–133
  spokespersons for, 85
  staff training in, 127
  as trend, 11
FoodPlay Productions, 145
Foodservice
  dietetic technicians and, 159
  dietitians' opportunities in, 123–128
  in health care, 129
  in schools, 130
Fripp, Patricia, 195
Functional medicine nutrition
  jobs in, 181–182
  market of, 179–182
  training for, 180–181
Funding, adequate, 45

G
Gada, Madhu, 203
Geriatric nutrition, 5
Giveaways, 231
Globalization, 6–7
  benefits of, 7
Goals
  networking and, 63
  of self-publishing, 206–207, 206t, 207t
  setting, 22
  in sports dietetics, 185
Grocery store. *See* Supermarkets

H
Hashimoto, Reiko, **33**
Hassard, Lynne, 159
Health care. *See also* Acute care; Medical
    nutrition therapy
  changes in, 5
  cost containment in, 135
  environment, 136–137
  expense reduction in, 135
  foodservice, 129
  marketing, 12, 135–142
  marketing in clinical setting of,
    137–141
  national, 23
  patient safety in, 137
  as trend, 11
Health fairs, 174
Healthy food
  culinary professionals and, 123–124
  marketing, 123–133
  on menus, 127–128
  new meaning of, 123–124
Heart disease, 5
Heterogeneity, 38–39
Hnida, David, 105
Hooper, Melissa, **175**
Hong Kong, dietitians in, 42
Hospitals
  dietetic technicians working in, 158
  promotion and, 149–151
Hotels, 128–129
Hotlines, 174
Hughes, Barbara Ann F., **74**
Hundredth Monkey Phenomenon, **10**
Hunt, Paula, **52**

I

Information age, opportunities in, 5–6
Inseparability, 38
Insurance companies, 74, 152
Integrated marketing, 19
International Standardized Book Number (ISBN), 208
Internet. *See also* Websites
  sales on, 209–210
Interpersonal skills, 63
Interviews
  giving, 105
  media, 93
  telephone, 106–107
  unexpected, 108–109
ISBN. *See* International Standardized Book Number
Israel, dietetics in, 23–24

J

Japan, dietitians in, 33–34

K

Kaisa, Tendai, 65
Key operating indicators (KOIs), 118–119, 118t
King, Kathy, 223
Knowledge, specialized, 39
Koch, Marlene, 202
KOIs. *See* Key operating indicators

L

Lebanon, dietitians in, 58
Letterheads, 97–98, 98f
Letters. *See also* Pitch letter; Promotion letters; Query letter
  biography, 247–248
  introductory, **248**
  referral, 247
  starting, 240
  steps to best-selling, 237, 240
Levinson, Yaakov, **23**
Libraries, 208
Licensing, requirements, 39
Lichten, Joanne, **30**
Life expectancy, as extended, 4–5
Links
  buying, 192
  linkbaiting and, 192
  natural, 193
  reciprocal, 191–192
  on websites, 191–193
Location, starting in new, **40–41**
Logos, 98–99
Long-term care
  consulting in, 264
  dietetic technicians in, 157
Luros-Elson, Ellyn, **45**

M

Management, selling to, 146
Managing editors, 207

Market research, 19
  analysis for, 21
  competition and, 56
  for marketing plan, 20–22
  in marketing plan, 115
  trends evaluated in, 20–21
Marketing. *See also* Marketing plan; Product marketing; Promotion; Target markets
  books, 205–211
  brochures, 213–216
  business ethics and, 83–87
  in business process, 3–4
  challenges in, 3–4
  to clients, 32
  in clinical setting, 137–141
  communication through, 27
  competition assessment for good, 55–59
  competition stimulating, 135
  as consultant, **32**
  consumer-oriented programs, 153
  consumers as helped by, 17
  as continuous process, 42
  conventions and, 243–246
  to current employer, 33
  customer satisfaction and, 18
  as defined, 17
  dietetic technicians, 157–160
  dietitians to supermarkets, 172–173
  food, 12
  food industry, 86, 123–133
  food products, 45
  health care, 12, 135–142
  healthy food, 123–133
  hospital-based promotion programs, 149–151
  individualized, 19
  to insurance companies, 74
  integrated, 19
  in larger economic picture, 4–5
  mix, 18
  networking and, 63–67
  for new location, **40**
  in new millenium, 3–7
  newsletters, 251–253
  nontraditional, 209
  nutrition in supermarket, 169–176
  to peers, 33
  in private practice, 151–152
  through proposals, 227
  as public speaker, 195–199
  in real world, **23**
  services, 35–42, 37t
  social, 19
  sports dietetics, 183–188
  of sports nutrition services, 153
  strategies, 18, 22–23
  successes, 135–136
  for supermarkets, 175–176
  terms, 18–19
  trade shows and, 243–246
  traditional, 208
  trends and, 10
  websites, 189–194
  wellness, 12, 143–154

worksite nutrition programs, 145–149, 150t
Marketing network, building, 39–40
Marketing plan
  budgeting/performance analysis/implementation section of, 119–120
  business plan v., 113
  effectiveness of, 120
  elements of, 114
  environmental analysis in, 114–115
  executive summary of, 114
  major product and target market of, 20
  market research for, 20–22, 115
  mission statement of, 20
  organizational support for, 20
  process of, 20
  promotion in, 117–118, 118t
  for public speaker, 195–196
  readers of, 113–114
  risk lowered with, 20–24
  situational SWOT analysis for, 115
  strategic assumptions in, 21–22
  strategies/objectives in, 116–117
  tactical marking programs in, 118–119
  target market/product line identified for, 114
  writing, 113–120
  before writing, 114
Marketing signal
  consumers use of, 36
  term, 36
  used for marketing services, 36, 37t, 38
Markets
  books taken to, 208
  challenger, 57
  followers, 59
  functional medicine nutrition's, 179–182
  leader, 57
  niche, 19, 35–36
  writing for public, 251–252
Media
  audience of, 105
  broadcast, 108t
  cable, 95
  concepts, 96–97
  good lead times for, 107
  news hook for, 105
  newsworthy, 104
  potential of, 103–111
  press kits and, 241–242
  print, 95, 108t
  proactive story placement in, 107–108
  public as reached by, 103
  radio, 95
  relations, 107
  rules of game in, 103–104
  as selected for promotion, 94–96
  skills as leveraged, 109
  success story, 109–111
  television, 95
  tracker, 105
  types of, 104
  unexpected, 108
  website, 94–95

Medical nutrition therapy, 136
Medicine. *See* Functional medicine
Murdock, Ann, **158**
Musk, Maye, **40**

N
Negotiations
    agreements, 69–74
    for contracts, 70–74
    discussion during, 69
    early moves in, 164–165
    fees and, 70
    give and take in, 165
    preparing for, 69
    purpose of, 74
    stages of, 163–164
    successful, 69–70
Networking, 29. *See also* Marketing
        network
    developing, 63
    etiquette, 64
    follow up in, 64
    goals and, 63
    groups, **64**
    interpersonal skills for, 63
    for job searching, 63
    marketing through, 63–67
    process of, 63–65
    self-promotion through, 90
    for websites, 189
News, media as worthy of, 104
News conferences, 93
Newsletters
    as communication tool, 252–253
    direct mail of, 251
    financial considerations and, 252
    marketing, 251–253
    outside help for, 251
    for public market, 251–252
    selling subscriptions to, 252
    subscription, 251
Newspaper columns
    content of, 260
    postscripts to, 260
    preparation for writing, 259
    process of writing, 260
    writing nutrition, 259–260
Niche businesses, 59
Nutrition. *See also* Functional medicine
        nutrition; Geriatric nutrition;
        Medical nutrition therapy; Nutrition
        genomic counseling; Sports
        nutrition services
    authors, 202–203
    care, 138–139
    care of outpatient, 141
    consulting services, 126–127
    cosmetics and, 65–66
    labeling, 174
    as marketed in supermarket, 169–176
    marketing services in, 135
    newspaper columns, 259–260
    outcome data, 141
    reimbursement for services in, 140–141
    screening, 138
    in South Africa, 12

support teams, 140
trends affecting, 153–154
worksite wellness programs in,
        145–149, 150t
Nutrition genomic counseling, 5
Nutritionists, corporate, 170

O
Objectives, 22
Opportunity, windows of, 56–57
Orbeta, Sanirose, **47**

P
Passion, 30
    pursuing, **28**
Patenaude, Jan, **193**
Pediatric weight control, 5
People skills, 30
Perishability, 38
Personal vision, creating, 27, 29
Pharmacies, 171
Physicians, writing to, 247–249, **248**
Pitch letter, 19
    target audience of, 240
    writing, 237, 238f, 239f, 240
Pleasure principle, 106
Plotkin, Robin, **124**
Point of sale, materials, 174
Popularity, of health-related ideas, 9
Population migration, 4
Portfolios, 99
Posters, 99
Poverty, 12–13
Press
    briefings, 93, 230
    kits, 93
    relations, 109
Press kits, 242f
    contents of, 241
    for corporate promotion, 242
    as developed, 241–242
    distributing, 241–242
    media coverage from, 241–242
    for media tour, 242
    outside folder of, 241
Press releases, 235f
    as communication tool, 236
    format guidelines for, 234, 236
    in public relations, 92
    for special events, 229–230
    topics for, 233
    types of, 233–234
    use of, 233
    writing, 233–236
Price(s)
    competitive analysis on, 75–76
    determining, 22
    increases, 80f, 81
    product, 76
    product marketing and, 44
    setting, 75–81
    strategies for determining, 76
    structures of competitors, 57
Private practice, marketing in,
        151–152
Product development, careers in,
        170–171

Product Life Cycle, 10–11, 10f
    curve, 21
    stages of, 11
Product marketing
    keys to successful, 43–45
    mix for, 44–45
    price and, 44
    promotion and, 44–45
    readings on, 46–47
    timing in marketplace for, 43
Productivity, 4
Products, 18. *See also* Product marketing
    characteristics of, 43
    competitive positioning of, 43–44
    developing new, 47
    failure, 45–46
    marketing, 43–48
    marketing strategies and, 22
    proprietary competitive advantages of,
        44
Professional agents, 196
Professional biography, writing, 218,
        223f, 224
Professional groups, joining/participating
        in, 33
Professional services, characteristics of, 39
Professional speakers. *See* Public speaking
Promotion, 19, 22. *See also* Advertising;
        Public relations
    aids for, 97–99, 101
    direct mail, 97
    direct-response, 19
    graphic/print materials for, 98–99
    health, 143–154
    hospital-based programs of, 149–151
    internal, 147, 149
    in marketing plan, 117–118, 118t
    media selection for, 94–96
    networking and, 90
    of personal assets, 31–32
    planning, 91
    plan's pieces, 91–92
    product marketing and, 44–45
    public speakers and, 197
    self, 90–91
    of service businesses, 89
    strategies, 89–91
    trade shows for, 97
Promotion letters
    content of, 247
    features of, 247–248
    follow up, **248**
Proposals, 99
    kinds of, 225–226
    long v. short, 225–226
    marketing through, 227
    preparing successful, 226–227
    questions for writing, 226
    reasons for writing, 225
    sole-source, 225
    structure of, 227
    unsolicited, 225
    writing, 225–227
Psychographics, 18
Public relations, 19
    activities of, 92
    campaigns, 92

celebrities and, 93
cosponsorship and, 93
as defined, 92
media interviews and, 93
press releases in, 92
resources, 96t
special events in, 93
Public speaking, 98
bureaus, 196
do's/don'ts of, 197–198
examples of, 199
marketing, 195–199
marketing plan for, 195–196
promotion pieces and, 197
selling game of, 198–199
Publicity
coverage of, 92
for special events as obtained, 229–232
Publisher, self-publishing and, 208
Publishing. *See* Self-publishing

Q
Query letter, 19
target audience of, 240
writing, 237, 238f, 239f, 240

R
Radio, 95
Recipe
analysis, 125–126
creating, 126
evaluation, 126
Relationships, building, 248–249
Reputation, **32**
Research. *See* Market research
Resorts, 128–129
Restaurants
chain, 128–129
independent, 128
Resumes, 98, 219f. *See also* Curriculum vitae
career as foundation of, 217
as package, 217–218
target of, 217–218
writing, 217–224
Richardson, Manette, **46**
Risks, calculated, 30

S
Scruggs, Alberta, 157
Search engines, 189–190
Self-confidence, 30
Self-marketing, **28**
learning, 11
preparing for, 31
as trend, 11–12
Self-promotion, 90–91
Self-publishing
acquisitions editor in, 207
authors who do, 205
books, 205–211
challenge of, 206
defining, 207–208
by dietitians, 205–206
goals of, 206–207, 206t, 207t

managing editors in, 207
as plausible option, 206
publisher and, 208
risks of, 210
sales director for, 208
Selling. *See also* Negotiations
as alternative, 163
books, 208–210
buying from, 166
on internet, 209–210
non-traditional, 166
presentation, 163–164
process of, 163–167
sales negotiations as changing in, 163
Service business, promotion strategies
for, 89
Service groups, **64**
Services, 18. *See also* Professional services
employment in, 35
marketing, 35–42
marketing signals use for marketing,
36, 37t, 38
Setnik, Jessica, **215**
Signs, 99
Skills, building, 29–31
Skimming, 76
Small business entities, 39
Snake oil pitches, 190
Sole-source proposals, 225
South Africa, dietetic professionals in,
12–13
Special events
celebrities for, 231
coordinator, 232
creating, 229–230
giveaways and, 231
marketing tools for, 231
press briefings for, 230
press release for, 229–230
publicity as obtained for, 229–232
sponsorship for, 230–231
Specialty sales, 209
Speech, power of, 29
Spence, A. M., 36
Spokespersons, 85
Sponsorship
benefits of, 230
cosponsorship and, 93
industry of, 230
opportunities for sponsor in, 230–231
securing, 230–231
for special events, 230–231
Sports dietetics
board certified specialist in, 183, **184**
expectations in, 184–185
goals in, 185
jobs in, 183–184
marketing, 183–188
resources for, 186t
target market in, 185
Sports nutrition services, marketing, 153
Storper, Barbara, **145**
Success, 100
Supermarkets
bottom line of, 172
community outreach programs
through, 173–174

dietitian careers with, 170–172
industry basics, 169–170
marketing for, 175–176
nutrition as marketed in, 169–176
programs with, 173
tours of, 175
websites, 175
SWOT analysis, 21, 21f

T
Taglines, 186
Tallmadge, Katherine, **147**
Target markets, 18, 185
of brochures, 213
of letters, 240
of marketing plans, 20
for products, 43
Technical competency, 39
Technicians. *See* Dietetic technicians
Television
media, 95
watching, 5
Tourism, culinary, 133
Trade name, 98
Trade shows, 97
exhibiting at, 243–244
follow-up after, 246
marketing during, 243–246
Trading down, 76
Trading up, 76
Training
employees, 51
for functional medicine nutrition,
180–181
Trends. *See also* Popularity
caring about, 9
defining, 9
evaluating, 20–21
future market, 58
liquid diet, 9
marketing and, 10, 153–154
next big, 11–12
nutrition/wellness affected by, 153–154
positive/negative, 9
in Product Life Cycle, 10–11
as started, 9–10

U
Unbundling, as market strategy, 45
Underbidding, 76
United Kingdom, dietitians in, 52–53

V
Value(s), 7
added, 76
creating, 51–51
perceived, 18, 75–76

W
Websites, 94–95
bonus, 193
copy written for, 190–191
links on, 191–193
marketing, 189–194
networking for, 189

Websites *(contd.)*
  search engines and, 189–190
  supermarkets, 175
  working from home and, 193–194
Weight. *See* Pediatric weight control;
    Weight loss
Weight loss, 5
Weiss, Liz, **109**
Wellness, 5
  breaking into, 147–149
  dietetic technicians working in, 157–158
  faith-based programs in, 154
  marketing, 12, 143–154
  nutrition aspects of, 154
  programs, 144
  statistics about, 144
  trends affecting, 153–154
Williams, Barbara, **28**
Wilson, Bob, 159
World knowledge indicators, 6t
Wright, Theresa, **78**
Writing, 31
  books, 201–204
  CVs, 218–224
  inverted pyramid style, 190
  keywords in, **190**
  marketing brochures, 213–216
  marketing plan, 113–120
  nutrition newspaper column, 259–260
  physicians, 247–249, **248**
  press releases, 233–236
  professional biography, 218, 223f, 224
  proposals, 225–227
  for public market, 251–252
  query letters, 237, 238f, 239f, 240
  resumes, 217–224
  as unbiased, 86
  for websites, 190–191

Y
Yahia, Najat, **58**

Z
Zied, Elisa, 202